Acupuncture and Osteopathy to Treat Musculoskeletal Pain of the Extremities:

the Mazzanti AcuOsteo Method®

Umberto Mazzanti MD, Acupuncturist, Osteopath DO MROI
Vice President
AMAB (Association of Medical Acupuncturists of Bologna)
Bologna, Italy
Vice Director
AMAB – Italian Chinese School of Acupuncture
Bologna, Italy
Treasurer
FISA (Italian Federation of Acupuncture Societies)
Bologna, Italy
Visiting Professor
NJUCM (Nanjing University of Chinese Medicine)
Nanjing, P.R. China
Inventor of Mazzanti AcuOsteo Method®

Carlo Maria Giovanardi MD, Acupuncturist
President
AMAB (Association of Medical Acupuncturists of Bologna)
Bologna, Italy

Director
AMAB – Italian Chinese School of Acupuncture
Bologna, Italy
President
FISA (Italian Federation of Acupuncture Societies)
Bologna, Italy
International Ambassador
SAR (Society for Acupuncture Research)
Winston Salem, NC
Visiting Professor
NJUCM (Nanjing University of Chinese Medicine)
Nanjing, P.R. China
Expert of Acupuncture
Alma Mater Studiorum University of Bologna
Bologna, Italy

Alessandra Poini MD, Acupuncturist
Board Member
AMAB (Association of Medical Acupuncturists of Bologna)
Bologna, Italy
Professor
AMAB - Italian Chinese School of Acupuncture
Board Member
FISA (Italian Federation of Acupuncture Societies)
Bologna, Italy

Giuseppe Tallarida MD, Acupuncturist
Professor
AMAB - Italian Chinese School of Acupuncture
Bologna, Italy

ELSEVIER

ELSEVIER
3251 Riverport Lane
St. Louis, Missouri 63043

ACUPUNCTURE AND OSTEOPATHY TO TREAT MUSCULOSKELETAL
PAIN OF THE EXTREMITIES: THE MAZZANTI ACUOSTEO METHOD®

ISBN: 978-0-323-83194-9

Executive Content Strategist: Lauren Willis
Content Development Manager: Ellen Wurm-Cutter
Content Development Specialist: Ranjana Sharma
Publishing Services Manager: Deepthi Unni
Senior Project Manager: Kamatchi Madhavan
Book Designer: Margaret Reid

Printed in Chinted in China by 1010 Printing International Ltd

Last digit is the print number: 9 8 7 6 5 4 3 2 1

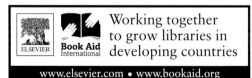

Disclaimer

This handbook about acupuncture and osteopathy is addressed to professionals, who according to the law, can administer acupuncture and osteopathy.

It can be a useful guide for other healthcare professionals such as physiotherapists, chiropractors, osteopaths, and medical doctors, duly trained and authorized by the law and the medical board and/or institution they belong to in the state where they practice their profession to insert acupuncture needles and perform osteopathic manipulative treatments.

This handbook on acupuncture and osteopathy aims to provide the professionals with further information on diagnosis, assessment, and treatment of injuries. The information contained in this book is not intended to and can never replace a correct diagnosis and medical evaluation made by professionals operating in this specific field and specialized in the subject treated.

In addition, it should be reminded that the insertion of acupuncture needle and treatment with hands-on osteopathic techniques are always associated with a potential risk. When performing any of the techniques described in this book, the professional must have full medical knowledge of the anatomy and physiology of the tissues to treat and must be fully aware of any medical contraindication that makes the treatment of the patient with acupuncture or osteopathy inadvisable.

The authors and publisher take no responsibility if the techniques described in this book are performed wrongly or improperly, or without asking and receiving preliminary medical advice.

It is worth reminding that a preliminary correct diagnosis and medical evaluation by professionals operating in this specific field and specialized in the subject treated is always mandatory.

The information in this book has been written and published in good faith with the aim of contributing to the medical profession. The authors and publisher take no responsibility for any errors or omissions in the text.

It is mandatory to be fully aware of the legislation in force in the country where practitioners work to comply with procedures and regulations concerning hygiene and safety when needles are inserted and skin is disinfected.

All videos were recorded in Italy between 2020 and 2023 in compliance with the legislation in force.

By that time, all patients had reached their majority. The models have given their consent to the publication of the photos and videos contained in the text.

Preface

This handbook is intended to set out with the application of a protocol patented on April 24, 2022, for the treatment of musculoskeletal pain of the limbs with acupuncture and osteopathy. This study aims to provide a guidance for practitioners when treating this specific type of pain.

As a medical doctor specializing in sports medicine and physical medicine and rehabilitation, I have been using this approach in my daily practice in Italy for more than 35 years. Patients' compliance has proven to be high, and the results have been far beyond my expectations. All the cases presented throughout the text are, therefore, drawn from my own practice, and the reader is invited to study them. They show how osteopathic manipulative treatment (OMT) is performed and how acupoints are chosen and combined.

It is quite unusual, that is to say a sort of exception, to be an MD or a practitioner at the same time professionally trained in acupuncture and osteopathy. For this reason, during my seminars or lectures delivered at national and international conferences, attendees have often asked me if I had written a book on this combined approach to obtain a deeper understanding of it.

Similarly, my masters, Giovanni Maciocia and Qiao Wenlei, have always encouraged and invited me to consider the idea of developing this project. In addition, after a lot of wavering, I finally made this decision when I had the chance to discuss it with Whitfield Reaves.

Once the decision was made, I actively involved a group of dear friends who are esteemed professionals to figure out a text that could be easy to read and use in daily practice, thanks also to the videos and images provided.

After introducing the fundamentals of acupuncture, the principles of OMT, and the main concepts of pain management, the authors dedicate each of the six chapters to the six major joints.

All of the chapters follow the same order, that is, a triple approach:

- The perspective of Western medicine: Western anatomy, differentiation of symptoms, orthopedic tests, and diagnosis
- Diagnosis in Chinese medicine
- Diagnosis in osteopathic medicine
- Treatment with acupuncture
- Treatment with OMT

By following this order, we make it possible for the reader to quickly make any comparison, if needed.

The use of this protocol is not in contradiction with whichever other approach a practitioner may decide to follow, and I hope this handbook can be useful to practitioners of different orientations.

For reasons of length, this book omits the discussion of spine pain, as well as MSK pain in the hands and feet. It is hoped that they will form the subject of a future book.

For didactic purposes and to make it easier for the reader, the authors have decided to always consider the right joint as the affected one, and therefore to be treated, whereas the left joint is always regarded as the unaffected. Consequently, all of the osteopathic maneuvers start with an explanation of where the patient and practitioner are positioned and then when reference is made to the joint or part of it, it will always be the right joint.

When it comes to the acupoints, the authors have followed this rule: if nothing is indicated after the acupoint, it means it is located on the affected side. Otherwise, the reader will find the word *opposite* in brackets, thus meaning that the point is located on the healthy side. If the word *bilaterally* is used, it means that the point should be needled on both sides, both affected and unaffected. The acupoints indicated for each condition are not formulae but only the possible points among which the practitioner can choose following the principles outlined in the protocol.

For specific categories of points, where there are couples of points to use, both terms, *affected* and *opposite*, have been mentioned to avoid any misunderstanding.

For terminology, preference was given to names of Greek or Latin origin, using acronyms when available.

Finally, every practitioner should rely only on the rules of Chinese and osteopathic medicine once the diagnosis has already been made following the rules of Western medicine and with imaging techniques, as and when necessary. As previously mentioned, each chapter includes the Western differentiation of symptoms, indicating the possible causes of pain according to the perspective of Western medicine.

Let me say that this handbook is not intended to be a replacement for a good book on Western clinical medicine: it is just meant to provide the reader with a short checklist of the possible causes of pain according to Western Medicine. This section is therefore of paramount importance, as practitioners should always know when a patient should be referred to a Western medical doctor and further imaging investigations are mandatory.

I sincerely hope that this book will be of practical use to practitioners, acupuncturists, and osteopaths from various countries to help them integrate their disciplines, thus making further progress in modern medicine when they strive to solve the tough issue of pain.

Umberto Mazzanti

Foreword

I have been in postgraduate courses on sports acupuncture with Dr. Umberto Mazzanti over the last few years. He is a very thoughtful and precise practitioner who displays enthusiasm for creative and effective techniques for treating pain and orthopedic dysfunction. Therefore it did not surprise me that my first reaction to Dr. Mazzanti's handbook of acupuncture was quite compelling. Clearly, his new publication will find itself favorably judged among the most important texts on orthopedic and anatomically based acupuncture. In addition, it will contribute to advancing assessment and treatment techniques from the core principles of Chinese medicine to a new integrated system of old and new. Indeed, Dr. Mazzanti's work is a big step in this process.

The *Acupuncture and Osteopathy to Treat Musculoskeletal Pain of the Extremities* highlights the use of the Mazzanti Acuosteo Method. In my first viewing of the material, I was very comforted with its use of high-density video showing needle techniques in the acupuncture tradition as well as specific orthopedic tests and osteopathic manipulation. Whether a first-time reader or a long-time practitioner, it immediately seemed relevant, comprehensive, and ready to become part of one's practice, regardless of the background. This handbook does a skillful job of integrating traditional and modern acupuncture with osteopathy.

The text was clear, and the diagrams and illustrations were quite useful for each of the extremities covered. Its comprehensive nature can be seen in the section on wrist pain, where assessment for inflammatory tendinopathy, tenosynovitis, or other related inflammatory conditions was outlined. Orthopedic testing was clearly described and illustrated, and when necessary, short but very clear and precise videos were offered. Moreover, each section contained "red flags" in Western medicine, diagnosis in Chinese medicine, etiology, and pathology. That certainly feels complete to my needs as a 40-year practitioner in orthopedic acupuncture.

I wondered at first if this was more relevant for the osteopathic physician. However, not long into the material came the acupuncture points, their locations, and the needle technique. Again, the videos were extremely helpful in viewing the author's suggested location and insertion angles, as well as depths.

In addition, it was very useful to read his order of needling, from distal points proximally to the core of the body. Called "options" in this text, numerous treatment perspectives are clearly delineated. For instance, the traditional point categories such as yuan-source points or "water" points are considered. Other options suggest using the opposite side or upper/lower mirroring by treating the ankle, for instance, for the wrist. Microsystems and empirical points complete the list. In the progression of these options, each step has a reason for use, an order to needle, and when or how to include the point in a specific injury or orthopedic condition. Yet also, quite importantly, Dr. Mazzanti makes room for the clinical experience of the practitioner to guide them with these choices in the treatment of each patient.

While some of the material may feel overwhelming to a new practitioner, there is ample opportunity for variation and adaptation, depending on the injury and the needs of the patients. In addition, photographs, illustrations, and videos seem to comfort the reader and give very clear direction and understanding as to what, where, and how!

This is a comprehensive text, rather than a handbook, as the name in the title implies. It could easily be used as a study guide for an entire course on orthopedic and sports acupuncture. Yet, the precision of each chapter would allow this to be a useful desk reference with the patient in pain when there is no clear path forward, an unclear diagnosis, and or questions about which points to use in treatment.

If you treat patients with injury and pain, which of course we all do in this profession, one could certainly benefit from this text on the Mazzanti Acuosteo Method. Some will need this, others may want it, but it will undoubtly help a practitioner dealing with patients and their injuries. I highly recommend it.

Whitfield Reaves, OMD, LAc

Acknowledgments

First of all, I would like to express my gratitude, deepest affection, and thankfulness to my dear friend, Carlo Maria Giovanardi, MD, Acupuncturist, President of the FISA (Italian Federation of Acupuncture Societies), and President of the AMAB (Association of Medical Acupuncturists of Bologna)—Italian Chinese School of Acupuncture. Meeting him changed my professional life's destiny as he introduced me to acupuncture and Chinese Medicine at the end of the 1970s. Ever since, and always together, we have walked the pathway leading to the foundation of the AMAB and its school. Together, we have traveled around the world to get to know the most important Maestros of Chinese Medicine to improve our knowledge and acquire new insights. We are still sharing our professional life and common projects for the future.

I would like to mention and deeply thank my Maestro, Giovanni Maciocia, who passed away in 2018. Since the beginning of the 1990s, he honored me with his friendship and shared his terrific knowledge with me. I will never forget his suggestions during the lectures he delivered at the AMAB, the training I received in his clinic in Amersham, and our long weekly discussions and debates over the phone: they were crucial to me. Drawing from his huge experience has meant a lot to me; I have acquired a deeper insight into Chinese Medicine and the techniques of how to use the acupoints. I want to share this knowledge with the readers of this book. With his books, Giovanni has been watershed contributing to the spreading and teaching of Chinese Medicine in the Western world. This is why I will always be indebted to him.

I am also extremely grateful to the author of the foreword to this book, Whitfield Reaves, OMD, LAc. The first time I met him dates back to 2018, when I was attending one of his seminars in Zurich. I had just finished reading his book *The Acupuncture Handbook of Sports Injuries and Pain*. It was so clear, his approach was so systematic, and his acupuncture method was so similar to mine. His lecture then was a driving force, a fundamental source of inspiration that pushed me to focus on a project I had been thinking about for so many years. The right time had come; after reading his book and attending his seminar, I finally decided to translate my own clinical practice into a manual integrating acupuncture and osteopathy. I am grateful to him for inspiring me, and I would like to acknowledge the role he has played in me making this decision.

I would also like to acknowledge and thank my Maestro, Qiao Wenlei, former professor of Chinese Medicine at Nanjing University of Chinese Medicine (NJUCM). I first met her in the early 2000s and subsequently multiple times from 2006 onwards during the Course of Clinical Training of Acupuncture of the AMAB students at the NJUCM; it was the first of many meetings to come, such as the continuing education seminars or lectures she was invited to deliver at our school. Her clear, simple, and practical way of teaching, along with her availability to share wide knowledge of Chinese Medicine, have a remarkable effect on my clinical approach to the patient and treatment.

I would also like to acknowledge and thank the individuals who volunteered to help me write this handbook. Without them, this project would have not been possible. They are not only very qualified professionals but also close friends who have treated this handbook with sincere affection and sympathy.

First of all, I would like to mention Alessandra Poini, MD, and Giuseppe Tallarida, MD, who coauthored this book in addition to Carlo Maria Giovanardi. They are acupuncturists and professors at the AMAB—Italian Chinese School of Acupuncture—who ensure the bright future of this institution. In addition to contributing with sections of the texts, they have supported me and given invaluable advice throughout these 3 years of hard work.

Franco Guolo, Osteopath, DO, Didactic Manager of the C.I.O. (Italian College of Osteopathy), Parma and I were schoolmates when we attended a course in osteopathy early in the 1990s. Thanks to his deep knowledge of osteopathy and amazing way of teaching, he was able to get into the spirit of this book. His advice was really invaluable when it came to explaining osteopathy and making it simple and accessible to the readers.

Maurizio Draghetti, MD, Orthopedic Specialist, Head of the V Orthopedic Unit at the Clinic—Casa di Cura "Villa Erbosa GSD," Bologna, and I have known each other since high school. He gave me precious advice on writing the sections dedicated to orthopedics.

I am grateful to Matteo Mignani and his assistant, Guido Pedroni, video makers in Bologna, who shot the videos that form an integral and substantial part of this text. Their professionalism turned a didactic room into a real set and the perfect location for our editorial project. Their patience supported me throughout this experience, and their advice and shooting skills were of paramount importance in showing the acupuncture and osteopathy techniques. Matteo Mignani also created the images of the acupuncture channels, patiently meeting my specific needs.

I would like to thank Giuseppe Maserati, an architect in Monza. Thanks to his professionalism, he prepared anatomical drawings based on my simple suggestions.

By patiently meeting all my requests, he provided images that made this book enjoyable.

I am also pleased to thank Nicola Mazzoni, graphics and logo designer in Bologna, who created "The Mazzanti AcuOsto Method" logo. He succeeded admirably in the aim of symbolizing the combined treatment of acupuncture and osteopathy.

In addition, I would like to thank Linda Woodard who first believed in my editorial project, and Kevonne Holloway, Lauren Boyle, Kristin R. Wilhelm, Patricia Geary, Alister Lewcock, and my content development manager, Ranjana Sharma, at Elsevier for their support and professionalism.

Finally, I would like to thank Dr. Alessandra Bonzi, translator, for thoroughly translating my manuscript and painstakingly revising it. Her invaluable support guided me throughout the whole preparation and revision of the manuscript. I would also like to thank Dr. Eugenia Biavati, Doctor of Philosophy in English Language and Literature at King's College London, for her linguistic advice.

Contents

Video Contents

All videos courtesy Umberto Mazzanti Sr., MD

Chapter 1

Introduction

The Fundamentals of Acupuncture for Musculoskeletal Pain in the Limbs

Musculoskeletal (MSK) pain is a very common symptom often leading to healthcare seeking. However, patients only tend to consult a medical doctor when pain is intense and disabling, thus interfering with daily living activities. On the contrary, when pain is long standing, but mild or dull, medical care is less often sought.

Ultimately, consultation with a specialist is usually required when pain relapses following uncommon work- or sports-related activities or changes in weather and outdoor temperature. The latter is often, but not exclusively, the case when arthritis is the condition to treat (see Appendix 6).

It goes without saying that according to the rules of Traditional Chinese Medicine (TCM), MSK pain from acute or chronic Excess conditions is more commonly reported in clinical practice than pain from chronic Deficiency conditions. This explains why this handbook will focus more on the former than the latter.

It is worth remembering that in TCM, MSK pain is often called Bi syndrome (painful obstruction syndrome), a term that underlies the presence of Qì stagnation and Blood stasis resulting from the penetration of external pathologic factors into the outer layers of the body.

In this handbook, we will also focus on MSK pain due to other causes, such as trauma or microtrauma.

Although we are completely aware of the distinction between the two terms, to make the use of this manual easier for the reader and for didactic purposes only, we will mainly use the generic term "MSK pain" to refer to either of them, whereas a distinction will only be made when dealing with specific conditions.

Finally, we would like to stress that "Chinese Medicine" MSK disorders, including arthritis-related diseases and osteopathic somatic dysfunctions, are often comorbid and may affect the same anatomical region.

ETIOLOGY

The whole set of causes of pain are classically distinguished as follows:
- External pathogenic factors (EPFs)
- Internal pathogenic factors (IPFs)
- Factors other than EPFs and IPFs

This handbook will deal with the causes more frequently observed in our clinical practice when managing MSK pain in the limbs, without providing a deeper insight into IPFs, such as emotions, dietary intakes, and pain in other body regions.

External Pathogenic Factors

Of the six EPFs, Wind, Cold, and Dampness are the ones most likely to cause MSK pain. EPFs first invade the Secondary channels, which are the most superficial, and then over the course of time, they may invade the Main channels and penetrate deeper to affect the Zang-Fu organs.

The main symptoms of invasion of EPFs in the MSK system are the following:
- Acute onset
- Exacerbation from seasonal changes or exposure to the same EPF
- Pain mainly on the body surface
- Relatively easy treatment with good results in a short time

Invasion by EPFs usually arises as a result of the following three causes:
- Preexisting internal weakness, either temporary or permanent, due to Qì and Blood deficiency
- Too-strong pathogenic factors
- Patient's lifestyle

Wind

External Wind is commonly associated with another EPF and is often the vehicle through which other factors invade the body. The Wind penetrates the superficial layers of the body, and through the Muscle and

Connecting channels, it reaches the muscles and joints, where it impairs Qì and Blood circulation.

When Qì stagnation and Blood stasis due to Wind are in the Muscle channels, the main symptoms are muscle pain and stiffness. Instead, when they are in the Connecting channels, the main symptoms are joint pain and stiffness, as well as a reduced range of joint movement.

Another sign of Wind penetration in the Secondary channels is that pain and stiffness move around the body, wandering from one group of muscles or a joint to another.

Cold

External Cold can enter the body in different ways, for example through the mouth or nose. In our context, the main way it reaches the muscles and joints is through the skin.

Invasion of External Cold, which is often associated with Wind, usually results from fashion trends, such as wearing too little clothing, or unhealthy habits, such as exposure to cold after sweating, air conditioning, excessively cold workplaces, or butchers' cold rooms. A relationship with the winter season is more rarely observed, since people tend to wear more clothes.

Cold penetrates the Muscle and Connecting channels and reaches the muscles and joints, where it causes Qì stagnation and Blood stasis.

When Qì stagnation and Blood stasis due to Cold are in the Muscle channels, the main symptoms are muscle pain, contracture, spasm, and stiffness. Instead, when they are in the Connecting channels, the main symptoms are joint pain and stiffness, as well as a reduced range of joint movement.

In either case, pain can be intense, it is generally unilateral and located in a well-defined area, and its symptoms are relieved when heat is applied. On the contrary, they get worse with exposure to cold weather.

Over time, if it is not expelled correctly or if the Wei Qi (Defensive Qi) is not strong enough to stop its penetration, Cold moves deeper into the body through the Main channels and reaches the internal organs (Zang Fu), where it mainly damages the Spleen and Kidney Yang-Qì.

This condition of Yang deficiency is also called Internal Cold.

Finally, a Yang deficiency can result in a deficient Wei Qi in the superficial layers of the body, which favors Cold penetration.

Dampness

Invasion of External Dampness usually results from living or working in damp environments, be they warm or cold.

Dampness penetrates the superficial layers of the body, and through the Muscle and Connecting channels, it reaches the muscles and joints. It is characterized by viscosity and stagnation and, therefore, causes Qì stagnation and Blood stasis in the MSK system.

When Qì stagnation and Blood stasis due to Dampness are in the Muscle channels, the main symptoms are muscle pain, numbness, and a feeling of heaviness. Instead, when they are in the Connecting channels, the main symptoms are joint pain, swelling up to the joint effusion, numbness, a feeling of heaviness and clumsiness.

In either case, pain is generally unilateral and located in a specific area, and its symptoms get worse with exposure to damp weather.

Over time, if it is not expelled correctly or if the Wei Qi (Defensive Qi) is not strong enough to stop its penetration, External Dampness moves deeper into the body through the Main channels and reaches the internal organs (Zang Fu), in particular the Stomach and Spleen.

This retention of Dampness can cause Stomach and Spleen Qì deficiency with disorders affecting their transportation and transformation functions and leading to accumulation of Internal Dampness, which may easily favor the invasion of External Dampness.

In addition, the long-term invasion of Damp Heat, above all if associated with Yin deficiency and Empty Heat, favors the onset of inflammation in the joints.

If compared to the other pathogenic factors, Dampness is more difficult to expel, and consequently, symptoms last for a longer time.

It should be remembered that internal Dampness can diffusively invade the muscles, thus causing widespread myalgia and a feeling of heaviness in the limbs.

Factors Other Than External Pathogenic Factors and Internal Pathogenic Factors

Overuse and Work- or Sports-Related Repetitive Strain Injury

Performing the same movement over and over again through work or sports activities may often cause local

Qì stagnation or, more rarely, Qì and Blood deficiency in a specific joint or anatomical district. It results in pain, strain, or weakness of MSK tissues (muscles, tendons, and ligaments).

Furthermore, the lack of Qì and Blood makes it more likely for the body to be prone to the invasion of EPFs.

Trauma and Sports Injuries

Falls, accidents, lifting too-heavy loads, either once or repeatedly, and sports injuries can cause excessive strain on the muscles, joint sprain, dislocation or fracture with swelling, and hematoma. They lead to pain and damage to muscle and joint tissues and result in Qì stagnation and Blood stasis with delayed healing and recovery.

Postsurgical Outcomes

In this specific context, we should also mention limb surgery, which can lead to a reduced range of joint movement and stiffness, even when it is well performed and successful. Surgery can cause Qì stagnation, Blood stasis, and damage to the channels. In addition, scar formation may obstruct the circulation of Qì and Blood in the channels (see Appendix 7). Although we will not be dealing with this issue, the surgical stress and how it disturbs the Shen should also be noted.

PATHOLOGY

As already mentioned, the types of MSK pain discussed in this handbook are from two different conditions, either Excess or Deficiency, with the former being the most observed in daily practice.

Excess conditions:
- Qì stagnation and/or Blood stasis

Deficiency conditions:
- Qì and/or Blood deficiency

Both conditions impair the circulation of Qì and Blood and prevent them from flowing smoothly and regularly.

Although it is obvious that the smooth flow of Qì and Blood in the body relies on the correct functioning and interrelationships of each Zang Fu, when it comes to MSK pain in the limbs, the Zang Fu are less involved than the Secondary channels and are affected at a later stage.

Qi Stagnation and/or Blood Stasis

These two patterns are often found to be associated with MSK pain and are a sign of obstruction to the local flow of Qì and Blood resulting from any of the causes previously mentioned.

In practice, the characteristics of pain due to Qì stagnation are quite different from those due to Blood stasis, which will be discussed later. However, they share some common features, meaning that whatever the condition is, pain:
- Often has an acute onset or is the exacerbation of chronic conditions
- Gets worse with pressure when applied on the painful site

Qì Stagnation

Pain presenting with the following characteristics is a symptom of mild obstruction to Qì flow.

It is described as:
- annoying
- associated with a feeling of distension
- radiating
- not well localized
- more disturbing in the morning or with onset of movement
- improving with mild physical activity, movement, and massage
- affected by mood

Blood Stasis

Pain presenting with the following characteristics is a symptom of severe obstruction to Blood flow.

It is described as:
- localized in a small area
- stubborn, constant, and persistent
- severe and sometimes unbearable
- stabbing
- getting worse when a patient starts moving
- showing no improvement with mild physical activity or movement
- getting worse or arising predominantly at night
- often associated with stiffness or with stiffness as the only symptom

Although the two patterns are often associated, for therapeutic purposes it is of paramount importance to identify the predominant one or the one that has led to the onset of the other.

This is a key issue whose importance will be highlighted in the chapter dedicated to Acupuncture treatment (see Section: The Five Options in Detail). Not only will the identification of the main pattern help us choose the most appropriate acupoints, but also and above all, it will help us decide whether needling (Qì stagnation) should or should not be associated with bleeding (Blood stasis). Further details are provided in Appendix 3.

Qì and/or Blood Deficiency

Also in this case, the two patterns are often found to be associated with MSK pain and are a sign of an impeded flow of local Qì and Blood, usually resulting from overuse or work- and sports-related repetitive strain injury (RSI).

In practice, the characteristics of pain due to Qì deficiency are quite different from those of pain due to Blood deficiency, which will be discussed later. However, they share some common features, meaning that whatever the condition is, pain:

- Has a gradual onset
- Is chronic, dull, and intermittent
- Is never too severe
- Improves with local pressure

Qì Deficiency

Pain presenting with the following characteristics is a symptom of Qì deficiency.

It is described as:

- Tolerable and associated with asthenia of the anatomical district involved
- Manifesting itself after physical activity—improving with rest—getting worse during the day (over time, Qì is consumed to perform daily activities, and consequently deficiency gets worse)

Blood Deficiency

Pain associated with tingling and cramps is a symptom of Blood deficiency.

Although the two patterns are often associated, for therapeutic purposes it is of paramount importance to identify the predominant one or the one that has led to the onset of the other.

This is a key issue whose importance will be highlighted in the chapter dedicated to Acupuncture treatment (see Chapter Section: The Five Options in Detail). Not only will the identification of the main pattern help us choose the most appropriate acupoints, but also and above all, it will help us decide whether needling (Qì deficiency) should or should not be associated with moxibustion (blood deficiency). Further details are provided in Appendix 5.

LOCATION OF PAIN

In TCM, MSK pain is mainly the obstruction of Qì and Blood flow in the channels due to invasion of EPFs, overuse, RSI, and trauma.

The Channels

The complex network of Main and Secondary channels is one of the unique features characterizing TCM.

As the word suggests, the Main channels are the most important ones: they have their own points, connect the superficial regions to the deeper layers of the body, and distribute the Qì and Blood received from the respective Zang Fu (Internal Organs) all over the body. In short, they maintain homeostasis and ensure that each Zang Fu works properly.

The Secondary channels come out from the Main channels. They run more superficially than the Main channels and are responsible for several functions, including the ability to move and defending the body from invasions of EPFs and traumas.

Each Main channel has its own network of Secondary Channels that can be activated through the acupoints located on the Main channels.

For didactic purposes, we will only focus on the Muscle and Connecting (Luo) Secondary channels. The underlying reason for our choice is that MSK pain mainly affects the channels and Zang Fu only when it is chronic. In particular, the Muscle and Connecting channels are involved more often than the Main channels, which may be affected at a later stage.

The Zang Fu are involved later, that is, in chronic conditions, that is to say when the EPFs have overcome the defense systems of the body, in particular the network of channels. At that stage, the conditions to be treated are arthritis-related and rheumatic diseases (see Appendix 6). Finally, it is worth mentioning that severe pain in the Secondary channels is a sign of Excess, while dull pain or weakness are signs of Deficiency.

Below, a description of the main features of the two Secondary channels which are the object of our study. It should also be said that the conditions related to the Muscle and Connecting channels almost always overlap when it comes to MSK disorders.

Muscle Channels

The Muscle channels are both energy channels and structures of muscles and tendons: they integrate the muscles and tendons into the system of the Main channels. Like Main channels, there are 12 Muscle channels but are located more superficially. They show a ribbon-like (not linear) pattern lying over the Main channels and roughly matching their pathway. They run within the most important muscles, tendons, and ligaments. At the level of the major joints, their bands shrink at the insertion points. They originate from the tips of the toes and fingers and flow upward toward the trunk and head. Fig. 1.1 shows the Gall Bladder Muscle channel.

Disorders of the Muscle channels may have various clinical manifestations, including pain in the muscles, tendons, and ligaments, contractures, spasms, stiffness, and numbness. Pain may radiate upward or downward along the affected channel, and this is a sign of Qì stagnation. Nevertheless, Blood stasis can also be observed in the Connecting channels, as it happens with muscle injuries following contusion or strain. Other symptoms depend on the pathogens involved, if any. It is worth mentioning now that to activate and treat the Muscle channels, we have to needle the Jing-Well, Ah Shi, and insertion points. For further information, see the chapter dedicated to Acupuncture treatment (see Section: The Five Options in Detail).

Connecting Channels

We use the term *Connecting channels* to refer to:
- Twelve "Transversal" Connecting channels, which originate from the Luo point and connect it to the Yuan point of the Internally-Externally related channel on the opposite side.
- Sixteen "Longitudinal" Connecting channels (hereinafter, they will be referred to as "proper" channels), which have a clear pathway and well-defined symptoms. They include:
  - Twelve channels that originate from the 12 Luo points of the Main channels, and two that

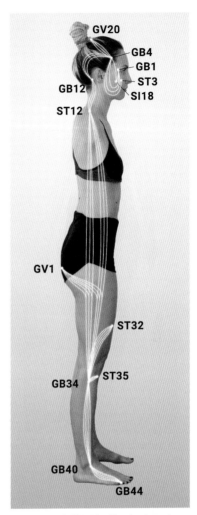

Fig. 1.1 Gallbladder Muscle channel.

originate from the Luo points of the Du Mai and Ren Mai
  - The Big Luo of the Spleen
  - The Big Luo of the Stomach

Fig. 1.2 shows the Gall Bladder Connecting channel "proper."
- Superficial Connecting channels, whose pathway is not well defined. Sun, Fu, and Xue Luo (Minute, Superficial, and Blood Luo) run in the space between the skin and muscles (Cou Li) and transport Qì and Blood to all the tissues.

They flow in all directions (vertically, horizontally, and crosswise), unlike the Main channels, which only

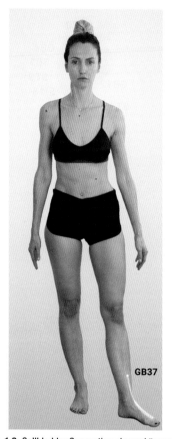

Fig. 1.2 Gallbladder Connecting channel "proper."

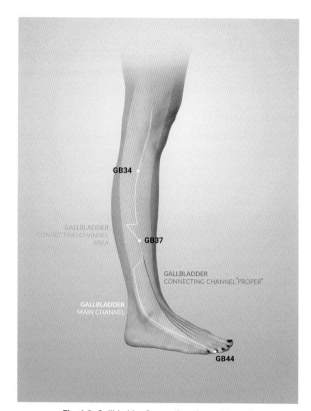

Fig. 1.3 Gallbladder Connecting channel "area."

flow longitudinally, and can be compared to a "sponge" that fills that space (Cou Li). In Western anatomy, this space is called *subcutaneoustissue*.

Let us see an example.

The Gall Bladder Connecting channel "area" (highlighted in light blue in Fig. 1.3) is the whole area where the Gall Bladder Connecting channels flow; it is the whole space from the skin to the muscles, where Fu, Sun, and Xue Luo run.

The Gall Bladder Connecting channel "area" is not limited to the area reached by the Gall Bladder Connecting channel "proper" (highlighted in blue in Fig. 1.3), that is, the dorsum of the foot.

The Gall Bladder Main channel (highlighted in white in Fig. 1.3) controls its Connecting channel "area," which extends over the whole pathway of the Gall Bladder Main channel up to the head at GB1.

The same applies to every Main channel and its Connecting channel "area." Disorders of the Connecting channels mainly manifest themselves as joint pain and stiffness. Pain is more localized, especially in a joint, and is a sign of Blood stasis.

Nevertheless, Qì stagnation can also be observed in the Connecting channels, as happens when joint stiffness improves with movement. Other symptoms depend on the pathogens involved, if any. It is worth mentioning now that to activate and treat the Connecting channels we have to needle the corresponding Luo point.

As each Connecting channel "area" represents its whole "subcutaneous tissue" and not only the Connecting channel "proper," we prefer needling the Luo point on the opposite side. The choice of the side does not affect treatment, because the subcutaneous tissue extends throughout the body and connects the right to the left side.

Furthermore, by proceeding this way, we can balance the two sides (right and left) and avoid needling too many points on the affected side. For further information, see the chapter dedicated to Acupuncture treatment (see Section: The Five Options in Detail).

ACUPUNCTURE TREATMENT
The Five Options: General Principles

The *Five Options* **is the name of the acupuncture approach we recommend for the treatment of acute and chronic MSK pain in the limbs due to Qì stagnation, Blood stasis, as well as Qì and Blood deficiency in the channels.**

These disorders may result from trauma, microtrauma, and overuse through work and sports. The *Five Options* can also be used in the case of invasion of EPFs: specifically, we are referring to acute conditions or acute exacerbations of chronic conditions, the so-called "Bi syndrome," also corresponding to osteoarthritis-related conditions, tendinitis, bursitis, and rheumatic diseases in Western medicine.

Although we are aware of this distinction, in general, we will refer to both of them using the term "MSK pain" for didactic purposes and a better understanding of the text. However, in some specific contexts, we will need to make a distinction between the two.

Therefore the aim of the treatment we suggest for MSK pain will be:

- To eliminate Qì stagnation and Blood stasis, mainly in the Muscle and Connecting channels
- To expel EPFs in case of Bi syndrome
- To tonify Qì and Blood Deficiency, mainly in the Muscle and Connecting channels

The Five Options offer the reader a systematic and simple method to select points and accessory techniques: these guidelines, though systematic, are a pathway for pain management. However, they are not meant to be strictly followed, since every practitioner has their own theoretical knowledge, clinical experiences, and therapeutic options. That is the reason why the different steps suggest different management options that allow practitioners to leave the marked pathway and then come back to conclude treatment. In this sense,

it is similar to choosing an itinerary to reach a place to visit and being instead offered many alternative routes.

The general lines of the therapeutic protocol of the Five Options will now be discussed and will be applied to each single condition covered by the section dedicated to the clinical practice. Repeating the protocol steps for each condition might sound unnecessarily pedantic, but our aim is to make it automatic for the practitioner to apply it in their clinical practice. Our teaching experience of more than 35 years has demonstrated how easy it is for less expert practitioners to follow their own therapeutic options and by doing so miss the target they want to achieve.

Our therapeutic approach increases practitioners' awareness of their own point selection: both acupoints and therapeutic options may be well known to our readers, but how to select and use them is something that should not be taken for granted. We have all studied acupuncture, but there are a number of different schools of thoughts and ways of teaching. Consequently, the therapeutic approach we are suggesting, that is, using less common acupoints and often overlooked treatment protocols, may be interesting and, to some extent, innovative. We hope that after reading the manual the selection of acupoints will be easier, though its application requires skill and precision.

Another practical aspect of the Five Options is to provide an effective and quick therapeutic strategy to manage severe pain, either acute or chronic, so as to get immediate relief during the therapeutic session.

We start with Option One, which deals with the selection of those distal points whose great dynamics and effectiveness in terms of therapeutic action provide immediate results. Option Two involves selection of local points, as they also have an immediate and specific action with regards to removal of Qì stagnation and Blood stasis, both causing local pain in muscles, tendons, ligaments, and joints. Options Three, Four, and Five aim to complete and stabilize the therapeutic results obtained with the first two options.

The aim is therefore to give the practitioner the widest range of options to be selected according to the patient's responses to treatment, since neither all the options nor all the steps are needed in all the cases.

Let us see how to establish a rule to select the points.

Option One is always the starting point. Soon after every step, that is, 1 to 5, testing the efficacy of the distal points before moving to the following step is mandatory: if the results obtained are satisfactory, the practitioner should skip the remaining steps and move to Option Two.

What is stated above for the distal points also applies to local points, that is, to Option Two: the recommended steps have to be followed until the desired effect is achieved.

Similarly, the use of the points listed under Options Three, Four, and Five is recommended when further treatment is necessary, and that depends on each specific case being treated, that is, on the patient's response.

We proceed this way to reduce the number of needles we use, in accordance with the principle that the fewer needles are used, the more effective they become and the more comfortable the session is.

The Five Options are specifically meant to set a therapeutic strategy from the Exterior to the Interior, which means from the surface to the required depth. Option One starts with treatment of the MSK pain to be resolved which, due to its nature, is located on the superficial layers of the body. Gradually, a deeper treatment is reached, with Option Four aimed at rebalancing the inner organs directly or indirectly involved in pain. Option Five's inclusion of microsystems will not be considered now, as Ear and Wrist-Ankle Acupuncture (WAA) can manage both superficial and deep conditions.

With the therapeutic protocol of the Five Options being immediately effective, treatment frequency ranges from once to twice a week according to pain intensity up to a total of five or six sessions; by then, pain should be either completely resolved or at least relieved by 75%. If necessary, treatment continues for another four sessions, which are to be administered once a week, until the pain disappears.

The kind of condition treated and the patient's overall health status are to be assessed to decide whether treatment should be prolonged to maintain the result obtained or avoid pain recurrence. If the expected results are not obtained, the whole clinical picture should be reconsidered and the patient should be referred to another specialist.

In clinical practice, MSK intense pain from acute and chronic Excess conditions is more frequently observed than dull pain from chronic Deficiency conditions. Therefore this handbook will focus more on how to manage conditions with intense pain, usually associated with limited range of motion (ROM).

The Five Options: Summary

Option One: Distal Points
First step: Jing-Well Points
Second step: Luo Points
Third step: Empirical Points
Fourth step: Opposite Extremity Points (upper/lower)
Fifth step: Categories of Traditional Points
Sixth step: Opening Points of the Extraordinary Vessels

Option Two: Local Points
First step: Painful Point(s) (Ah Shi)
Second step: Anatomically Mirrored Point(s)

Option Three: Adjacent Points
First step: Adjacent Points

Option Four: Etiological Points
First step: Points According to Patterns
Second step: General Points

Option Five: Microsystems
First step: WAA
Second step: Ear Acupuncture

Below is a general overview of the Five Options followed by an in-depth analysis of each step—to provide readers with a complete picture of our therapeutic protocol.

The Five Options Step-By-Step

Option One: Distal Points
The first treatment of musculoskeletal pain in acute and chronic conditions consists of six steps to select distal points.

Results should be assessed after needling each single point and following the order of the list.

Before starting treatment, the practitioner should accurately locate the point or painful area, as well as identify the channels involved.

Distal points can immediately relieve patients' symptoms, such as pain, and also improve restricted ROM, as well as reduce inflammation or swelling.

Each of the first five steps making up Option One recommends needling or bleeding only one point at a time: a few seconds after insertion and before moving to the next point, the practitioner can evaluate effectiveness by assessing pain relief on palpation and on movement, and improvement in ROM.

Testing the efficacy of the distal point of each single step before moving to the following step offers the following advantages:

1. It confirms correctness of the choice made.
2. If the result obtained is very satisfactory, the practitioner can skip the following steps of Option One and move to Option Two.
3. Last but not least, the patient realizes their condition can be successfully treated, the effectiveness of treatment is thus reinforced, and the patient's motivation to continue with the sessions increases alongside benefit from therapy.

By doing so, the practitioner understands which points are the most effective according to their physiology, therapeutic actions, and indications.

The distal points we suggest are the following:

First Step: Jing-Well Points
Aim: To activate the Muscle channels using the Jing-Well point on the affected side.

Second Step: Luo Points
Aim: To activate the Connecting channels using the Luo point on the unaffected side.

Third Step: Empirical Points
Empirical points are acupoints or extrapoints needled on the opposite side of pain. Both tradition and practice have demonstrated their effectiveness in the treatment of signs and symptoms reported by patients. However, not all the conditions described in this manual envisage the use of these points.

Fourth Step: Opposite Extremity Points (upper/lower)
The point to be used is on the unaffected side, on the corresponding joint of the opposite extremity on the paired channel according to the six stages.

It may or may not be an acupoint or a tender point. The anatomically mirrored point is also chosen. It may or may not be tender on palpation and is located on the opposite extremity on the unaffected side, in an area which corresponds to the pain site, although it is not on the channel according to the six stages.

Fifth Step Categories of Traditional Points
Points are selected from the Five Shu Transporting points or the Specific Categories of points according to their physiological functions, actions, and indications.

Regarding the Five Shu Transporting points, the Jing-Well points are of utmost importance, as already mentioned above (first step). However, the importance of the Shu-Stream point needled on the same side of pain should also be mentioned, since it is useful to couple it with the Shu-Stream point on the paired channel according to the six stages on the opposite side of pain.

It is important to note that, so far, we have been following the insertion order outlined earlier, and we have assessed the result obtained after each single needling or bleeding, in terms of both pain relief on palpation and on movement and improvement in ROM.

However, based on our experience, the following distal points of this step do not have the same dynamic and immediately effective characteristics; that is why in our practice, we prefer to proceed with the local points of Option Two, and only afterward, we go back to the distal points left behind.

We act this way because the local points of Option Two are also immediately effective in the removal of Blood stasis and Qi stagnation.

Among the Five Shu Transporting points, another point that is likely to be useful is the Jing-River point to be needled on the same side of pain or bilaterally.

The Jing-River point is used to expel EPFs from joint, bones, and tendons as well as prevent EPFs from reaching the Interior. In addition, it is also used to prevent exacerbation from seasonal changes or exposure to EPFs.

Regarding the Specific Categories of points, in the second step we have already mentioned the fundamental importance of the Luo points. It is now worth emphasizing the role of the Xi-Cleft and Yuan-Source points. The former can remove Blood stasis, especially in the Yin channels, and are needled on the same side of pain. The latter should be used in chronic pain conditions due to Deficiency to tonify both Qi and Blood of the channels running through the affected area, and they should be needled on the same side of pain.

Finally, there are other Specific Categories of points that, in general, affect the anatomic structures and

Vital Substances involved in MSK pain, such as the Hui-Gathering points of sinews, bones, Qì and Blood or the Back-Shu points, the Front-Mu points, and the Hui points of the Zang Fu that contribute to rebalance the Zang Fu in Excess/Deficiency patterns.

Sixth Step: Opening Points of the Extraordinary Vessels

The Extraordinary Vessel to use is chosen based on the patient's symptoms and pain site. The Extraordinary Vessel affected is activated by using its opening point together with the coupled point to enhance the effect of treatment in a specific area.

However, Extraordinary Vessels are not commonly used in the treatment of limb MSK disorders. Among those, Du Mai, Yang, and Yin Qìao Mai are more often used. When we think an Extraordinary Vessel is involved, we prefer to needle it before all the other points, if possible.

Option Two: Local Points

Local treatment always involves accurate localization of the point or the painful site.

In acute and chronic conditions with intense pain, local points are always associated with Qì stagnation and Blood stasis and can be needled or bled. Soon after using them, we can assess how effective our choice has been.

First Step: Painful Point(s) (Ah Shi)

Local points eliciting tenderness on palpation are the Ah Shi points called tender and trigger points in Western medicine and, less frequently, they can correspond to the acupoints. If pain is well localized and very intense, it is a sign of Blood stasis and consequently, we prefer to bleed the point to move blood and remove stasis.

This *modus operandi* enables us to test the effectiveness of our treatment on palpation and on movement immediately after bleeding.

If pain is more widespread, radiating, and less intense, it is a sign of Qì stagnation and therefore we would rather use the needling technique. However, needle insertion into tissues will elicit pain and thus may prevent us from assessing both immediate effectiveness of our treatment on palpation and on movement and improvement in ROM.

In chronic conditions mainly due to Qì and Blood deficiency, the local "point(s)" are used to direct Qì

and Blood flow to the painful site. Needles should be inserted more superficially than in the case of Qì stagnation and Blood stasis.

Local moxa can be useful to tonify Qì and Blood in the affected tissue.

Second Step: Anatomically Mirrored Point(s)

Located on the unaffected side, the corresponding anatomically mirrored point(s) can be needled in acute and chronic Excess conditions with intense pain. The point(s) may or may not be tender on palpation.

Option Three: Adjacent Points

Adjacent points are located at a variable distance from the painful site. Their physiological characteristics, actions, and indications explain their effect on the affected area.

First Step: Adjacent Points

Adjacent points stimulate both the "longitudinal" flow of Qì along the channels involved and its "horizontal" movement between the three Yang and three Yin channels on the affected area. They are selected based on the target area they affect according to classical indications.

Among the adjacent points, the insertion points of the Muscle channels are of paramount importance, as they specifically promote the longitudinal flow of Qì along the affected channel.

Practitioners do not need to test their effectiveness immediately after insertion since they are complementary points selected to promote Qì flow and their needling does not necessarily result in immediate pain relief and improvement in ROM.

Option Four: Etiological Points

Intense MSK pain in acute and chronic conditions is always associated with Qì stagnation and Blood stasis regardless of their cause.

Dull MSK pain or muscular weakness observed in chronic Deficiency conditions is due to the lack of Vital Substances that the Zang Fu should produce.

First Step: Points According to Patterns

Etiological points are the acupoints that contribute to remove local Qì stagnation and Blood stasis to treat acute and chronic pain from Excess conditions.

If pain from Qì stagnation and Blood stasis is caused by invasion of EPFs—mainly Wind, Cold, and

Dampness—into the MSK tissues, practitioners should select the acupoints that make it possible to expel them.

If the Zang Fu do not produce enough Vital Substances for adequate tissue nutrition, we should select those acupoints that stimulate production of Qì and Blood and promote their flow in the channels running through the painful site. This is the case in chronic Deficiency conditions with dull pain, weakness, or numbness or in the resolution phases of pain.

Second Step: General Points

General points are those acupoints belonging to the categories of Traditional Points such as the Hui-Gathering points of sinews, bones, Qì, and Blood. In general, they affect the anatomical structures and Vital Substances involved in MSK pain. Among them, Back-Shu points, Front-Mu points, and Hui points of the Zang Fu contribute to rebalance impaired Zang Fu when they are coupled with specific Shu Transporting points selected based on the pattern to treat, be it Excess or Deficiency.

Option Five: Microsystems

In Chinese Medicine, some microsystems can be very effective in the treatment of MSK pain. We recommend using the WAA and Ear Acupuncture since they are not only effective but also simple and easy to apply.

First Step: Wrist and Ankle Acupuncture

It is based on the selection of six points in the wrist and another six points in the ankle. These points are used to treat conditions localized in six longitudinal and symmetrical regions of the body. The six points each of the wrist and the ankle are used to treat disorders affecting the upper and lower limbs, respectively. Practitioners can choose one or more points corresponding to the superficial and deep body areas they want to treat.

WAA is characterized by the positioning of the needle, which is inserted tangential to the skin and secured in place by an adhesive plaster. We generally use this microsystem at the end of the session or after Option Two, if we are not satisfied with the result obtained.

Should the patient be unable to locate exactly the most painful site or should this area be rather wide and consequently involve more channels, then the WAA can be very useful to relieve secondary pain and highlight the main pain on a single channel. In this specific case, we would rather use it at the beginning of the session, that is, Option One. Further details are provided in Appendix 1.

Second Step: Ear Acupuncture

Specific points on the ear are stimulated to promote healing of the corresponding painful areas, systems, and internal organs involved from the perspectives of both Chinese and Western medicine. For example, when treating shoulder pain, at least one specific ear point is used that corresponds to the area where the Ah Shi point(s) is located (the shoulder), the system involved (subcortex), and the internal organ involved (the Liver). Further details are provided in Appendix 2.

We generally use this microsystem at the end of the session or after Option Two, if the outcome obtained so far is not satisfactory.

The Five Options in Detail

Option One: Distal Points

First Step: Jing-Well Points

Activate the Muscle channel involved using the Jing-Well point on the affected side. Soon after needling or bleeding, assess improvement in pain and ROM.

In our clinical practice, when managing intense MSK pain, treatment usually starts with activation of the Muscle channel running through the painful area.

This very easy technique is based exclusively on the use of the Jing-Well point on the affected side; it is very effective and remarkable improvements in terms of pain reduction, and increased ROM can be observed few seconds after needling.

As it is less painful, bleeding of the Jing-Well point is preferable to needle insertion. Moreover, and this is the most important reason for choosing to bleed the Jing-Well point, intense and well-localized MSK pain, both acute and chronic, results from Blood stasis and therefore bleeding is the most appropriate treatment.

We opt for needling the Jing-Well point when:

- Qì stagnation prevails with less intense and more widespread pain radiating along the Muscle Channel.
- Blood stasis, pain, and ROM do not show significant and immediate improvement after bleeding.

In addition, the bleeding technique can also be used in case of bilateral pain since it neither prevents patient's movements nor makes them uncomfortable.

The distal phalanx of the finger or toe should be kept gently firm even when the Jing-Well point is needled: we use a 0.25 × 25 mm needle or a 0.20 × 15 mm needle.

The bleeding technique is discussed in detail in Appendix 3.

After bleeding or needling, once the expected outcome in terms of pain reduction on palpation and a wider ROM has been achieved, practitioners can proceed to the next steps of Option One to further improve results.

We would like to reiterate that bleeding the Jing-Well point is our first choice in the treatment of intense MSK pain in acute and chronic Excess conditions, especially if associated with inflammation (sign of Heat) or local swelling (sign of Heat or Dampness). The reason is that the bleeding technique not only removes Blood stasis, but it also clears Heat and resolves Dampness. In addition, bleeding the Jing-Well is highly effective and therefore strongly recommended, even if pain is due to a more severe injury to muscle or tendon tissues, such as strains and sprains.

Second Step: Luo Points

Activate the Connecting channel using the Luo point on the unaffected side. Soon after needling, assess improvement in pain and ROM.

Clinical Notes

- Identify the Muscle channel(s) running through the painful site.
- Bleed or needle the Jing-Well point on the affected site in acute and chronic Excess conditions with intense pain from Blood stasis or Qì stagnation.
- More Jing-Well points can be used if the condition affects more Muscle channels.
- In case of significant improvement in pain and ROM, proceed to the next steps and options bearing in mind that the number of points to use can be reduced.
- If no significant result is obtained after bleeding or needling, remove the needle inserted in the Jing-Well point, reassess the correspondence between the Muscle channel selected and the painful area, and try with another Jing-Well point.
- Should no significant result be obtained, remove the new needle and proceed to the second step of Option One.

In our clinical practice, we are used to continuing treatment by activating the Connecting channels covering the painful site when managing intense MSK pain, either acute or chronic, from Excess conditions.

The Luo point removes local Qì stagnation and Blood stasis. The technique is easy as it only involves using the Luo point. Our preferred method is to needle the Luo point on the unaffected side.

Needling of the unaffected side is explained by the anatomy and physiology of the Connecting channels (see Section: LOCATION OF PAIN, The Channels, Connecting Channels).

Needling the contralateral Luo point is not mandatory. As a matter of fact, it can be needled on the same side or on the opposite side; however, we prefer the latter option for an immediate balancing of the right and left sides.

Just as the previous point, the Luo point is also very effective, and its manipulation can result in a significant improvement in pain and ROM after a few seconds.

Needle Technique. The Luo point on the unaffected side is needled, or alternatively **on** the side that is more tender on palpation.

There is no contraindication to the change of side; if we needle the unaffected side and are not satisfied with the result, we can remove the needle and insert it onto the affected side, and vice versa.

When we treat limb in chronic Deficiency conditions with dull pain, weakness, or numbness, or the resolution phases of pain, we use the well-known Luo-Yuan point combination: first, as main point, we needle the Yuan point of the affected side and then, as secondary point, the Luo point on the Internally-Externally related channel on the opposite side.

Third Step: Empirical Points

Both tradition and daily practice suggest using these points. They are acupoints or extrapoints that have proved to be effective in the treatment of patients' symptoms. We prefer to needle them on the unaffected side. Immediately after needling, assess pain relief on palpation and on movement and ROM.

We use this technique to treat acute or chronic pain from Excess conditions.

There are several categories of empirical points passed down by the tradition, and others, more recent, that can be included in the new therapeutic options.

Our experience leads us to use both acupoints and extrapoints located along or outside the pathway of a

- Identify the Connecting channels covering the painful area.
- Use the Luo point on the unaffected side to treat acute and chronic pain from Excess.
- Use the Yuan point of the Main channel running through the painful area as the main point to treat chronic Deficiency conditions with dull pain, weakness, or numbness, or in the resolution phases of pain; as secondary point, use the Luo point of the Internally-Externally related channel on the opposite side.
- More Luo points can be used if the affected area covers more Connecting channels.
- Even if a significant improvement in pain and ROM was observed, treatment should continue as indicated by the following steps and options, although the number of points to select should be reduced.
- If no significant result is obtained, remove the needle from the Luo point and reassess the correspondence between the Connecting channels and the painful area and then try with another Luo Point.
- Should no significant result be obtained, then remove the new needle and proceed to the third step of Option One.

Main channel, following the guidelines contained in classical texts and our masters' indications.

Needle Technique. Empirical points belong to Option One; therefore, after needling, both pain relief on palpation and on movement, as well as improvement in ROM, should be immediately observed. Needle manipulation should be more intense and longer than with the other points. The patient is required to actively move the affected area: if severe pain prevents them from doing so, then they should be helped by the practitioner or physician assistant to induce restricted motion passively and repetitively. Such stimulation should be repeated two to three times during the session.

In acute and chronic Excess conditions the needle is inserted on the unaffected side.

Fourth Step: Opposite Extremity Points (upper/ lower)

The point(s) used corresponds to the painful site but is located on the unaffected side. The

- Use empirical point(s) on the opposite side of the affected area only in acute and chronic Excess conditions. Alternatively, needle the side that is more tender on palpation and if the outcome is not satisfactory, remove the needle and try the other side.
- Even if a significant improvement in pain and ROM was observed, treatment should continue as indicated by the following steps and options.
- Should no significant result be obtained, remove the needle from the empirical point(s) and proceed using the fourth step of Option One.

point(s) are to be searched in the corresponding joint (Fig. 1.4) on the lower limb if the painful site is on the upper limb, and vice versa. The point(s) are located on the paired channel according to the six stages. The corresponding point may or may not be an acupoint or a tender point. After insertion, immediate improvement in pain and ROM should be assessed.

We use this technique to treat acute or chronic pain. The technique consists of needling the limb of the opposite extremity, upper for lower and vice versa, on the unaffected side. Needling the opposite side is not mandatory; needling the same side can be as effective as needling the opposite side, but we prefer the latter to balance the right and left sides sooner. Alternatively, the side which is more tender on palpation can be needled.

There is no contraindication to the change of side: if we needle the opposite (unaffected) side and are not satisfied with the result, we can remove the needle and insert it onto the same (affected) side, and vice versa.

Some authors recommend treatment on the affected side in case of chronic Deficiency conditions with dull pain, weakness, or numbness or in the resolution phases of pain.

Steps One and Two have shown that the first thing to do is to choose the points on the channel(s) running through the affected area, both on the same and opposite sides.

Now, we are referring to points located on channels that do not run through the affected area but are

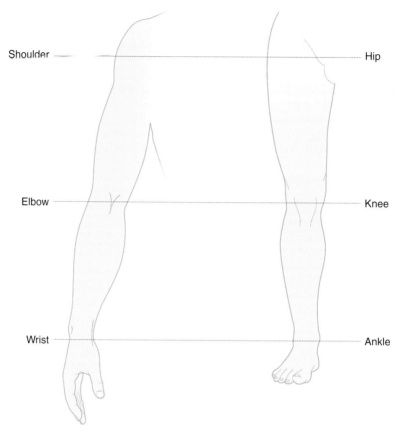

Fig. 1.4 The corresponding joint on the limbs.

strictly related to the others since they are paired channels according to the Six Stages.

This technique has demonstrated to be more effective for the Yang channels due to the "anatomical continuity" of their pathway in terms of energy flow when they reach the head. In addition to that, we also use it when the Yin channels are involved on account of their indirect interconnection in the trunk and in depth.

Selection should also be made considering that each limb is composed of three major joints: shoulder, elbow, and wrist (upper limb) and hip, knee, and ankle (lower limb). According to the mirror concept, points are chosen on the opposite side because there is a correspondence between shoulder and hip, elbow and knee, and wrist and ankle. That is why we select acupoints located on or near the corresponding mirrored joints of the upper limb for the lower extremity, and vice versa. The technique is easy and can be

extended so as to choose the tender point in the joint area, even if it is not an acupoint. In addition, the *mirror concept* can be applied to muscle pain, for example, deltoid pain on the pathway of the Large Intestine channel can be treated by needling the painful point on the proximal end of the quadriceps on the pathway of the Stomach channel, and vice versa (Box 1.1).

A final consideration regarding the anatomical mirroring concerns the choice of the point, to be made by taking into account not only its belonging to the paired channel according to the Six Stages but also its anatomical correspondence, though this a rare situation. For example, in the presence of anterior ankle pain along the pathway of the Stomach channel, practitioners should also needle a point on the dorsum of the wrist, approximately along the pathway of the Triple Burner, meaning that the point is not located on the Yangming stage coupled with the Stomach channel,

BOX 1.1 POINTS OF THE PAIRED YANG CHANNELS ACCORDING TO THE SIX STAGES: CORRESPONDENCE BETWEEN JOINTS IN THE UPPER AND LOWER LIMBS

Joint	Six Stages	Arm	Leg
Shoulder	Yangming	LI15	ST31
	Shaoyang	TE14	GB30
	Taiyang	SI10	BL54
Elbow	Yangming	LI11	ST35, ST36
	Shaoyang	TE10	GB34
	Taiyang	SI8	BL40
Wrist	Yangming	LI5	ST41
	Shaoyang	TE4	GB40
	Taiyang	SI5	BL60

Clinical Notes

- Locate a point, corresponding to the affected joint, on the paired channel according to the Six Stages.
- This point may or may not be an acupoint or a tender point.
- The choice of the point could also be made taking into account not only its position on the paired channel according to the Six Stages but also its anatomical mirroring.
- Use these points—in general, one or two—on the opposite side and extremity of the affected area in acute and chronic Excess conditions with intense pain.
- The points along the pathway of the Yang channels are more effective than those on the Yin channels.

but it is found on the Shaoyang stage coupled with the Gall Bladder channel. This point may or may not be an acupoint or a tender point.

Needle Technique. The use of points on the opposite side and extremity on the paired channel according to the Six Stages, or simply on the anatomically mirrored side, belongs to Option One; therefore their needling should result in immediate pain relief on palpation and on movement. Consequently, after insertion, a mild manipulation is performed to assess improvement in terms of pain and active ROM. If severe pain prevents the patient from doing so, then they should be helped by the practitioner or physician assistant to induce restricted motion passively and repetitively.

As already mentioned, when describing the other steps of Option One, we expect immediate improvement in the parameters of our interest and, if that is the case, needles are left in situ and we proceed to the next step. Should no significant result be obtained, remove the needles and proceed to Option Two, because the following steps of Option One are unable to provide immediate results.

Fifth Step: Categories of Traditional Points

The points used are the Five Shu Transporting points or some points of the Specific Categories. They are selected based on their physiological functions and therapeutic indications. Several different combinations are possible and left to the choice of each practitioner.

Immediate effectiveness after needling can be assessed only when the Jing-Well, Luo, and Shu-Stream points are used, since the other specific acupoints are not so immediately effective. However, they are equally useful in that they complete treatment according to the patterns, Zang Fu, and tissues involved.

The Five Shu Transporting Points

Jing-Well points

They are the first of the Five Shu Transporting points and, as already said (see Section: The Five Options in Detail, Option One: Distal Points, **First Step: Jing-Well Points**), are our first choice when treating acute and chronic MSK disorders with intense pain in Excess conditions.

Ying-Spring points

They are the second of the Five Shu Transporting points. According to the Five-Element theory, the Jing-River points are "Water" points on the Yang channels, while they are "Fire" points on the Yin channels. Consequently, they both have a strong action and are used to clear Heat in conditions characterized by inflammation or swelling of tissues.

Shu-Stream points

They are the third of the Five Shu Transporting points and are extremely important in the treatment of acute and chronic Excess conditions.

In these points:

- EPFs can move internally and penetrate deeper into the Main channels.
- The Wei Qi gathers.

Consequently, they are used to treat pain, prevent EPFs from reaching the Interior or to expel them if they have already reached this level. That is the reason why they are needled to treat Painful Obstruction Syndrome (Bi syndrome), especially from Wind and Dampness. It should be noted that those located on the Yang channels have a more dynamic effect than those on the Yin channels.

According to the Five-Element theory, the Shu-Stream points are "Wood" points on the Yang channels and therefore are used to expel external Wind; being "Earth" points on the Yin channels, they are used to resolve internal and external Dampness. Finally, they are mostly used to treat Yin Organs as they correspond to the Yuan points in the Yin channels, that is why they could also be used in chronic Deficiency conditions, as we will see later.

The Shu-Stream point(s) can be needled alone on account of the physiological characteristics and clinical indications outlined above. In the presence of MSK pain, our approach combines two Shu-Stream points on the paired channel according to the Six Stages, selected according to the affected area.

Needle Technique. The first to be needled is the Shu-Stream point of the channel involved on the affected side and then, as secondary point, the Shu-Stream point of the coupled channel according to the Six Stages on the opposite side.

These points belong to Option One and consequently, immediately after insertion, both pain relief on palpation and on movement and improvement in ROM should be observed. Therefore, after insertion, mild manipulation should be performed after which improvement in pain and ROM should be assessed (Box 1.2).

Jing-River points

They are the fourth of the Five Shu Transporting points.

From these points EPFs are deviated to joints, bones, and tendons where they settle and can remain for a long time without penetrating deeper and affecting

---

Clinical Note

- Differently from what we have been doing so far with points of Option One, if we are not satisfied with outcomes in terms of improvement in pain and ROM, we prefer to leave needles in situ in consideration of the specific physiological functions and clinical indications of these points.

BOX 1.2 SUMMARY OF THE SHU-STREAM POINT COMBINATIONS

Channels	Affected side	Opposite side
Lungs	LU9	SP3
Large Intestine	LI3	ST43
Stomach	ST43	LI3
Spleen	SP3	LU9
Heart	HT7	KI3
Small Intestine	SI3	BL65
Bladder	BL65	SI3
Kidneys	KI3	HT7
Pericardium	PC7	LR3
Triple Burner	TE3	GB41
Gall Bladder	GB41	TE3
Liver	LR3	PC7

the internal organs, thus giving rise to local pain and inflammation. That is why they are used to expel EPFs from joints, bones, and tendons and prevent EPFs from reaching the Interior. Another important characteristic is that their needling prevents exacerbation from seasonal changes or exposure to EPFs. It should be noted that we usually use only those points located on the Yang channels, as they are more effective than those on the Yin channels. Finally, according to the Five-Element theory, the Jing-River points of the Yang channels are "Fire" points that can clear internal and external Heat. Consequently, they are useful in the treatment of conditions with inflammation or swelling of tissues.

He-Sea points

They are the fifth of the Five Shu Transporting points and where the Qì of the channel slowly enters a deeper level to join energy circulation in the body. The He-Sea points are less dynamic, and their action develops gradually. They are generally used to treat chronic Deficiency conditions with dull pain.

Specific Categories of Points
The Luo points

In cases of acute and chronic pain from Excess conditions, they are the second step to complete Option One, since each Luo point activates its corresponding Luo Connecting channels. The Luo points and their use in the treatment of chronic Deficiency conditions have already been discussed in detail before (see Section: The Five Options in Detail, Option One: Distal Points, Second **Step: Luo Points**).

BOX 1.3 SUMMARY OF THE LUO-YUAN POINT COMBINATION

Channels	Yuan	Luo
Lungs	LU9	LI6
Large Intestine	LI4	LU7
Stomach	ST42	SP4
Spleen	SP3	ST40
Heart	HE7	SI7
Small Intestine	SI4	HE5
Bladder	BL64	KI4
Kidneys	KI3	BL58
Pericardium	PC7	TE5
Triple Burner	TE4	PC6
Gall Bladder	GB40	LR5
Liver	LR3	GB37

The Yuan-Source points

We recommend using the Yuan-Source point(s) in chronic Deficiency conditions with dull pain, weakness or numbness, or in the resolution phases of pain, to tonify Qì and Blood of the channel running through the painful site.

Needle Technique. Needling is to be performed on the affected side. In this case, we can associate the Yuan point with the Luo point, that is to say the well-known Luo-Yuan point combination. First, as main point, we needle the Yuan point on the affected side and then, as the secondary point, the Luo point on the Internally-Externally related channel on the opposite side (Box 1.3).

The Xi-Cleft or Accumulation points

These points are where the Qì of the channel gathers and goes deeper. They are mostly used for the treatment of acute pain due to Blood stasis, in particular in the Yin channels. Those in the Yang channels are less used because they are less effective.

Needle Technique. The Xi-Cleft points are deep points and thus longer needles, in general 0.30 × 40 mm, are used to reach the best anatomical location.

The Back-Shu and Front-Mu points

These points treat both associated Zang Fu and corresponding tissues according to the Five-Element theory. Full details can be found under the second step of Option Four (see Section: The Five Options in Detail, Option Four: Etiological Points, Second **Step: General Points**).

The Hui-Gathering points

Traditionally, these are the points associated with anatomical structures or Vital Substances upon which

they act positively. They will be discussed in detail under the second step of Option Four (see Section: The Five Options in Detail, Option Four: Etiological Points, Second **Step: General Points**).

Sixth Step: Opening Points of the Extraordinary Vessels

The opening point of the affected Extraordinary Vessel is needled together with the opening point of the coupled Extraordinary Vessel identified according to symptoms and site of the painful conditions.

The Extraordinary Vessels play a key role in the regulation of Qì and Blood flow in the body. Therefore they are used to reinforce the action of our treatment, or **to** direct its effects towards a target area with the main aim to remove Qì stagnation and Blood stasis. However, they are not frequently used in the treatment of musculoskeletelal disorders of the limbs, since those more often involved are Du Mai, Yang, and Yin Qìao Mai. A specific indication for the use of the Extraordinary Vessels is when the painful area is wide and covers more channels. If this is the case, needling them first enables practitioners to reduce location of pain for a better identification of the Main channel involved.

Du Mai

The pathway of the Du Mai, also known as Governing Vessel, is complex. According to some authors, it can be divided into a Main channel and two branches, an anterior and an internal. For our didactic purposes, we are describing only its main posterior one.

The Du Mai originates in the middle of the pelvis, in between the kidneys, and emerges to the body's surface at GV1. It runs upward, along the midline of the body, up the back, to the nape and head, where it reaches the front. Then, it enters the inner aspect of the upper lip at GV28. GV14 is the meeting point of all Yang channels. A branch originating from GV16 enters the brain and then reaches GV20.

Its "proper" Connecting channel originates from GV1 and ascends the paravertebral region in two parallel branches. Then, it splits and connects bilaterally to the lumbar and dorsal *Hua Tuo Jia Ji*, cervical "Jia Ji," and the main Bladder channel.

It is classically used to manage back pain, but in our practice, we also use it to treat epicondylitis and shoulder pain.

Yang-Qìao Mai

It originates from BL62, outside the heel, ascends along the lateral aspect of the lower extremity, low back, trunk, and head to terminate at the inner canthus of the eye at BL1. One of its branches reaches the shoulder running from SI10 to LI15.

In Excess conditions, muscles of the lateral aspect of the leg and thigh are tight, while those of the medial aspect of the leg and thigh are flaccid, and vice versa in Deficiency conditions.

It is mainly used in Excess conditions with spasms, tightness, and muscle pain affecting the lateral aspect of the leg and thigh. It can also be useful to treat Excess shoulder pain and when pain affects a whole side of the body, that is, shoulder, lateral thoracolumbar spine, and lower extremity. Finally, it can be useful in the treatment of postural imbalance with foot pronation.

Yin Qìao Mai

It originates from KI2, inside the heel, and ascends along the medial aspect of the lower extremity, the inguinal region, and the anterior side of the body to reach the head at BL1.

In Excess conditions, muscles of the medial aspect of the leg and thigh are tight, while those of the lateral aspect of the leg and thigh are flaccid, and vice versa in Deficiency conditions.

It is mainly used in Excess conditions with spasms, tightness, and muscle pain affecting the medial aspect of the leg and thigh, and the inguinal region. It can also be useful in the treatment of postural imbalance with foot supination (Box 1.4).

Needle Technique. When an Extraordinary Vessel is involved, we prefer to activate it by needling it before all of the other points, if possible. First of all, we needle the opening point of the Extraordinary Vessel involved and then the opening point of the coupled Extraordinary Vessel. We also recommend using both opening and coupled points monolaterally: the opening point on the affected side and the coupled point on the unaffected side. For example, if lateral pain radiates along the right lower extremity on the Yang-Qìao Mai, first we will needle the opening point BL62 on the right and then the coupled point SI3 on the left. Opening and coupled points can also be used bilaterally (Boxes 1.5 and 1.6).

BOX 1.4 THE USE OF EXTRAORDINARY VESSELS IN PAIN MANAGEMENT

Extraordinary Vessels	Excess Conditions
Du Mai	Stiffness and cervical pain
Yang-Qìao Mai	• Spasms, tightness, and muscle pain on the lateral aspect of the leg and thigh • Pain affects a whole side of the body
Yin Qìao Mai	• Spasms, tightness, and muscle pain on the medial aspect of the leg and thigh • Pain in the inguinal region

BOX 1.5 OPENING AND COUPLED POINTS OF THE EXTRAORDINARY VESSELS TO TREAT LIMB DISORDERS

Extraordinary Vessel	Opening Point	Coupled Point
Du Mai	SI3	BL62
Yang-Qìao Mai	BL62	SI3
Yin Qìao Mai	KI6	LU7

BOX 1.6 POINTS OF THE EXTRAORDINARY VESSELS TO TREAT LIMB DISORDERS

Extraordinary Vessel	Points
Du Mai	GV14 Cervical Jia Ji
Yang-Qìao Mai	BL62 BL61 BL59 GB29 SI10 LI15 LI16
Yin Qìao Mai	KI2 KI6 KI8

Option Two: Local Points

First Step: Painful Point(s) (Ah Shi)

Treatment of the painful point(s) or site is a fundamental step to manage pain and aims at removing

- Identify the Extraordinary Vessel running through the painful site and traditionally indicated for the treatment of the patient's symptoms.
- Use the Extraordinary Vessel when the painful area is wide and affects more channels.
- Use the opening point on the same side of pain and the coupled point on the opposite site, even if some colleagues prefer bilateral needling of both points.
- To activate the Extraordinary Vessel, needle it first, if possible.
- Use no more than two Extraordinary Vessels.

Qì stagnation and Blood stasis, and expelling EPFs, if any.

Soon after needling or bleeding, immediate pain relief and improvement in ROM should be observed.

Local treatment starts with the precise identification of the painful point(s) or site and assessment of the channels involved. The treatment rationale is simple and consists of removing Qì stagnation and Blood stasis from the channels and regulating the function of the affected tissues, such as muscles, tendons, ligaments, and joints where the inflammatory process is often located.

As already seen, we expect significant pain reduction after using distal points; however, if the outcome is not satisfactory, treatment of local points almost always contributes to further improvement. Local points can be bled or needled to treat acute and chronic pain from Excess conditions or limited ROM. Their effectiveness can be assessed immediately. Local points painful on palpation are called Ah Shi points, or tender and trigger points in Western medicine.

Trigger points are points of local tenderness radiating pain to a wide and well-defined area far from the trigger point itself. Therefore the practitioner may be led to mistakenly locate the site where pain arises and consequently the area to be treated.

Ah Shi points do not always correspond to acupoints, but when some points eliciting local tenderness in the painful site are determined by palpation,

these should also be needled in addition to common acupoints.

Our first aim is to determine by palpation the painful point(s), the so-called "Ah Shi point(s)," corresponding to Qì stagnation and Blood stasis in muscles, tendons, ligaments, and joints.

Very intense and well-localized pain is a sign of Blood stasis: should this be the case, we recommend bleeding the point to remove Blood stasis.

The bleeding technique allows immediate assessment of treatment effectiveness on palpation and on movement. Less intense pain, either widespread or radiating along the pathway of the channel, is a sign of Qì stagnation. In this case, we recommend needling the points to remove Qì stagnation. However, this technique may prevent us from immediately testing effectiveness of our treatment, due to the onset of pain from needle insertion because of the type of tissue or area involved, for example, a joint that should be mobilized to assess ROM.

In chronic conditions from Qì and Blood Deficiency, pain is neither severe nor well localized. Instead, we observe dull pain, weakness, or numbness. Needling aims to direct Qì and Blood flow to the affected areas to nourish tissues. Needles should be inserted more superficially than in case of Qì stagnation and Blood stasis. To tonify Qì and Blood in the affected tissues, it may be more effective to use a moxa stick to warm the area or acupoints. Alternatively, a moxa on the needle can be applied, where it is possible, to combine the therapeutic action of Heat, that is, directing Qì and Blood flow, with the "proper" effect of needling.

Needle Technique. The bleeding technique is easy to apply: the Ah Shi point(s), or less often the acupoint, is pricked quickly and superficially with a sterile lancet. A lancet is used if pain is pricking or localized in a small area, whereas we use a plum blossom needle if the painful area is wider. If the body area to treat is suited for cupping, this therapy should be associated to further promote Blood flow, otherwise tissues should be gently pinched with the thumb and index finger to elicit blood drops. Further details are provided in Appendix 3.

With regards to the number of drops to elicit, we prefer to follow the classical rule, that is, we make it bleed until blood turns from dark red, a sign of Blood stasis, to bright red, a sign of definite removal of Blood stasis.

The bleeding technique can also be used in case of bilateral pain since it neither prevents the patient's movements nor causes pain.

In the few cases where the expected immediate result is not observed in terms of improvement in Blood stasis and, consequently, in pain and ROM, the local Ah Shi point(s) or acupoint(s) can be needled. In general, the needle is inserted perpendicularly to the required depth to reach the site of Qì stagnation and Blood stasis, for example, a ligament or an osteotendinous junction.

When we needle the point(s), we generally use 0.25 × 25 mm or 0.30 × 40 mm needles according to the affected area.

If the expected result in terms of pain relief on palpation and on movement and wider ROM is obtained after bleeding or needling, we proceed to Option Three. Alternatively, if we are not satisfied with the outcome, we proceed to the second step of Option Two.

We would like to stress the importance of the bleeding technique according to our experience. As a matter of fact, it is necessary to bleed the local Ah Shi point(s) to manage MSK intense pain, both acute and chronic as well as from Qì stagnation and Blood stasis. This is particularly true when pain is associated with inflammation, which reveals the presence of Heat, or local swelling, which reveals the presence of Heat or Dampness.

Among other things, the bleeding technique is in fact indicated to clear Heat and resolve Dampness. Our experience teaches us that it is specifically effective and useful also in case of musculotendinous injury, such as a muscle or ligament tear.

In the case of Pain Obstruction Syndrome (Bi syndrome), where the invasion of EPFs has led to Qì stagnation and Blood stasis causing MSK pain, auxiliary techniques may be used at local level to promote removal of stasis and stagnation so as to improve therapeutic outcome. Most frequently, invasions of Wind, Cold, and Dampness are observed, less often Heat.

The following treatment options are recommended:
- Wind: cupping therapy or needle cupping
- Cold: a moxa stick or moxa on the needle
- Dampness: bleeding, moxa, and cupping
- Heat: bleeding and a plum blossom needle

The auxiliary techniques are discussed in detail in Appendices 3–5.

Clinical Notes

- Locate the Ah Shi point(s) that may or may not be acupoint(s).
- First treatment is bleeding in case of Blood stasis and needling in case of Qì stagnation.
- First of all, use the Ah Shi point(s) on the affected area to treat acute and chronic pain from Excess conditions.
- More points around the most painful one can also be bled.
- Additional needles may be inserted around the needle inserted perpendicular to the most painful point.
- Should needling of the painful point(s) increase pain, which is quite a rare occurrence, remove the local needle, and proceed to the Step Two of Option Two.
- Moxa can be used to expel and warm Cold, as well as resolve Dampness, and bleeding to clear Heat and dry Dampness.
- It should be kept in mind that once the needles are inserted, their effectiveness in terms of pain and ROM can no longer be tested.

Second Step: Anatomically Mirrored Point(s)

Use the point(s) on the unaffected side that correspond exactly to the Ah Shi point(s) on the anatomically mirrored side of the affected area. The point(s) can be needled in acute and chronic Excess conditions with intense pain. The point(s) to select may or may not be an acupoint or tender on palpation. Soon after insertion, immediate improvement in pain and ROM should be assessed.

This therapeutic option is used if the results obtained with the treatment of the painful point(s) (Ah Shi) are not satisfactory. In addition, we recommend using it only to treat acute and chronic pain from Excess conditions.

If the anatomically mirrored point(s) are not tender on palpation, we suggest moving a little farther away from the anatomically mirrored point to locate another point, reasonably close and tender.

Under specific clinical situations, multiple tender points can be identified on the anatomically mirrored opposite side and selected for treatment.

Needle Technique. The needling technique is easy; the point(s) to needle is the anatomical mirror of the Ah Shi point(s) and is located on the unaffected side.

The needle is usually inserted perpendicularly to the skin and the pecking and rotating stimulation is applied, even though it is more painful and uncomfortable. The depth of needle insertion to the target tissue should be previously established and not exceeded.

Moderate to strong point stimulation should be applied lasting 10 to 20 seconds until Deqì is obtained. Then, the patient is asked to actively move the affected area to assess improvement in pain and ROM. If severe pain prevents them from doing so, then they should be helped by the practitioner or physician assistant to induce restricted motion passively and repetitively. If the outcome meets expectations, the needle can be either left in or removed and treatment can continue following Option Three.

On the contrary, if there is no significant and immediate improvement in pain and ROM, the needle should be removed and another anatomically mirrored point should be chosen, up to a maximum of two points. Again, if the expected result in terms of pain and ROM is obtained, the needle can either be left in or removed and treatment continued according to Option Three, otherwise the needle should ultimately be removed and treatment continued following Option Three.

When using this technique, the needle may be removed after stimulation; consequently, this type of treatment can also be used in case of bilateral pain, since it does not prevent the patient's movements nor makes them uncomfortable.

In general, we use 0.25 × 25 mm or 0.30 × 40 mm needles according to the anatomical area affected.

Clinical Notes

- Locate the exact point(s) on the unaffected side that is the anatomical mirror of the Ah Shi point(s) on the affected side.
- The point may or may not be tender on palpation or be an acupoint.
- Precise location and needle depth are required.
- Use a maximum of two corresponding points on the opposite unaffected side.
- If the expected result is not obtained, remove the needle and proceed to Option Three.

Option Three: Adjacent Points

Adjacent points are located near the painful point(s) or site and on account of their characteristics they act on the affected area and are therefore complementary to the points used so far.

Assessment of immediate improvement in pain and ROM is not required after needling, since effectiveness is not immediate, unlike distal and local points.

Adjacent points are selected according to the different therapeutic principles:

- The "horizontal" movement of Qì
- Insertion points of the Muscle channels
- Target area
- Orthopedic tests
- Energetic actions of the points

The "Horizontal" Movement of Qì. Stimulating the "horizontal" movement of Qì means promoting the flow of Qì between the three Yang and three Yin channels on the affected area (the "longitudinal" movement of Qì is the one along a channel); this will result in enhanced power of the distal and local points in removing obstructions due to Qì stagnation and Blood stasis from the channel affected.

For example, if we are managing shoulder pain at TE14, we will use both SI10 and LI15. Although this principle is better applied to the movement between channels with the same Yang or Yin polarity, we also use it when a point adjacent to an Ah Shi point on a Yang channel is located on a Yin channel, and vice versa. For example, if pain is located on the wrist at LI5, we will use both TE4 and LU9.

The Insertion Points of the Muscle Channels. They stimulate the "longitudinal" movement of Qì along the channels.

We choose the insertion points surrounding pain when it radiates upward and downward along the pathway of the Muscle channel affected by MSK pain. For example, if deltoid pain is located on the Muscle channel of the Large Intestine at LI14 and radiates upward to the shoulder and downwards to the elbow, we can use LI15 in the shoulder and LI11 in the elbow. These points help the flow of Qì upward and downward, thus ensuring the free and smooth circulation in joints and promoting the expulsion of EPFs, if there are any.

Target Area. An acupoint affects a well-defined area according to classical indications. For example, when we manage shoulder pain at SI10, both SI11 and SI13 controlling scapula and shoulder can be used.

Orthopaedic Tests. Western diagnosis allows identification of the muscles, tendons, ligaments, and joints affected by the MSK pain to be treated. To reach this goal, practitioners can use points located on the injured structures. For example, LI16 corresponds to the musculotendinous junction of the supraspinatus muscle, whereas SI12 to its belly.

Energetic Actions of the Points. It should be kept in mind that these are complementary points selected to promote Qì flow in the affected area.

For example, TE5 is useful for wrist pain, whereas LI4 is useful for fingers, **and** both of them promote the flow of Qì.

Needle Technique. A mild stimulation is applied at the depth of insertion previously established. More points can be chosen according to therapeutic principles selected, extent of the painful area, and pain radiating upward or downward.

If pain is radiating, we usually needle the point reached by pain or those points located on the pathway of radiating pain. In the latter case, it would be more correct for didactic purposes to call these points local rather than adjacent points. Needle insertion is perpendicular to the affected area, or oblique, and we generally use 0.25 × 25 mm or 0.30 × 40 mm based on the affected area.

Clinical Notes
....

- Select the points surrounding the painful area according to the most appropriate therapeutic principles.
- We recommend choosing those points corresponding to more therapeutic principles.
- More points can be used, but **no** more than four.

Option Four: Etiological Points

Treatment consists of needling those acupoints that, if associated with distal and local points, contribute to remove Qì stagnation and Blood stasis or to tonify Qì and Blood in acute and chronic conditions.

Assessment of immediate improvement in pain and ROM is not required after needling, since effectiveness is not immediate, unlike distal and local points.

Qì stagnation and Blood stasis are often due to trauma, repetitive microtrauma, overuse, or invasion of EPFs. Less frequently, they result from internal imbalance caused by IPFs that accumulate following imbalance of the Zang Fu.

In case of intense pain, the etiological points are those acupoints that help remove Qì stagnation and Blood stasis due to Excess conditions.

In case of dull pain, weakness, or numbness, we recommend using those acupoints that stimulate production of Qì and Blood by the Zang Fu, the lack of which prevents adequate nutrition of tissues.

It is worth reminding that the lack of Vital Substances in the MSK tissues may predispose to strains and sprains, and favor the invasion of EPF.

In conclusion, we can affirm that treatment of the Zang Fu imbalance is often useful in the management of MSK pain in Excess and Deficiency conditions.

First Step: Points According to Patterns

Etiological points according to patterns are the acupoints that contribute to remove Qì stagnation and local Blood stasis, whatever their cause is, EPF and IPF included. Furthermore, they contribute to tonify Qì and Blood.

In case of intense, acute, or chronic pain from Excess conditions, the etiological points usually belong to the Five Shu Transporting points or the Specific Categories of points. This means that they lack those physiological activities and dynamic effects, pertaining to the Jing-Well, Luo, and Shu-Stream points, required for immediate removal of Qì stagnation and Blood stasis, or expulsion of IPFs and EPFs. Therefore, once needled, it is not necessary to test their effectiveness in terms of pain improvement and increased range of motion (Box 1.7).

In case of dull pain, weakness, or numbness from chronic Deficiency conditions, the etiological points are those acupoints that enhance production of Qì and Blood by the Zang Fu to nourish tissues. Under these circumstances, we find it more effective to stimulate the Liver; since it controls correct Blood flow in musculotendinous tissue, and treats and prevents pain and disorders of muscles, tendons, ligaments, and joints (Box 1.8).

BOX 1.7 POINTS FOR EXCESS CONDITIONS

Qì stagnation	LI4, LR3, GB34
Blood stasis	BL17, LI11, PC6, SP6, SP10
Phlegm	ST40, SP9, CV12, CV 9, BL20
Cold	GV14, Du4, BL23, CV6, CV4, ST36, all of them with moxa
Dampness	BL20, SP6, SP9, ST36, GB34
Wind	BL12 with cupping, BL17, BL18, GV14 with cupping, GB31, GB39
Heat	LI4, LI11, ST43, GV14 with bleeding cupping

BOX 1.9 INTERNAL ORGANS AND THEIR CORRESPONDING ACTION ON QÌ AND BLOOD

Zang	Corresponding Actions on Qì and Blood
Liver	Harmonizes the free flow of Qì and Blood, Stores Blood
Spleen	Produces and controls Blood
Kidneys	Hold Qì
Lungs	Contribute to production and distribution of Qì all over the body
Heart	Contributes to production and distribution of Blood all over the body and controls blood vessels

BOX 1.8 POINTS FOR DEFICIENCY CONDITIONS

Qì/Blood deficiency	ST36, SP6, CV4, CV6, CV12, LR8
Liver, Spleen, and Kidney deficiency	LR8, SP6, ST36, KI3, GB34, BL18, BL20, BL23, CV4

Second Step: General Points

General Points usually belong to the Specific Categories of points and contribute to expel EPF and IPF. In addition, they act on the anatomical structures, Vital Substances, and Zang Fu involved in MSK pain and help rebalance impaired physiological activities in Excess and Deficiency conditions.

The Back-Shu and Front-Mu points. These points act on the related Zang Fu and on the corresponding tissues according to the Five Elements.

The Back-Shu points are useful to reinforce effectiveness of treatment to rebalance Zang Fu in Excess and Deficiency conditions; they are combined with the Five Shu Transporting points, especially the Shu-Stream points which represent the classical combination.

According to the tradition, the Back-Shu points are used in chronic Deficiency conditions to tonify Vital Substances, and in acute and primarily chronic Excess conditions to expel IPFs. The Front-Mu points are mainly selected to manage acute conditions, but almost exclusively in the treatment of internal diseases to expel IPFs. The only exception worth mentioning here is the Front-Mu point of the Stomach CV12, to

be selected to enhance the production of Qì and Blood in chronic Deficiency conditions.

The Back-Shu points we use more frequently are BL18 corresponding to the Liver, BL20 to the Spleen, and BL23 to the Kidneys; these points control and act on tendons, muscles, and bones, respectively.

It should be remembered that Back-Shu and Front-Mu points also treat Qì and Blood impairment along their corresponding channels.

The *a priori* mistake to assume there is a direct relationship between pain on a channel and an organic dysfunction with associated pattern should not be made. In the same way, recurrent pain or repeated trauma in the same anatomic region crossed by a channel should not be necessarily attributed to a specific Zang Fu pattern.

In our clinical experience, neither direct nor indirect involvement of Zang Fu in MSK pain is frequent. Despite that, if the patient's medical history highlights one or more patterns of the Zang Fu, though not related to pain onset, we prefer using some etiological points for general rebalancing of the patient. To reach this goal, Back-Shu and Front-Mu points are among the most useful ones. Needless to say, the most appropriate point can be combined with an acupoint selected from the Five Shu Transporting points or Specific Categories of points (Boxes 1.9 and 1.10).

Needle Technique. Regarding the Back-Shu points, there are different ways to needle them according to different anatomical and therapeutic principles and depending on the diseases to treat.

The needle is inserted at an angle from oblique to transverse and downwards, following the pathway of

BOX 1.10 BACK-SHU POINTS, INTERNAL ORGANS, AND CORRESPONDING TISSUES, ACCORDING TO THEIR FIVE ELEMENTS

Back-Shu Point	Zang Fu	Tissue
BL13	Lungs	Skin
BL15	Heart	Vessels
BL18	Liver	Tendons
BL20	Spleen	Muscles
BL23	Kidneys	Bones

BOX 1.11 THE HUI-GATHERING POINTS, THEIR CORRESPONDING TISSUES, VITAL SUBSTANCES AND ZANG FU

Hui-Gathering Points	Tissue, Qì, Blood, and Zang Fu
GB34	Sinews
BL11	Bones
GB39	Marrow
LU9	Vessels
CV17	Qì
BL17	Blood
LR13	Zang
CV12	Fu

the Bladder Channel. By doing so, Qì flow is enhanced throughout the body, specifically in the target Zang Fu. This option is particularly suitable for the Back-Shu points in the upper back where the muscle mass is reduced and consequently points are more superficial. Practicality is another reason for choosing this technique: limb MSK pain often requires needle insertion with the patient lying supine for about 25 to 30 minutes. This method enables practitioners to insert needles in the Back-Shu points and then leave them in situ with the patient lying on them.

We recommend using 0.25 × 25 mm or 0.30 x 40 mm needles according to the anatomical area affected. A mild rotating stimulation is applied to the Back-Shu points. Unlike the other acupoints where needles are usually left in for about 25 to 30 minutes, needles can be left in the Back-Shu points for a shorter time, about 10 to 15 minutes. The reason for such a difference lies in the type of stimulation: by needling these points, the nerve structures from the vertebral canal are almost directly stimulated due to their proximity. Therefore their action is both direct and indirect on the autonomic and peripheral nervous system.

The Hui-Gathering Points. Traditionally, these are the points associated with the anatomical structures, Vital Substances, and Zang Fu, on which they act to regulate their impaired functions. That is why some of them, such as the Hui-Gathering points of sinews, bones, Qì and Blood, can help treat MSK pain. More frequently, we use GB34; not only is it the Gathering point of sinews and, in general, it treats tendons and may therefore be used as a secondary point for tendonitis, but the classical indications also suggest that it promotes the smooth flow of Liver Qì. Because of its action, it is an important point to relax the

sinews whenever there are contractions of the muscles, cramps, or spasms, and to move Qì stagnation and remove Blood stasis. On these grounds, GB34 is an important point in the treatment of Painful Obstruction Syndrome (Bì Syndrome).

Finally, it should be kept in mind that the Hui-Gathering points of the Zang Fu can be used as general points, since they contribute to reinforcing the effectiveness of treatment of MSK pain and rebalancing the Zang Fu, both in Excess and in Deficiency conditions (Box 1.11).

Option Five: Microsystems
We recommend associating the WAA and Ear Acupuncture with the abovementioned acupoints, since these techniques potentiate the effects of the acupoints, in addition to being effective and simple to apply. Further details of both techniques are provided in Appendices 1 and 2.

The Fundamentals of Osteopathy for Musculoskeletal Pain in the Limbs

According to the World Health Organization, osteopathy relies on manual contact for diagnosis and treatment. Special emphasis is put on the structural and functional integrity of the body, regarded as an integrated whole and a self-healing mechanism.

Osteopathy is a hands-on therapy that aims to influence all the systems of the body including muscles, bones, and the nervous system, as well as circulatory and immune functions to encourage good health.

- Use the etiological points since they help:
  - Reduce in Excess conditions with Qì stagnation and Blood stasis or in the presence of IPFs and EPFs
  - Tonify in Deficiency conditions with Qì and Blood deficiency.
- A direct or indirect relationship between Zang Fu imbalance and MSK pain onset or recurrence should not be taken for granted.
- However, if the patient's medical history highlights noticeable Zang Fu impairment, we recommend using one or two points for rebalancing.
- In addition, a combination of Back-Shu and Hui-Gathering points of the tissues and Vital Substances involved in MSK pain from Excess or Deficiency is required.
- Treatment of Zang Fu and Vital Substances implies selecting among a large number of diagnostic and therapeutic options, and each practitioner makes their choice based upon their experience. That is why there is no standard protocol to follow.
- The points on the Bladder channels and located on the upper back should be used with the utmost care; when needles are inserted perpendicularly and with the patient in the prone position, there is a high risk of pleural puncture. Therefore we would recommend oblique to transverse needling orientation.

Osteopathic manipulative treatments (OMTs) include hands-on manipulations of different body structures to increase systemic homeostasis and total patient well-being.

At the end of the 19th century, Andrew Taylor Still first introduced the concept of Osteopathic Medicine and somatic dysfunction.

Born in 1828 in Virginia, United States, after acquiring medical training he started questioning traditional medicine and, above all, drug abuse. He believed that osteopathic medicine could offer more to the patient and therefore formulated his principles of osteopathy. In 1892, he founded the American School of Osteopathy, and 2 years later, he established the *Journal of Osteopathy*. He died in 1917 at the age of 89.

It was William Garner Sutherland (1873–1954) who first presented the Cranial Concept in 1929.

Fascinated by the study of the cranial bones, he noticed that they had an inherent motion to them and were strictly interconnected and, at the same time, connected to the sacrum through the meninges.

Craniosacral mobility is one of the peculiar features characterizing osteopathy. This technique is often used to treat internal medicine diseases, pediatric patients, and spine disorders.

This handbook only deals with MSK pain of the upper and lower limbs, with special attention to the osteopathic dysfunctions of the shoulder, elbow, wrist, hip, knee, and ankle, that is to say the joints more frequently treated in clinical practice.

The only way to diagnose a somatic joint dysfunction is to assess the passive movements of its two articular ends in relation to one another and compared with the same joint on the healthy side.

When quantity and quality of the reciprocal movement of the two articular ends are altered, then there is a somatic dysfunction.

THE BARRIER CONCEPT

The barrier is the limit to joint motion and can be either physiologic or pathologic. In defining barriers, quality and ROM of the involved joint should be assessed. In the next sections the following barriers will be covered:

- Anatomical barrier: the limit of maximum passive motion imposed by the anatomic structure
- Physiological barrier: the limit of active motion
- Elastic barrier: the limit of passive motion
- Restrictive barrier: the dysfunctional limit of motion

The neutral point of a joint is a balance point of myofascial tension that allows active and passive mobility of little amplitude.

The neutral point is the theoretical point to refer to when assessing active and passive ROM, both physiologic and dysfunctional, of the two joint ends under examination.

SOMATIC DYSFUNCTION

Somatic dysfunction is an osteoarticular disorder causing impaired or altered function of related components of the somatic system: skeletal, articular, and myofascial structures, and related vascular, lymphatic, and neural elements. Somatic dysfunction can be treated using OMT.

Specifically, performing tests in the correct way is of paramount importance.

The presence of a somatic dysfunction is a sign of limitation to movement, that is, restriction in joint ROM. Somatic dysfunction is often compared to a "blocked" joint. It is often believed that only a severe trauma can lead to a dysfunction, thus underestimating poor posture, microtraumas due to work- or sports-related repetitive movements, physical, social, and environmental features, as well as emotional stress.

THE DIAGNOSTIC PROTOCOL

To identify evidence of somatic dysfunction, specific tests are performed to assess the ROM of each single joint forming the anatomo-functional structure involved, and then to compare it with the respective contralateral joint.

Consequently, at this stage the totality of movement of the anatomic structure affected (for example, knee flexion and extension) is not assessed. And since such motion results from the sum of movements of each single joint (patellofemoral, tibiofemoral, and tibiofibular joints), each joint will be evaluated individually.

The passive movement of the two joint ends is assessed, distal versus proximal, for motion restriction and for dysfunctional parameters.

Somatic dysfunction is called after the direction in which motion of the articular end is freer. Motion will be more limited, that is, more restricted, in the opposite direction (restrictive barrier).

Then, all the joints functionally involved in the *dynamics* of movement of the anatomical unit affected should be tested, even if they are asymptomatic. For example, when treating knee pain, both hip and ankle joints should be assessed.

It is therefore evident how important it is for the practitioner to acquire sensitivity to palpation to be able to identify those dysfunctional parameters defining a somatic dysfunction.

OSTEOPATHIC MANIPULATIVE TREATMENT

Mobility tests assess dysfunctional parameters, meaning restriction in motion of a joint end in relation to the other end. The aim of OMT is to restore normal (functional) joint mobility. The main osteopathic techniques are the so-called musculoskeletal, myofascial, cranial, and visceral techniques.

This handbook only deals with MSK techniques, which include:

- High velocity-low amplitude (HVLA) techniques—"thrust": the practitioner applies a rapid final force of brief duration—the "Thrust"—over a short distance, to move the dysfunctional joint end in the direction it would not move in (restrictive barrier).
- Articulatory techniques: the practitioner use a gentle manipulation force to move the dysfunctional joint end in the direction it would not move in (restricted motion).
- Muscle energy techniques (METs): the dysfunctional joint end is pulled or pushed by the patient while the practitioner introduces an equal counterforce (isometric-contraction) in the direction of a better mobility.
- Soft tissue technique: the goal is to relax and lengthen a muscle.

All the dysfunctions revealed by the tests of the joints should be treated, even if no signs of disease are observed. For example, when managing knee pain, both hip and ankle dysfunctions need to be treated.

A STEP-BY-STEP APPROACH

The Barrier Concept

Correct joint mobility reveals the physiological condition of a joint. The **main difference** between active and passive ROM is the fact that the **active movement is carried out by the patients themselves, whereas the passive movement is carried out by the practitioner**. Understanding this difference is the key to introduce the barrier concept.

The Anatomical Barrier

The total range of motion (ROM) of a joint is the limit of maximum passive motion imposed by the anatomic structures. It is limited by the integrity of joint structures and components, such as bones, ligaments, muscles, joint capsule, and fasciae. The limit of the total ROM is called the anatomic barrier.

Exceeding the anatomic barrier causes fractures, dislocations, or soft tissue injuries, such as ligament tears.

Within the total ROM is located the neutral point (see Fig. 1.5).

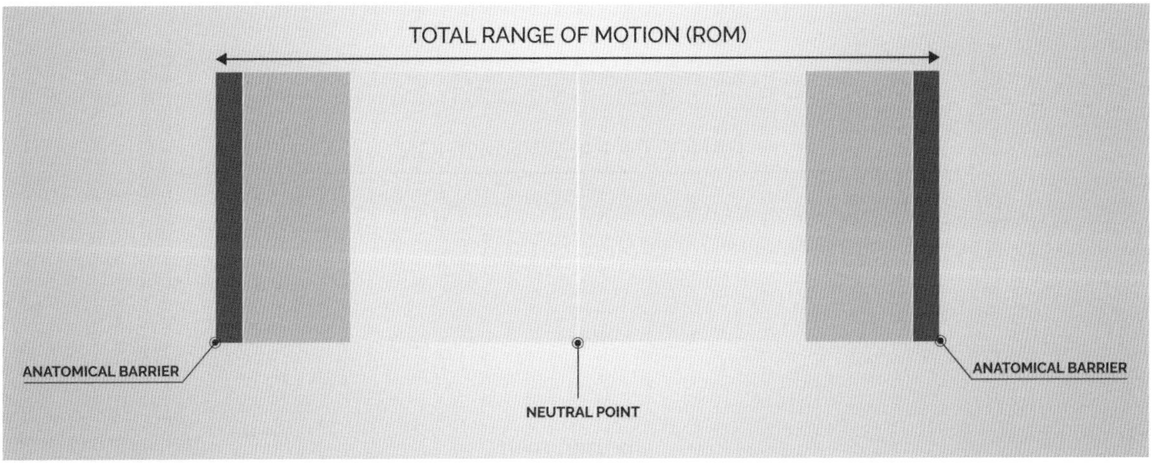

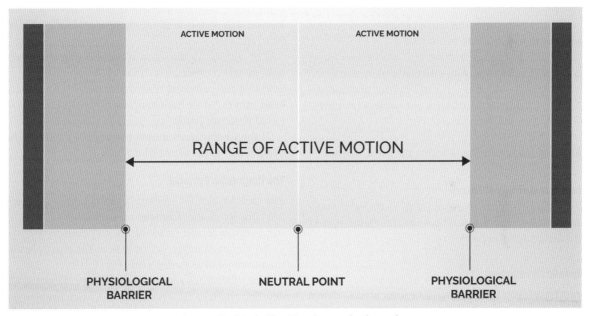

Fig. 1.5 Anatomical barrier, total ROM, and neutral point.

Fig. 1.6 Physiological barrier and range of active motion.

The Physiological Barrier

Within the total ROM, there is the range of active motion, which is the movement voluntarily produced by the patient.

Active ROM is more limited than passive ROM, and its end point is called the physiological barrier (see Fig. 1.6).

The Elastic Barrier

Within the total ROM, there is a range of passive motion achieved when the practitioner applies a force on the joint. The limit of the range of passive motion is called the elastic barrier. The range of passive motion includes the space between the elastic barriers, which

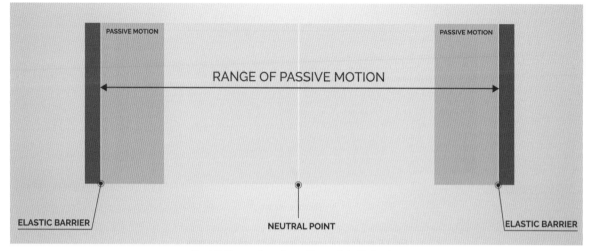

Fig. 1.7 Range of passive motion and elastic barrier.

means it also includes the range of active and passive motion of the joint.

The aim of the osteopathic test is to assess range and quality of motion of an articular end in relation to the other end, which is held still by the practitioner. Motion is then compared with the same joint movement on the opposite side (see Fig. 1.7).

According to the recent scientific literature, the thrust should be safely performed within the elastic barrier.

Paraphysiological Space

The paraphysiological space (Fig. 1.8) is a small amount of potential space between the elastic barrier and the anatomical barrier.

Somatic Dysfunction

Somatic dysfunction is a diagnostic term used to define the altered range of movement of a joint. When impaired or altered function of a joint structure is observed, the first signs to appear are vasodilation, edema, pain, and muscular contracture, which alter myofascial tensions.

Somatic dysfunction is associated with loss of active and passive ROM in all directions, but one direction will be more restricted.

Consequently, we can say that the active and passive movements are all restricted, but the most important restrictive barriers of active and passive

motion will be found in the more restricted direction (see Fig. 1.9).

The somatic dysfunction is named after the direction in which motion is freer. For example, when assessing the proximal tibiofibular joint, if the fibular head moves better backward, then the dysfunction is called *posterior fibula*.

If the fibular head moves better forward, then the dysfunction is called *anterior fibula*.

The Diagnostic Protocol

The examination for "somatic dysfunction" is the central concept of the diagnostic process. Position of the hands varies according to the test to perform.

To see an example, let us look at the test to assess the proximal tibiofibular joint (Fig. 1.10).

The patient lies supine, with the knee flexed at 90 degrees, and foot flat on the bed. The practitioner sits on the foot to stabilize the leg.

To perform the test correctly, hand positioning is paramount.

Before performing any movement, the practitioner should "feel" the patient's bony structures. First, a progressive pressure is applied on the soft tissues until the bone level is reached. Afterward, the movement of an articular end is assessed in relation to the other end by pushing or pulling first in a direction and then in the opposite direction.

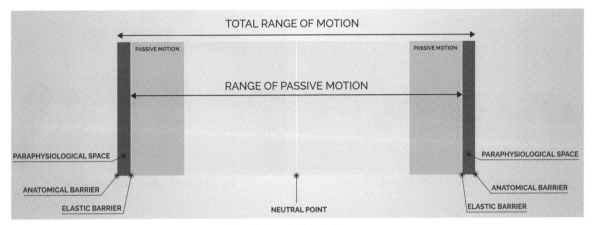

Fig. 1.8 Paraphysiological space.

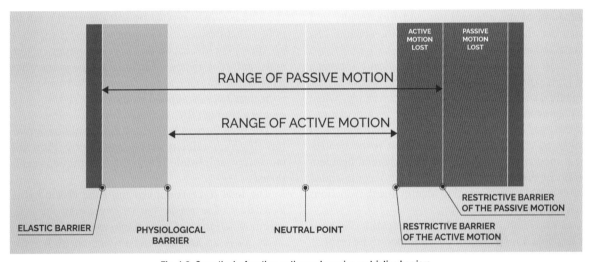

Fig. 1.9 Somatic dysfunction, active and passive restrictive barriers.

The direction of the articular end changes according to the biomechanics of each single joint. Movement will always start from and go back to the neutral point of that joint.

The other crucial step is to keep still that joint end, which is regarded as the reference joint. For example, if the fibular motion is being tested, the hand that is not on the fibula should hold the tibia still, otherwise it would not be possible to appreciate the relative fibular motion. In the beginning, it is not always easy to appreciate the movements of the articular ends in relation to one another. A possible explanation is that we are used to performing orthopedic tests, which have taught us to assess macromovements. Instead, the osteopathic tests will teach us to appreciate gentle micromovements with limited elasticity.

Once range and quality of motion have been appreciated and compared with the contralateral side, if motion in a direction is restricted, then there is a dysfunction.

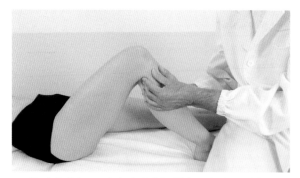

Fig. 1.10 Anteroposterior test of the fibula—starting position.

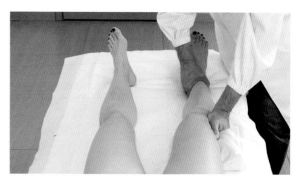

Fig. 1.11 Anterior fibula treatment—thrust.

Finally, OMT can be performed to restore the physiological motion of the joint.

To sum up, the examination for "somatic dysfunction" is the key concept of the diagnostic process; palpation of the affected area and functionally and anatomically related components of the somatic system is the only way to assess it.

Consequently, the osteopathic diagnostic approach to MSK pain is based on the identification of all the somatic dysfunctions of a joint. For example, when managing knee pain, not only will all the articulations of the knee be assessed, but also those of the hip and ankle. So, regardless of the condition to be treated, be it medial meniscus tear, medial collateral ligament strain or tear, or any other, all of the recommended tests should be performed to identify the dysfunctions that occur more frequently.

It is therefore evident that the osteopathic diagnosis is developed regardless of the condition to be treated.

Osteopathic Manipulative Treatment

The aim of OMT is to restore the physiological motion of the joint, meaning moving the restrictive barrier as far into the direction of motion loss as is possible, that is, as close as possible to the physiological and elastic barriers.

High Velocity-Low Amplitude Techniques—"Thrust"

This technique reverses the direction of the dysfunctional parameters of the affected articular end, with the aim to restore physiologic motion. Put simply, it consists in moving the affected articular end in the direction it would not move in.

Procedure. The practitioner positions the affected bone end so as to engage the restrictive barrier. The practitioner positions the affected bone end so as to engage the restrictive barrier. Then, firm and painless pressure is slowly applied on soft tissues to reach the bony structures.

After joint decoaptation (soft separation of joint ends) and rebalancing (searching for the point where tensions of muscles and ligaments are balanced), a corrective force is applied to move the dysfunctional segment through the restrictive barrier.

The final force of brief duration should be applied rapidly (high velocity [HV]) and over a short distance (low amplitude [LA]): this technique is called *thrust*.

The final force is applied until the elastic barrier is reached. The elastic barrier represents the space within which the practitioner can exert a force to passively move an articular end in relation to the other end without damaging the articular tissues.

Depending on the joint involved, thrust manipulation may or may not generate the distinctive popping sound.

Let us put theory into practice with an example of correction of the anterior fibula, which means anterior sliding of the tibia is better than posterior sliding.

The patient is supine with the knees extended. The practitioner holds the ankle of the affected leg with the right hand, while the left thenar eminence is over the fibular head (Fig. 1.11).

After joint decoaptation and rebalancing, the thrust is performed by vertically pushing the fibular head downward with the left hand.

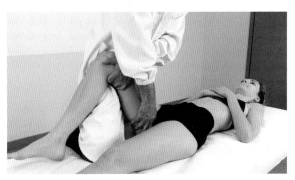

Fig. 1.12 Tension of the obturator membrane treatment.

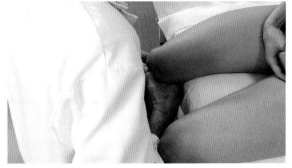

Fig. 1.13 Anterior medial meniscus—starting position.

Soft Tissue Techniques

The goal is to relax and lengthen muscles and membranes and involves stretching movements across or along muscular fibers and membranes. These techniques can be performed before the thrust or as a stand-alone technique on account of its mechanical effect.

To see an example, let us examine how to treat tension of the obturator membrane.

The patient lies supine. The practitioner brings the affected hip into flexion with slight abduction (Fig. 1.12). With the thumb of the right hand, the practitioner palpates for the tender point on the obturator membrane.

The practitioner progressively reduces abduction until tenderness disappears and then holds this position for 90 seconds.

Articulatory Techniques

It is the practitioner's action that achieves correction. This procedure is an extended mobility test for diagnostic purposes. It aims to restore joint physiological function and motion symmetry, as well as resolve pain. It can also be used as preparation for the HVLA technique.

To see an example, let us look at the treatment of the anterior medial meniscus.

The patient sits on the bed, legs off the edge. The practitioner sits on the patient's foot holding the affected leg in internal rotation. Then, the practitioner grasps the knee joint with both hands and places the thumbs on the anterior horn of the medial meniscus.

While standing up, the practitioner extends and externally rotates the leg, always keeping the thumbs still on the anterior horn to force the meniscus to move backward (see Figs. 1.13 and 1.14).

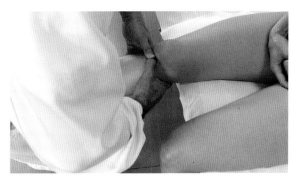

Fig. 1.14 Anterior medial meniscus—final position.

Muscle Energy Techniques (METs)

It is an active technique in which the patient is asked to actively use their muscle's own energy. Motion starts from a specific position and moves in a specific direction, both of which vary according to the joint involved. At the same time, the practitioner introduces an equal counterforce.

The practitioner places the affected joint end so as to engage the restrictive barrier. Then, the patient is asked to perform a muscle contraction in the direction where there is more freedom of motion.

Let us examine how to treat posterior fibular head. A reminder that posterior dysfunction means that backward sliding of the fibula is better than forward sliding.

The patient is supine close to the bed edge with the knee flexed at 90 degrees and foot flat on the bed.

The practitioner sits on the foot to stabilize the leg and holds the tibia with the right hand while the

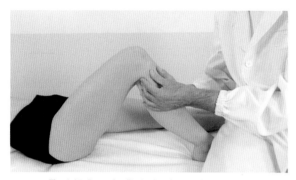

Fig. 1.15 Posterior fibular head—starting position.

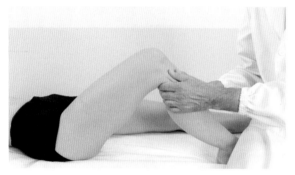

Fig. 1.16 Posterior fibular head—final position.

thumb, index finger, and middle finger of the left hand grasp the fibular head.

The patient is asked to flex the knee against the practitioner's fingers, while the practitioner exerts an equal counterforce. The position is held for 3 seconds and followed by a 3-second period of postisometric relaxation. Afterward, the practitioner pulls the head of the fibula forward to engage a new restrictive barrier. Then, the patient is asked again to flex the knee against the practitioner's fingers. This sequence should be repeated three times (see Figs. 1.15 and 1.16).

In conclusion, the key point of the osteopathic therapeutic process is the treatment not only of the somatic dysfunctions of the joint affected but also of those which are functionally and anatomically related, even if asymptomatic.

For example, when managing knee pain, both hip and ankle dysfunctions need to be treated. In conclusion, regardless of the condition to manage, all the dysfunctions identified should be treated.

BIBLIOGRAPHY

Osteopatia Audouard M. *l'Arto Inferiore*. Editore Marrapese; 1989.

Deadman P., Al-Khafaji M., Baker K., Manuale di Agopuntura, Ed. italiana a cura di Grazia Rotolo e Giulio Picozzi, CEA (Casa Editrice Ambrosiana), 2000

Giusti R. *Glossary of Osteopathic Terminology*. 3rd ed. American Association of Colleges of Osteophatic Medicine; 2017.

Greenman PE. *Principles of Manual Medicine*. 2nd ed. Williams & Wilkins; 1996.

Guolo F. *Atlante di Tecniche di Energia Muscolare*. Piccin; 2014.

Legge D. *Close to the Bone*. Sydney College Press; 2010.

Maciocia G. *The Foundations of Chinese Medicine*. 2nd ed. Churchill Livingstone, Elsevier; 2005.

Maciocia G. *The Channels of Acupuncture*. Churchill Livingstone, Elsevier; 2006.

Maciocia G. *The Practice of Chinese Medicine*. 3rd ed. Elsevier; 2022.

Nicholas AS, Nicholas EA. *Atlas of Osteophatic Thechniques*. Lippincott Williams & Wilkins; 2012.

Qiao W. *Wrist and Ankle and Balance Acupuncture*. Italian Chine School of Acupuncture-A.M.A.B (Association of Medical Acupuncturist of Bologna) Seminar; 2007.

Reaves W, Bong C. *The Acupuncture Handbook of Sports Injuries & Pain*. third edition. Hidden Needle Press; 2013.

Romoli M. *Auricular Acupuncture Diagnosis*. Churchill Livingstone Elsevier; 2009.

Tan RT., Dr. Tan's Strategy of Twelve Magical Points. Edited by Besinger JW, San Diego, California, 2003

Qì-cai Wang. *Secondary Channels and Collaterals*. People's Medical Publishing House; 2007.

Yajuan Wang. *Micro-Acupuncture in Practice*. Churchill Livingstone Elsevier; 2009.

Liansheng Wu, Qì Wu. *Yellow Emperor's Canon of Internal Medicine, Chinese-English Addition*. China Science and Technology Press; 2005.

Tixa S. *Atlas d'Anatomie Palpatoire, tome 2, Membre Inferior*. 3rd ed. Elsevier Masson; 2005.

Tixa S, Ebenegger B. *Atlas de Techniques articulaires ostéopathiques, tome 3, Les Membres*. 2nd ed. Elsevier Masson; 2016.

Yi-ling W. *Collateral Disease Theory in Practice*. People's Medical Publishing House; 2008.

Qinghui Z, Changquan L, Xinshu Z. *Wrist-Ankle Acupuncture*. Publishing House of Shanghai University of Traditional Chinese Medicine; 2002.

Chapter 2

The Shoulder

Supraspinatus and Infraspinatus Tendonitis, Tendonitis of the Long Head of the Biceps, and Acromioclavicular Joint Disorders

Supraspinatus and infraspinatus tendonitis, and tendonitis of the long head of the biceps (LHB) are types of tendinopathy causing inflammation of the tendons and their protective synovium sheathing.

They are of mechanical origin and occur as the consequence of work- or sports-related repetitive shoulder movements, which cause the tendon to rub against the underlying bony surfaces.

Similarly, acromioclavicular (AC) joint disorders occur as a consequence of work- or sports-related repetitive shoulder movements or may result from distracting injury to the shoulder.

Local pain can radiate distally to the arm or proximally to the scapula and toward the neck.

Anatomy and Biomechanics According to Western Medicine

JOINTS AND MUSCLES

The shoulder complex is composed of four bones (the humerus, scapula, clavicle, and sternum) and four joints.

The anatomical or true joints are the following:
- The glenohumeral (GH)
- The AC
- The sternoclavicular (SC)

The physiological or false joint is the scapulothoracic (ST), which is an articulation of the scapula with the thorax. In this area the interposition of muscles and a bursa between the scapula and the rib cage enables the scapula to "slide" over the underlying rib cage.

The humerus is a long bone. Its proximal articular surface, which is called the head of the humerus,

is shaped like a smooth hemisphere, is covered with cartilage, and is encircled by a groove (the anatomical neck). The tuberosity located lateral to the anatomical neck at the proximal end is called the greater tuberosity, whereas the lesser tuberosity is located inferior to the head, on the medial part of the humerus. Between the two tuberosities is located the bicipital groove.

The head of the humerus articulates with the glenoid fossa of the scapula.

The scapula is a triangular-shaped bone with a superior base and an inferior apex and is placed on the posterosuperior aspect of the thoracic cage. On the posterior surface is the scapular spine that is continuous with a robust bony process called the acromion. On the lateral angle of the scapula is the glenoid cavity, a shallow depression that has a fibrocartilaginous structure on its margin called the glenoid labrum and that articulates with the head of the humerus. In addition, a robust bony structure called the coracoid process projects from the upper margin of the scapula. The acromion articulates with the clavicle.

The clavicle is a sigmoid-shaped long bone lying horizontally. On the medial border, there is a facet for articulation with the manubrium of the sternum; on the lateral flat border, there is a facet for articulation with the acromion.

The sternum lies in the anterior midline of the thoracic region. With its upper side, the manubrium, it articulates with the clavicle on each side.

The muscles attaching to and acting on the four joints of the shoulder complex can be divided into:
- Intrinsic muscles (supraspinatus, infraspinatus, subscapularis, deltoid muscle, teres minor, and teres major)

- Extrinsic muscles (serratus anterior, subclavius, latissimus dorsi, elevator scapulae, rhomboid major, rhomboid minor, and trapezius)

The rotator cuff consists of four muscles and their tendons. They are the supraspinatus, the infraspinatus, the teres minor, and the subscapularis muscles. The first three allow the shoulder to extrarotate, whereas the fourth allows it to intrarotate.

The supraspinatus arises from the supraspinous fossa of the scapula and attaches to the greater tuberosity of the humerus.

The infraspinatus arises from the infraspinous fossa of the scapula and attaches to the greater tuberosity of the humerus.

The teres minor arises from the lateral border of the scapula and attaches to the greater tuberosity of the humerus.

The subscapularis arises from the subscapular fossa of the scapula and attaches to the lesser tuberosity of the humerus (Figs. 2.1A and 2.1B).

ANATOMICAL LANDMARKS

The most useful anatomical landmarks are listed in the following (Figs. 2.2A and 2.2B):

- The manubrium of the sternum: its fossae articulate with the medial ends of the clavicles and the costal cartilage of the first and second ribs.
- The clavicle: the rounded sternal end articulates with the sternum to form the SC joint, while the other flat end articulates with the acromion to form the AC joint.
- The acromion: it is a bony process of the scapula, which extends anteriorly and articulates with the clavicle.
- The scapula: it is placed on the posterosuperior aspect of the thoracic cage and articulates with the humeral head.
- The LHB tendon: it originates at the supraglenoid tubercle, runs intraarticularly over the humeral head and follows the bicipital groove distal to the GH joint.
- The first rib: it is the most curved and usually the shortest, broadest, and flattest of the ribs.
- The humeral head: it is the proximal end of the humerus and articulates with the glenoid fossa of the scapula.

- The scapular spine: it is a bony prominence which crosses the whole posterior surface of the scapula horizontally.

JOINT MOVEMENTS

The Physiological Movements of the Shoulder

Biomechanics of the shoulder is very complex due to the multiple joints involved in its great range of motion.

The shoulder joint has three degrees of freedom, which means it can move the upper limb in the three planes of symmetry of the body: sagittal plane, frontal plane, and transverse plane (Fig. 2.3).

The neutral position of the shoulder is with the upper limb close to the trunk in slightly internal rotation.

- Flexion:
  Upper limb forward and upward in the sagittal plane of the body.
- Extension:
  Upper limb backward and upward in the sagittal plane of the body.
- Abduction:
  Upper limb raises laterally away from the midline in the frontal plane of the body.
- Adduction:
  Upper limb moves toward the midline in the frontal plane of the body.
  There are two methods to assess external and internal rotation.
- External rotation in the sagittal plane of the body:
  The arm is abducted and the elbow flexed, both to 90 degrees. Then, the forearm moves upward.
- External rotation in the transverse plane of the body:
  The arm is in neutral position, elbow at 90 degrees, and forearm in neutral position. Then, the forearm moves outward.
- Internal rotation in the sagittal plane of the body:
  The arm is abducted and the elbow flexed, both to 90 degrees. Then, the forearm moves downward.
- Internal rotation in the transverse plane of the body:
  The arm is in neutral position, elbow at 90 degrees, and forearm in neutral position.

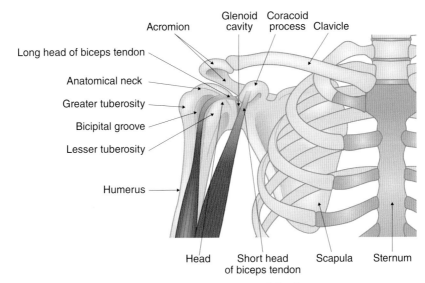

Fig. 2.1A The shoulder anatomy: anterior view.

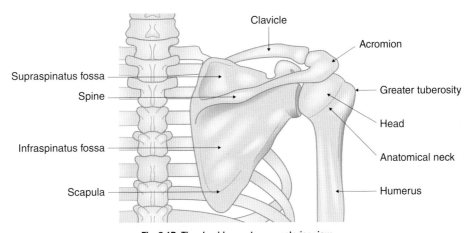

Fig. 2.1B The shoulder anatomy: posterior view.

Then, the forearm moves inward or backward.

The normal range of motion of the shoulder from neutral position:

- To full flexion is 0 to about 180 degrees
- To full extension is 0 to about 50 degrees
- To abduction is 0 to about 180 degrees
- To adduction is 0 to about 45 degrees

From the neutral position where the arm is abducted and the elbow flexed both at 90 degrees:

- To full external rotation, 0 to about 90 degrees
- To full internal rotation, 0 to about 70 degrees

From the neutral position where the elbow is flexed at 90 degrees:

- To full external rotation, 0 to about 45 degrees

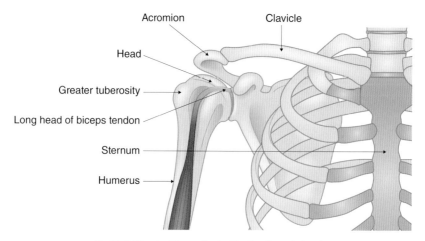

Fig. 2.2A The shoulder anatomical landmarks: anterior view.

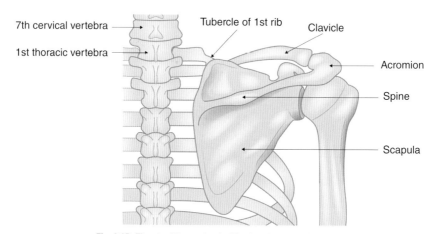

Fig. 2.2B The shoulder anatomical landmarks: posterior view.

- To full internal rotation, 0 to about 55 degrees (inward) and 45 degrees (behind the back)

Diagnosis in Western Medicine

SUPRASPINATUS TENDONITIS

It is a common and disabling condition mostly seen after middle age. It is a cause of shoulder pain and is characterized by the inflammation of the supraspinatus tendon, which can progressively lead to

degeneration and calcification of the tendon. It is said to be multifactorial in its etiology and often occurs as the consequence of overuse, repetitive strain injury, or work- and sports-related overhead shoulder movements. The tendon of the supraspinatus may also impinge under the acromion as it passes between the acromion and the humeral head.

The most common symptoms are the following:

- Pain, which gets worse with movement, especially with abduction

Planes of symmetry of the body

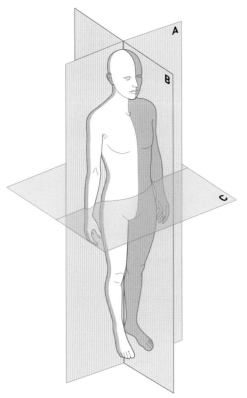

Fig. 2.3 The shoulder: planes of motion: (A) frontal plane, (B) sagittal plane, and (C) transverse plane.

- Pain on the anterolateral shoulder, which may radiate proximally to the neck and distally to the deltoid
- Night pain when lying on the affected side
- Restricted range of motion in abduction due to pain of variable intensity
- Positive Jobe's test
- Positive Yocum's test in case of impingement

Jobe's Test

It is used to assess supraspinatus tendonitis.

The patient sits or stands (Fig. 2.4).

The practitioner stands opposite the patient.

The patient is asked to abduct the arms to 90 degrees with a forward angle of 30 degrees, to extend the elbows, and to internally rotate the limbs.

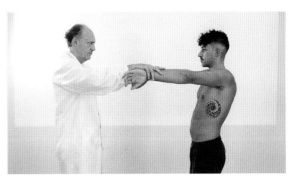

Fig. 2.4 Jobe's test.

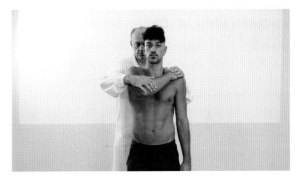

Fig. 2.5 Yocum's test.

Then, the practitioner applies pressure on the forearms, while the patient attempts to maintain the position against the practitioner's resistance.

The test is considered positive if the patient reports shoulder pain or weakness on the affected side (Video 2.1).

Yocum's Test

It is used to assess supraspinatus tendon impingement between the humeral head and the coracoacromial ligament.

The patient sits or stands (Fig. 2.5).

The practitioner stands behind the patient.

The patient is asked to place the right hand on the left shoulder and raise the elbow against the practitioner's resistance.

The test is considered positive if the patient reports shoulder pain (Video 2.2).

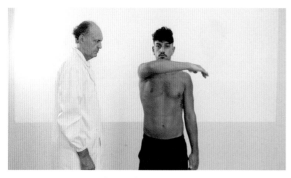

Fig. 2.6 Cross-arm test.

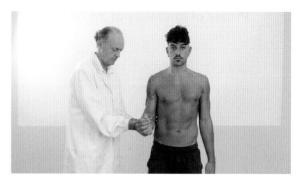

Fig. 2.7 External rotation strength test.

ACROMIOCLAVICULAR JOINT DISORDERS

Disorders is an umbrella term that encompasses several conditions. AC disorders can be due to trauma, such as subdislocation of the AC joint or degenerative conditions, such as osteoarthritis.

The most common symptoms are the following:
- AC pain and swelling
- Pain that gets worse with movement toward the unaffected limb
- Pain throughout the range of motion in abduction
- Positive cross-arm test
- Positive piano key sign after AC dislocation

Cross-Arm test

It is used to assess AC joint disorders.

The patient sits or stands (Fig. 2.6).

The practitioner stands opposite the patient.

The patient is asked to lift the right arm to the front to 90 degrees and then actively adduct it.

The test is considered positive if the patient reports shoulder pain (Video 2.3).

INFRASPINATUS TENDONITIS

It is a type of tendinopathy including those degeneration processes of the tendon, which are sometimes associated with calcification.

It is said to be multifactorial in its etiology and often occurs as the consequence of overuse, repetitive strain injury, or work- and sports-related overhead shoulder movements.

The most common symptoms are the following:
- Shoulder pain in the deltoid region

- Joint stiffness
- Positive external rotation strength test

External Rotation Strength Test

It is used to assess infraspinatus tendonitis.

The patient sits or stands with the right arm in neutral adduction (Fig. 2.7).

The practitioner stands close to the patient's right side.

The practitioner flexes the elbow to 90 degrees and maintains this position with the left hand, while holding the wrist in neutral position with the right hand.

The patient is asked to rotate the shoulder externally against resistance from the practitioner's hand.

The test is considered positive if rotation results to be painful or weak (Video 2.4).

TENDONITIS OF THE LONG HEAD OF THE BICEPS

It is considered as one of the most common causes of anterior shoulder pain, but diagnosis is often difficult because it is frequently associated with rotator cuff disorders.

The most common symptoms are the following:
- Acute pain, sometimes disabling
- Pain perceived on palpation of the muscle or tendon, and when stretching
- Pain radiating to the muscle belly, sometimes up to the elbow
- Restricted range of motion in abduction due to pain

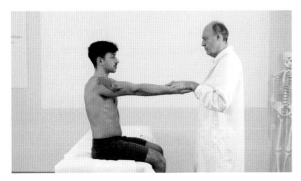

Fig. 2.8 Palm-up test.

- Muscular atrophy may be associated in the phases of chronic pain
- Positive palm-up test

Palm-Up Test

It is used to assess tendonitis of the LHB.

The patient sits with the shoulders flexed at 90 degrees, forearms supinated, and elbows extended (Fig. 2.8).

The practitioner stands opposite the patient and applies a counterforce against the patient who is asked to lift the arms.

The test is considered positive if the patient reports pain in the bicipital groove; pain indicates tendon malposition (Video 2.5).

JOINT PAIN, ARTHRITIS, AND STIFFNESS

Patients with shoulder arthritis and postsurgical outcomes usually complain of pain, weakness, and restricted range of motion.

Shoulder arthritis is a condition rarely encountered. Among the most common causes of shoulder arthritis are fractures, rheumatoid arthritis, septic arthritis, and primary osteoarthritis.

Diagnosis is based on the patient's medical history, clinical findings, and radiographic examinations.

The most common complications that may occur after surgery or as a result of fracture include:

- Shoulder stiffness with possible loss of motion (flexion, extension, pronation, and supination)
- Late-onset osteoarthritis

- Failed fusion
- Persistent pain

Frozen shoulder, also called adhesive capsulitis, is an inflammatory disease which leads to significant loss of motion of the GH joint.

Its etiology remains unknown, though it can also result from trauma or surgery.

The early symptoms are usually mild, but they get worse over time.

The frozen shoulder typically develops in three stages:

- First stage—freezing stage: any movement of the shoulder causes pain. Patient can still move the limb but slowly loses range of motion.
- Second stage—frozen stage: pain slightly decreases, but the range of motion is markedly restricted.
- Third stage—thawing stage: the shoulder slowly improves with either a complete return to normal or close to normal strength and motion which may occur after months, if not years.

RED FLAGS IN WESTERN MEDICINE

The presence of heat (calor), redness (rubor), swelling (tumor), pain (dolor), and loss of function (function laesa) determines the need for diagnostic investigations.

Shoulder trauma is a common occurrence. Among the signs and symptoms of fracture or dislocation are swelling and/or deformity of the limb. A fracture affects the continuity of a bone, whereas a dislocation involves a joint.

Patients with rheumatoid arthritis of the shoulder usually complain of pain throughout the range of motion; the shoulder is usually affected in the later stages of the disease. Both fatigue and general discomfort can also be observed.

Special attention should be paid if concomitant symptoms are observed, such as numbness, tingling, paresthesia (abnormal sensation), muscle weakness, decreased tendon reflexes, and pain, mainly at night.

Abnormalities uncovered on history taking or physical examination may require medical evaluation, laboratory tests, and imaging investigations, such as x-rays, US, CT, and MRI.

RED FLAGS	PAIN	INSPECTION	OTHER SIGNS	NEUROLOGICAL SIGNS	RECOMMEN-DATIONS
Inflammation	Pain	Redness, swelling, and heat		Functional deficit	Physician evaluation Imaging investigations
Fracture	Spontaneous pain	Deformity and swelling	Movement beyond normal range of motion	Functional deficit	Physician evaluation Imaging investigations
Dislocation	Pain with movement	Deformity and joint swelling	Hematoma	Functional deficit	Physician evaluation Imaging investigations
Rheumatoid arthritis	Pain with or without movement	Redness and swelling	Fatigue and general discomfort	Functional deficit	Physician evaluation Imaging investigations Laboratory tests
Herniated disc or cervical radiculopathy	Cervical pain radiating to the elbow			Paraesthesia, hypoesthesia, tingling and lack of deep tendon reflexes	Physician evaluation Imaging investigations
Myocardial infarction	Pain that affects the shoulder and the left chest, and may radiate to the arm and inferior neck		Cold sweat, shortness of breath, chest pressure		Emergency medical treatment
Biliary colic	Pain affecting the right shoulder and concomitant pain in the right hypochondrium or the abdomen		Positive Murphy's sign, fever, difficult palpation of the abdomen		Emergency medical treatment

Diagnosis in Chinese Medicine

In Chinese Medicine, musculoskeletal (MSK) pain results from the obstruction of Qì and Blood circulation or inadequate Qì and Blood for the nourishment of the secondary channels, especially the Muscle and Connecting channels.

The Muscle and Connecting channels more often involved in shoulder disorders are listed below:
- Large Intestine
- Lung
- Small Intestine
- Triple Energizer

The channels affected vary according to pain location:
- Large Intestine: pain is on the anterolateral side, with pathologies being supraspinatus tendonitis, AC joint disorders, and tendonitis of the LHB.
- Lung: pain is on the anterior side, the pathology is tendonitis of the LHB.
- Small Intestine: pain is on the posterior side, with pathologies being infraspinatus tendonitis and supraspinatus tendonitis.
- Triple Energizer: pain is on the posterolateral side, the pathology is infraspinatus tendonitis.

What matters most is to identify the affected channel where pain is located.

Sometimes, it is not so easy to determine it, and consequently, the following data concerning the Muscle channels involved in shoulder movements should be acquired for a better identification.
- Abduction: LI, TE, and SI
- Adduction: LU, HT, and PC
- Internal rotation: LU, HT, and PC
- External rotation: SI and TE
- Flexion: LU and LI
- Extension: SI and TE

The information so acquired on the channel that is likely to be involved, that is, pain location and related movement restriction, can also be integrated with the results from Western Medicine orthopedic tests to identify which muscle, tendon, and joint are affected in the case of:
- Supraspinatus tendonitis
- AC joint pain
- Infraspinatus tendonitis
- Tendonitis of the LHB

ETIOLOGY

Shoulder pain is usually caused by:
- *Overuse, repetitive strain injury.* Through work (house painter) or sports (pitcher); performing the same movement over and over again causes local Qì stagnation or Qì and Blood deficiency.
- *Trauma, sports injuries.* If mild, they cause local Qì stagnation. If severe, they cause local Blood stasis.
- *Cold.* Local invasion of Cold causes Qì stagnation and Blood stasis with contractures of muscles and tendons and consequent pain and stiffness aggravated by exposure to Cold.

If Cold is not expelled, stasis can become chronic. This condition predisposes:
- The channels to other invasions of Cold
- The patient to sensitivity to seasonal changes thus creating a vicious circle

Previous accidents often predispose the shoulder to more frequent invasions of external pathogenic factors (EPFs), especially Cold.

PATHOLOGY

The Muscle and Connecting channels are often affected by Qì stagnation and Blood stasis:
- Qì stagnation manifests itself with widespread pain radiating along the pathway of the Muscle channels and could be associated with muscle contracture and stiffness of the trapezius, also perceived upon palpation.
- Blood stasis, usually occurring in the Connecting channels, manifests itself with more intense pain localized in the joint or, more frequently, at the site of muscle insertion with consequent limited range of motion or joint stiffness.

As already mentioned in the discussion of fundamentals of acupuncture for MSK pain in the limbs (see Chapter 1), the term "Connecting channels" includes not only the Connecting channel "proper" but also the Connecting channel "area" that covers the whole pathway of the Main channel.

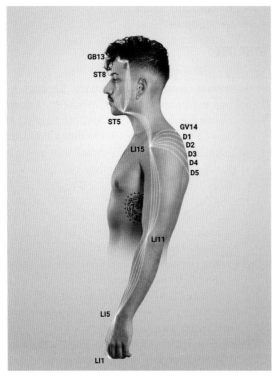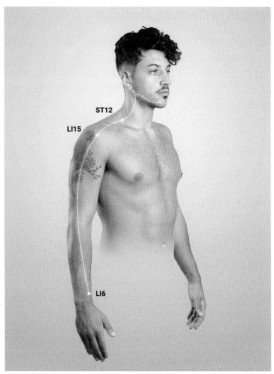

Fig. 2.9 The pathways of the Large Intestine Muscle and Connecting "proper" channels.

SUPRASPINATUS TENDONITIS AND ACROMIOCLAVICULAR JOINT DISORDERS

To identify the Muscle and Connecting channels affected, we check location and characteristics of MSK pain, palpate the affected area, test the range of motion for each shoulder movement, and perform orthopedic tests to elicit pain.

The Pathways of the Large Intestine Secondary Channels

In case of supraspinatus tendonitis and AC disorders, the Large Intestine Muscle and Connecting channels are involved.

The pathway of the Large Intestine Muscle and Connecting channels explains pain on the anterolateral side of the shoulder, which could radiate distally to the deltoid or proximally to the trapezius and scapula up to the higher tract of the upper back (Fig. 2.9).

The Pathways of the Small Intestine Secondary Channels

In case of periarthritis of the shoulder due to supraspinatus disorders, the Small Intestine Muscle and Connecting channels may be involved.

The pathway of the Small Intestine Muscle and Connecting channels may explain pain on the supraspinatus fossa of the scapula where the supraspinatus arises, and its belly resides (Fig. 2.10).

INFRASPINATUS TENDONITIS

To identify the Muscle and Connecting channels affected, we check the location and characteristics of MSK pain, palpate the affected area, test the range of motion for each shoulder movement, and perform orthopedic tests to elicit pain.

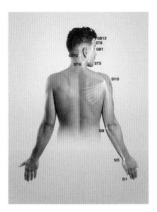
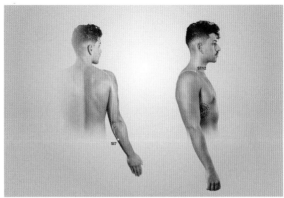

Fig. 2.10 The pathways of the Small Intestine Muscle and Connecting "proper" channels.

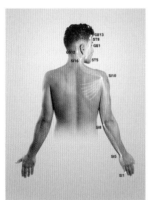
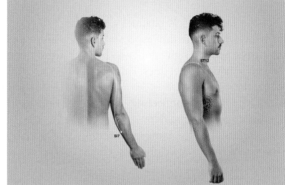

Fig. 2.11 The pathways of the Small Intestine Muscle and Connecting "proper" channels.

The Pathways of the Small Intestine Secondary Channels

In case of infraspinatus tendonitis the Small Intestine Muscle and Connecting channels are involved.

The pathway of the Small Intestine Muscle and Connecting channels explains pain on the posterior aspect of the shoulder, which could radiate proximally to the scapula and distally to the posteromedial aspect of the arm (Fig. 2.11).

The Pathways of the Triple Energizer Secondary Channels

In case of infraspinatus tendonitis, the Triple Energizer Muscle and Connecting channels may be involved.

The pathway of the Triple Energizer Muscle and Connecting channels could explain pain on the back of the shoulder, specifically on the osteotendinous junction of the infraspinatus to the humerus. Pain could radiate proximally to the scapula and distally to the posterior aspect of the arm (Fig. 2.12).

TENDONITIS OF THE LONG HEAD OF THE BICEPS

To identify the Muscle and Connecting channels affected, we check the location and characteristics of MSK pain, palpate the affected area, test the range of motion for each shoulder movement, and perform orthopaedic tests to elicit pain.

The Pathways of the Lung Secondary Channels

In case of tendonitis of the LHB, the Lung Muscle and Connecting channels are involved. It should also be kept in mind that since the Lung Muscle channel

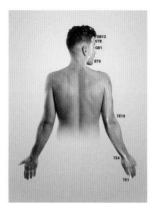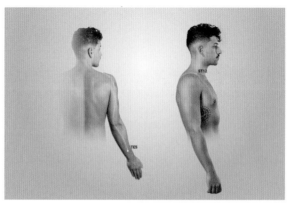

Fig. 2.12 The pathways of the Triple Energizer Muscle and Connecting "proper" channels.

reaches point LI15, the Large Intestine channels may also be involved.

The pathway of the Lung Muscle channel cannot perfectly explain pain on the anterior aspect of the shoulder because it does not run right along the LHB, which is what the Lung Main channel does. Pain could radiate distally along the biceps.

The pathway of the Lung Connecting channel "proper" does not ascend to the shoulder.

Since we are now referring to the Lung Connecting channel "area," we regard the Lung Connecting channels as channels involved (Fig. 2.13).

The Pathways of the Large Intestine Secondary Channels

In case of tendonitis of the LHB, the Large Intestine Muscle and Connecting channels may be involved.

An explanation for the involvement of the Large Intestine channels can be found in the anatomical location of point LI15, which is positioned next to the humeral bicipital groove where the tendon of the LHB runs (Fig. 2.14).

Diagnosis in Osteopathic Medicine

The examination for "somatic dysfunction" is the central concept of the diagnostic process: palpation of the affected area and functionally/anatomically related components of the somatic system is the only way to assess it.

Consequently, the osteopathic diagnostic approach to MSK shoulder pain is based on the identification of joint somatic dysfunctions not only of the shoulder but also of the elbow and wrist.

Regardless of the condition to be treated, be it supraspinatus or infraspinatus tendonitis, AC joint disorders, tendonitis of the LHB, arthritis of the shoulder, or surgical outcomes, all of the recommended tests should be performed to identify the dysfunctions that occur more frequently.

It is therefore evident that the osteopathic diagnosis is developed regardless of the condition to be treated, and consequently, the osteopathic tests recommended for the shoulder, elbow, and wrist will not be repeated when the "injuries" are treated.

TESTS FOR THE MAIN SOMATIC DYSFUNCTIONS

The only way to diagnose the somatic dysfunctions of a joint is to assess the passive movements of its articular ends in relation to one another and compare them with the same movements of the joint on the healthy side. Testing of all shoulder joints is required.

On the same plane of motion, passive mobility is quantitatively and qualitatively equal on both sides of a theoretical neutral point that represents the reference point.

When balance is lost and range and quality of motion are not the same in both directions, then there is somatic dysfunction.

Test of the Sternoclavicular Joint

A test is performed to assess the most common clavicular dysfunctions:
  1. Posterior clavicle
  2. Anterior clavicle

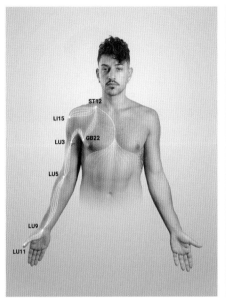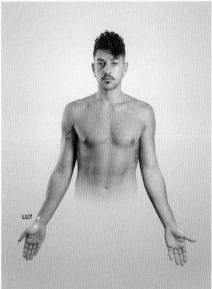

Fig. 2.13 The pathways of the Lung Muscle and Connecting "proper" channels.

Bilateral Posterior Test of the Clavicle

The patient sits.

The practitioner stands behind the patient to assess the right shoulder: the fingers are placed on both clavicular medial ends and the forearms on the anterior side of the shoulders.

The practitioner counterbalances the backward force applied on the clavicular medial ends with the chest while slightly pulling the lateral ends of the clavicles with the forearms laterally and pushing its medial ends with the fingers backward.

By doing so, the practitioner appreciates the movements with the finger pads and then compares the range and quality of motion of both joints.

If the clavicle on the affected side slides more easily posteriorly than the clavicle on the unaffected side, then there is posterior dysfunction, and if it does not slide easily posteriorly, then there is anterior dysfunction (Fig. 2.15; Video 2.6).

Tests of the Acromioclavicular Joint

Tests are performed to assess the most common clavicular dysfunctions:

1. Anterior rotation of the clavicle
2. Posterior rotation of the clavicle

Anterior Rotation Test of the Clavicle

The patient sits.

The practitioner stands behind the patient to assess the right shoulder with the left fingers placed on the clavicular lateral end.

The practitioner pulls the patient's elbow backward to appreciate the range and quality of motion of anterior rotation and then compares them with posterior rotation (Figs. 2.16 and 2.17). If the clavicle moves more easily forward than backward, then there is anterior rotation dysfunction (Video 2.7).

POSTERIOR ROTATION TEST OF THE CLAVICLE

The patient sits.

The practitioner stands behind the patient to assess the right shoulder with the left fingers placed on the clavicular lateral end (Figs. 2.18 and 2.19).

The practitioner pushes the patient's elbow forward to appreciate the range and quality of motion of posterior rotation and then compares them with anterior rotation. If the clavicle moves more easily backward than forward, then there is posterior rotation dysfunction (Video 2.8).

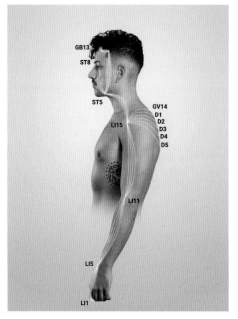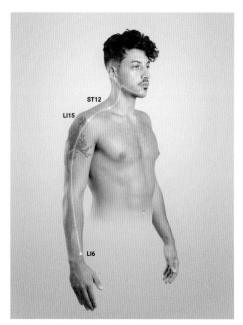

Fig. 2.14 The pathways of the Large Intestine Muscle and Connecting "proper" channels.

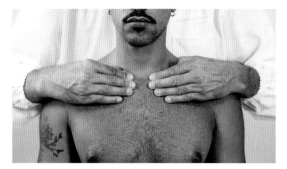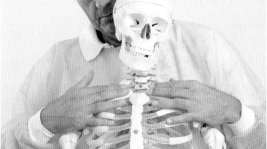

Fig. 2.15 Bilateral posterior test of the clavicle.

Tests of the Glenohumeral Joint

Tests are performed to assess the most common humeral head dysfunctions:

- Anterior humeral head
- Superior humeral head

Anteroposterior Test of the Humeral Head

The patient sits.

The practitioner stands behind the patient to assess the right shoulder. The left fingers hold the acromion, while the right fingers make the humeral head slide first forward and slightly medially and then backward and slightly laterally, to appreciate the range and quality of motion of the two movements (Fig. 2.20). If the humeral head slides more easily forward than backward, then there is anterior dysfunction, and vice versa (Video 2.9).

Vertical Test of the Humeral Head

The patient sits.

The practitioner stands behind the patient to assess the right shoulder: the left fingers hold the acromion, with the sensing pads placed on the humeral head. The practitioner pushes the elbow downward with the right hand and then pulls it upward to make the humeral head slide (Fig. 2.21).

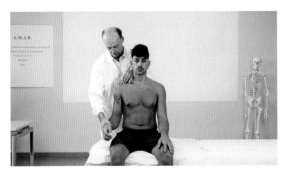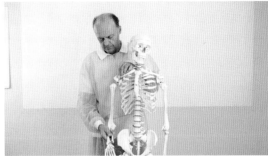

Fig. 2.16 Anterior rotation test of the clavicle: starting position.

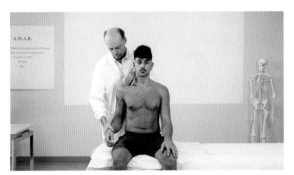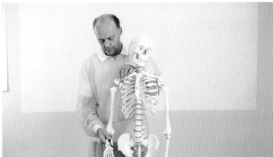

Fig. 2.17 Anterior rotation test of the clavicle: final position.

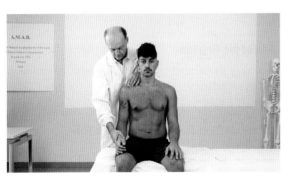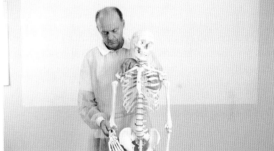

Fig. 2.18 Posterior rotation test of the clavicle: starting position.

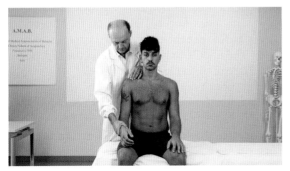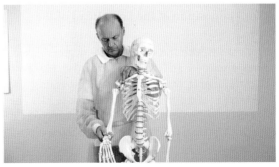

Fig. 2.19 Posterior rotation test of the clavicle: final position.

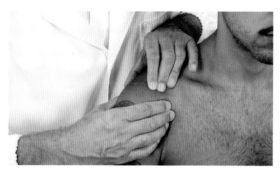 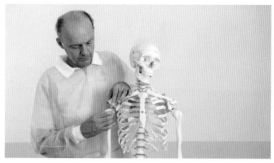

Fig. 2.20 Anteroposterior test of the humeral head.

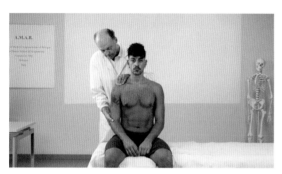 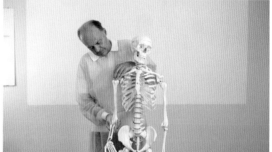

Fig. 2.21 Vertical test of the humeral head.

The range and quality of motion of the two movements are then compared. If the humeral head slides more easily upward than downward, then there is superior dysfunction (Video 2.10).

Test of the Long Head of the Biceps

A test is performed to assess the most common dysfunctions of the LHB:
- Medial malposition
- Lateral malposition

Test for Malposition of the Long Head of the Biceps

The patient sits with the shoulders 90 degrees flexed, forearms supinated, and elbows extended.

The practitioner exerts a counterforce against the patient who is asked to lift the arms (Fig. 2.22). The test is considered positive if the patient reports pain in the bicipital groove, which indicates tendon malposition (Video 2.11).

Test of the First Rib

A test is performed to assess the most common first rib dysfunction:
- Elevated first rib

Bilateral Test for Elevated First Rib

The patient sits.

The practitioner stands behind the patient.

With the index and middle fingers of both hands, the practitioner palpates the first rib at the C7 level in front of the anterior border of the trapezius:
- The index finger is placed on the superior surface of the tubercle close to the trapezius.
- The middle finger is placed on the superior surface of the body close to clavicle.

The practitioner pushes the ribs downward and then compares the range and quality of motion of the two movements (Fig. 2.23). If a rib does not move downward, then there is elevated dysfunction of the first rib, both anteriorly and posteriorly (Video 2.12).

Treatment With the AcuOsteo Method: The Choice of an Integrated Approach

The therapeutic approach of the AcuOsteo Method aims to treat MSK injuries that do not require consultation with a surgeon or a physician.

Once this fundamental aspect has been defined, treatment envisages the use of acupuncture and osteopathy according to their diagnostic and therapeutic approaches.

We would like to stress that at this point in diagnostic assessment, we do not have to follow the rules of Western Medicine, except for some specific cases, such as arthritis of the shoulder, posttraumatic and postsurgical pain, and stiffness, which will be covered later.

In addition, we should not be misled by diagnostic imaging investigations and should rely only on the rules of Chinese and osteopathic medicine, which means selecting points according to symptoms and channel pathways and treating all of the somatic dysfunctions encountered.

For didactic purposes, treatment with acupuncture will precede osteopathic treatment, whereas in clinical practice the order is reversed since it may be difficult to perform osteopathic manipulations once the needles have been inserted.

An exception to this methodology is represented by those morbidities where marked stiffness prevents joint mobilization as required by osteopathic manipulations. Specifically, we are referring to the frozen shoulder, the outcomes after immobilization following surgery, fractures, and shoulder dislocation.

In these cases, we suggest first using acupuncture, especially the bleeding techniques, and then, at the end of the session and after removing the needles, osteopathy.

In any case, it is always the practitioner's clinical experience that will guide them along the most appropriate pathway to treat each patient's condition.

Osteopathic manipulation in the treatment of "somatic dysfunction" is the central concept of the therapeutic process to treat the affected joints and functionally/anatomically related components of the somatic system.

Consequently, the osteopathic manipulative approach to MSK shoulder pain focuses on the treatment of joint somatic dysfunctions not only of the shoulder but also of the elbow and wrist.

Regardless of the condition to be treated, be it supraspinatus or infraspinatus tendonitis, AC disorders, tendonitis of the LHB, arthritis of the shoulder, or postsurgical outcomes, all of the dysfunctions diagnosed should be treated.

It is therefore evident that the osteopathic therapeutic approach does not vary with the condition to

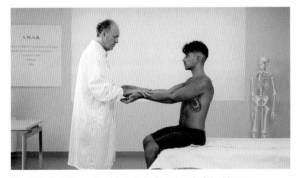

Fig. 2.22 Test for malposition of the long head of the biceps.

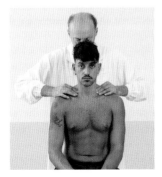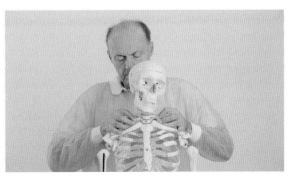

Fig. 2.23 Bilateral test for elevated first rib.

be treated, and thus the osteopathic manipulations described for the shoulder, as well as those for the elbow and wrist, will not be repeated under the paragraphs dedicated to the "injuries."

ACUPUNCTURE TREATMENT

Supraspinatus Tendonitis and Acromioclavicular Joint Disorders

The Five Options and Selection of Acupoints

The approach we suggest is widely described in the section dedicated to the Fundamentals of acupuncture for MSK pain in the limbs (see Chapter 1).

The most important aspect is the identification of the Ah Shi point(s) to determine which channels are affected. In this specific case, the Large Intestine Muscle and Connecting channels are involved.

It is worth reminding that the Large Intestine Muscle channel runs in all the portions of the supraspinatus muscle: osteotendinous junction, tendon, musculotendinous junction, and muscle belly. It should also be kept in mind that since the Large Intestine Main channel reaches point SI12, which corresponds to the supraspinatus muscle belly, the Small Intestine channels could also be involved.

In practice, both the Large Intestine and Small Intestine Muscle channels run along the supraclavicular fossa where the supraspinatus arises and its belly resides. Therefore, when a combination of two points (LI and SI) is presented, the first point to be needled or bled is the LI point, whereas the SI point is the second option in case the results are not satisfactory. Once the most effective channel is identified, the selection of distal points continues along it.

Pricking pain localized on the anterolateral aspect of the shoulder is a sign of Blood stasis to be treated with the bleeding technique, whereas widespread pain radiating along the arm is a sign of Qì stagnation to be treated with the needling technique.

It is worth reminding that the distal points should be needled one at a time and their effectiveness in terms of pain and range of motion tested after each insertion. The same applies to the local points.

Finally, since both options 1 and 2 consist of several steps, it is important to highlight how selection should be made. Specifically, the practitioner might wonder if all or some of the steps should be followed. The rule

we follow is simple: when the result achieved is satisfactory, the remaining steps should be skipped, and the practitioner should move to the following option. Similarly, the use of the points recommended under options 3, 4, and 5 should be carefully evaluated according to the case being treated.

The points and accessory techniques we recommend using are listed below.

Order of Needling

Option One: Distal Points

First Step: Large Intestine and Small Intestine Muscle Channels

LI1 and SI1. These Jing-Well points activate the Large Intestine and Small Intestine Muscle channels, and they remove Qì stagnation and Blood stasis with needling and bleeding techniques, respectively.

Second Step: Large Intestine and Small Intestine Connecting Channels

LI6 and SI7 (Opposite Side). These Luo points activate the Large Intestine and Small Intestine Connecting channels, and they remove Qì stagnation and Blood stasis in acute or chronic conditions from Excess (Figs. 2.24 and 2.25).

Our technique consists of needling LI6 from oblique to transverse in proximal direction along the pathway of the Large Intestine Main channel (Video 2.13).

LU7 and HT5 (Opposite Side) These Luo points activate the Lung and Heart Connecting channels. They are also used in chronic Deficiency conditions with dull pain to tonify Qì and Blood in their respective internally-externally related channels. In this case, we associate Yuan point LI4 with Luo point LU7, and Yuan point SI4 with Luo point HT7, that is to say, the well-known Luo-Yuan point combination: first, as the main point, we needle the Yuan point on the affected side and then, as a secondary point, the Luo point on the internally-externally related channel on the opposite side.

Our technique consists of needling LU7 from oblique to transverse in a proximal direction along the pathway of the Lung Main channel (Figs. 2.26 and 2.27; Video 2.14).

Third step: Empirical Points

ST38 (Opposite Side) This is the empirical point classically recommended to treat pain and motion restriction.

According to our experience, it is worth remembering that it is effective in the treatment of shoulder

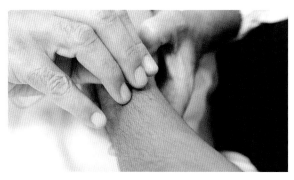

Fig. 2.24 Needling of the LI6: starting position.

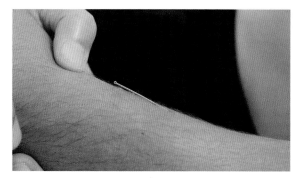

Fig. 2.25 Needling of the LI6: final position.

conditions when pain is localized on the Stomach channels alone, especially if there is restricted range of motion in abduction.

Our technique consists of needling ST38 on the opposite side of the affected area in acute and chronic Excess conditions with intense pain. Alternatively, the most tender point side on palpation can be needled: if the outcome is not satisfactory, the needle should be removed and inserted on the other side.

Zongping (Opposite Side). This empirical point is located 1 cm distal and lateral to ST36, that is, between the Stomach and Gall Bladder Main channels.

Zongping is used on the opposite side of the affected area in acute and chronic Excess conditions with intense pain. Alternatively, the most tender point side on palpation can be needled; if the outcome is not satisfactory, the needle should be removed and inserted on the other side.

Fourth step: Opposite Extremity (Upper/ Lower)

ST31 (Opposite Side) It is located in the hip joint, which corresponds to the shoulder joint on the paired channel according to the Six Stages.

ST36 (Opposite Side) Although located distal to the hip joint, it is used more often because it mobilizes more energy than the previous point.

BL53 and BL54 (Opposite Side) They are located in the hip joint which corresponds to the shoulder joint on the paired channel according to the Six Stages.

BL40 (Opposite Side) Although located distal to the hip joint, it is used because it mobilizes more energy than the previous point.

Our technique involves needling the opposite extremity (lower/upper) on the opposite side in acute

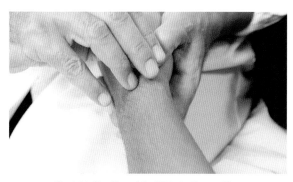

Fig. 2.26 Needling of the LU7: starting position.

and chronic conditions. Alternatively, the most tender point side on palpation is selected on the same or opposite side.

Fifth Step: Categories of Traditional Points

LI3 (Affected Side) and ST43 (Opposite Side), SI3 (Affected Side) and BL65 (Opposite Side) A good combination includes the Shu-Stream points on the paired channel, according to the Six Stages.

First, we needle the Shu-Stream point on the channel involved on the affected side and then the Shu-Stream point on the coupled channel on the opposite side and opposite extremity (upper/lower).

We use this technique in acute and chronic Excess conditions to treat pain and expel or prevent invasion of EPFs.

LI5 and SI5 The Jing-River points are used in acute or chronic Excess conditions due to the invasion of an EPF and they are needled to promote its expulsion from their respective channels. They are also useful to

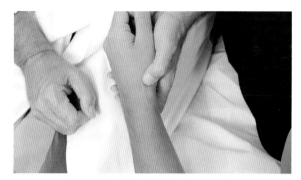

Fig. 2.27 Needling of the LU7: final position.

prevent pain exacerbation from seasonal changes or an invasion of EPF.

LI7 and SI6 The Xi-Cleft points are specifically used in acute conditions to treat Blood stasis in their respective channels. However, they are more effective in the *Yin* rather than in the *Yang* channels: that is why we would rather avoid using them to treat this condition.

LI4 and SI4 We recommend using these Yuan-Source point(s) in chronic Deficiency conditions with dull pain, in case of weakness, or in the resolution phases of supraspinatus tendonitis and AC joint disorders, to tonify Qì and Blood in their respective channels.

In this situation, we can also associate the Yuan point LI4 with the Luo point LU7 and the Yuan SI4 with the Luo point HT5, which is the well-known Luo-Yuan point combination. First, as the main point, we needle the Yuan point on the affected side and then, as a secondary point, the Luo point on the internally-externally related channel on the opposite side.

Sixth Step: Extraordinary Vessels

SI3 (Affected Side) and BL62 (Opposite Side) SI3 is the opening point of the Governing Vessel (Du Mai), while BL62 is the coupled point and opening point of the Yang Qiao Mai. The Governing Vessel is treated when cervical pain with concomitant irritation of the corresponding cervical roots is suspected. In this case, we associate BL60 and BL10 with either the cervical Jiaji C4–C5–C6–C7 on the affected side or the most tender point on palpation.

First, as the main point, the opening point of the Governing Vessel is needled on the same side and then, as a secondary point, the coupled point on the opposite side.

As cervical pain is rarely observed, treatment of the Governing Vessel is not often required and only the cervical Jiaji are to be needled if tender on palpation.

Option Two: Local Points
First Step: Painful Point(s) (Ah Shi)

Ah Shi Point(s) Palpation of the anterolateral GH joint reveals either the most painful point(s) (Ah Shi) corresponding to Blood stasis and therefore to be bled or an area of widespread pain corresponding to Qì stagnation and requiring needling. Pain could radiate distally to the anterolateral aspect of the arm.

When the bleeding technique is chosen, the cupping therapy should be used to bleed the Ah Shi point(s) and LI15 (Figs. 2.28 and 2.29; Video 2.15).

When needles are inserted, we choose the most painful point(s) (Ah Shi).

To treat supraspinatus tendonitis and impingement, the needle is inserted perpendicularly to the required depth until the tendon sheath or the osteo-tendinous junction to the humerus is reached.

To treat AC disorders, two needles are inserted, from oblique to transverse, on the two sides of the joint, which is located roughly halfway between LI15 and LI16. The first needle is inserted forward directed backward and slightly medially, while the second needle is inserted backward directed forward and slightly laterally. The needles should penetrate the joint and this may prove to be difficult.

We usually use 0.25 × 25 mm or 0.30 × 40 mm needles: the diameter and length of the needle to be used depend on the preference of the acupuncturist and the patient physique.

LI15 It can be considered the most important local point to treat shoulder disorders as it is the meeting point of the Large Intestine, Lung, Stomach, and Bladder Muscle channels. In addition, at this point the Large Intestine Main channel meets the Yang Qiao Mai Extraordinary channel. We also use it because it is an insertion point of the Large Intestine Muscle channel in the shoulder, as we will see later. In anatomical terms it corresponds to the osteotendinous junction of the supraspinatus to the humerus. That is why it is specifically used to treat insertional tendonitis of the supraspinatus.

It could be bled together with the Ah Shi point(s), as already mentioned above.

The needle is inserted perpendicularly to the required depth to reach the osteotendinous junction using a 0.25 × 25 mm or 0.30 × 40 mm needle: the diameter and length of the needle to be used depend on the patient's physique. If the pain radiates to the

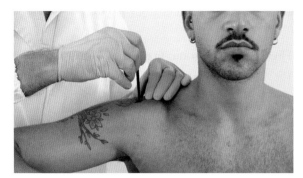

Fig. 2.28 Bleeding of the Ah Shi point(s) and LI15: starting position.

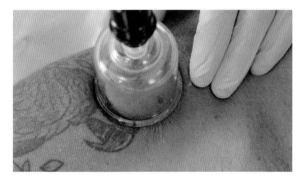

Fig. 2.29 Bleeding of the Ah Shi point(s) and LI15: final position.

deltoid, this point can be needled obliquely to transversely with the needle directed toward the elbow.

Both in acute and chronic conditions a moxa stick on the painful point(s) and LI15 can be useful to promote the flow of Qì and Blood. We can also use it to treat invasion of EPFs, Cold in particular.

However, attention should be paid since too much heat can increase the ongoing inflammatory process.

LI16 It can be considered a local point to treat supraspinatus tendinitis due to sub-AC impingement, because in anatomical terms this point corresponds to its musculotendinous junction.

Needle insertion is very important: the needle should be inserted at about 0.5 cm medial to the classical location of the point, from oblique to transverse, to pass under the AC bony arch directed anterolaterally, toward LI15, to reach the superficial layers of the muscolotendinous junction. Needle insertion should be smooth; the needle should enter and slide in easily.

More attempts are likely needed before proper positioning is achieved, as the tip of the needle will easily hit the bony surfaces.

We use a $0.30 \times 40\,mm^2$ needle to reach an insertion depth ranging from 1 to 1.5 cm. Electroacupuncture stimulation can be taken into consideration and used between LI15 and LI16.

SI12 It can be considered a local point in case of supraspinatus disorders when taut bands are found within the muscle belly and consequently, the point is tender on palpation. If the sizes of the taut bands allow us, two needles can be inserted.

The needle is inserted perpendicular and adjacent to the spine of the scapula into the trapezius until it reaches the supraspinatus sheath. Alternatively, needles can be inserted deeply until they reach the intermediate layers of the taut bands. We use a $0.25 \times 25\,mm$ or a $0.30 \times 40\,mm$ needle: the diameter and length of the needle to be used depend on the preference of the acupuncturist and the patient physique.

Electroacupuncture stimulation can be taken into consideration and used between these two points. Alternatively, the $0.30 \times 40\,mm$ needles are inserted from oblique to transverse along the taut band with a twisting and rotating manipulation.

To ensure the accuracy and precision of local needle placement and manipulation, we prefer the sitting position, paying attention to the risk of fainting. Then, the patient is asked to lie supine except for treatment with electroacupuncture, which is administered with the patient lying on the unaffected side.

Second Step: Anatomically Mirrored Points (Opposite Side)

The points to be needled are located on the opposite side and should correspond as precisely as possible to the anatomical mirror of the Ah Shi point(s) to be treated. The point(s) may or may not be tender on palpation.

To ensure the accuracy and precision of needle placement and manipulation, we prefer the sitting position, paying attention to the risk of fainting.

Option Three: Adjacent Points

First Step: Adjacent Points

LI14 It is located on the deltoid insertion distal to the humerus, exactly where pain can radiate to the shoulder. In this specific case, it can be considered a local point. The needle is inserted perpendicularly to promote the longitudinal flow of local Qì.

Jianqian, TE14, and SI11 They help promote the horizontal flow of local Qì.

LI15 It is the insertion point of the Large Intestine Muscle channel in the shoulder and as such it promotes the longitudinal flow of local Qì.

SI10 It is the insertion point of the Small Intestine Muscle channel in the shoulder, and as such it promotes the longitudinal flow of local Qì.

Option Four: Etiological Points

First Step: Points According to Patterns
LI4 and LR3 (Bilaterally) They promote the flow of Qì and help remove Blood stasis. Since LR3 is the Shu/Yuan point of the Liver, it also helps nourish muscles and tendons.

ST36 (Bilaterally) It is used to tonify Qì and Blood in chronic Deficiency conditions or the phases of pain resolution that can turn into muscle weakness.

Second Step: General Points
GB34 (Bilaterally) It is the Hui-Gathering point of Sinews and is specifically used for supraspinatus tendonitis. In addition, it promotes the flow of Qì thus contributing to remove Blood stasis.

BL17 (Bilaterally) It is the Hui-Gathering point of Blood and is used to remove Blood stasis.

BL18 (Bilaterally) It treats all Excess and Deficiency conditions of the Liver that may favor the onset or duration of musculotendinous symptoms. It harmonizes the flow of Qì and Blood and enhances the treatment of tendons and muscle.

Option Five: Microsystems

First Step: Wrist and Ankle Acupuncture
Upper 5 It roughly corresponds to the pathway of the Large Intestine channels; it also controls the upper back and the cervical paravertebral regions (Fig. 2.30).

Upper 5 also controls upper limb mobility.

Second Step: Ear Acupuncture (Fig. 2.31)
Local point: Shoulder
Zang Fu point: Liver
General points: Subcortex and Shenmen
Acute or Chronic Pain From Excess
Intense Pain or Range of Motion Reduced by Pain Principle of treatment: to remove Qì stagnation and Blood stasis and expel EPFs, if any (Box 2.1).

Chronic Pain due to Deficiency
Dull Pain or Muscle Weakness Principle of treatment: to tonify Qì and Blood, strengthen tissues, and

avoid pain exacerbation from physical activities or invasion of EPFs (Box 2.2).

Therapeutic Program, Frequency of Sessions

The frequency of sessions depends on the clinical condition of the patient. If the condition is acute or chronic with intense pain, we recommend sessions twice a week for 2 weeks and then once a week for another 2 weeks. If improvement is observed, sessions are then scheduled once a week until complete pain relief or at least reduction by 80% to 90%. If not, the whole clinical picture should be reconsidered, and the patient should be referred to another specialist.

If the condition is chronic with dull pain, we recommend sessions once a week for 4 weeks. Afterward, and if the patient continues to improve, sessions are then scheduled once a week until complete pain relief or at least reduction by 80% to 90%.

Infraspinatus Tendonitis

The Five Options and Selection of Acupoints
The approach we suggest is widely described in the section dedicated to the Fundamentals of acupuncture for MSK pain in the limbs (see Chapter 1).

The most important aspect is the identification of the Ah Shi point(s) to determine which channels are affected. In this specific case, the Small Intestine Muscle and Connecting channels are involved. It should also be kept in mind that since point TE14 corresponds to the osteotendinous junction of the infraspinatus to the humerus, the Triple Energizer channels could also be involved.

Therefore, when a combination of two distal points (SI and TE) is presented, the first point to be needled or bled is the SI point, whereas the TE point is the second option in case if results are not satisfactory. Once the most effective channel is identified, the selection of distal points continues along it.

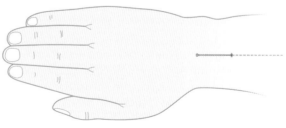

Fig. 2.30 Upper 5.

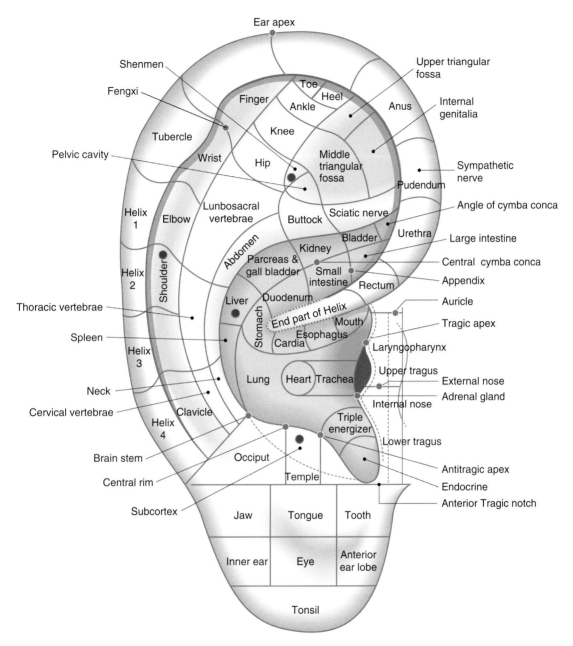

Fig. 2.31 Ear acupuncture.

Pricking pain localized on the posterior aspect of the shoulder is a sign of Blood stasis to be treated with the bleeding technique, whereas widespread pain radiating along the triceps is a sign of Qì stagnation to be treated with the needling technique.

It is worth reminding that the distal points should be needled one at a time and their effectiveness in terms of pain and range of motion tested after each insertion. The same applies to the local points.

BOX 2.1 ACUTE OR CHRONIC PAIN FROM EXCESS ACUPUNCTURE TREATMENT

Option 1 Distal points	• Jing-Well points LI1 and S1 • Luo points LI6 and SI7 (opposite side) • Empirical points ST38 and Zongping (opposite side) • Points according to the 6 Stages ST31 or ST36 and BL53, BL54 or BL40 (opposite side) • Shu-Stream points LI3 and SI3 (affected side) and Shu-Stream points ST43 and BL65 (opposite side) • Jing-River points LI5 and SI5
Option 2 Local points	• Ah Shi • LI15 • LI16 • SI12 • Anatomically mirrored point(s) (opposite side)
Option 3 Adjacent points	• LI14 • Jianqian • TE14 • SI11 • Insertion points LI15 and SI10
Option 4 Etiological and general points	• LI4 and LR3 (bilaterally) • GB34 (bilaterally) • BL17 (bilaterally) • BL18 (bilaterally)

Option 5
Microsystems
	• W-A acupuncture
	  • Upper 5
	• Ear acupuncture (opposite side)
	  • Shoulder
	  • Liver
	  • Subcortex and Shenmen

BOX 2.2 CHRONIC PAIN FROM DEFICIENCY ACUPUNCTURE TREATMENT

Option 1 Distal points	• Yuan points LI4 and SI4 • Luo points LU7 and HT5 (opposite side) • Points according to the Six stages ST31 or ST36 and BL53, BL54 or BL40 (opposite side) • Jing-River points LI5 and SI5
Option 2 Local points	• Ah Shi • LI15 • LI16 • SI12
Option 3 Adjacent points	• LI14 • Jianqian • TE14 • SI11 • Insertion points LI15 and SI10
Option 4 Etiological and general points	• ST36 (bilaterally) • GB34 (bilaterally) • LR3 (bilaterally) • BL18 (bilaterally)

Option 5
Microsystems
	• W-A acupuncture
	  • Upper 5
	• Ear acupuncture (opposite side)
	  • shoulder
	  • Liver
	  • Subcortex and Shenmen

Finally, since both options 1 and 2 consist of several steps, it is important to highlight how selection should be made. Specifically, the practitioner might wonder if all or some of the steps should be followed. The rule we follow is simple: when the result achieved is satisfactory, the remaining steps should be skipped, and the practitioner should move to the following option. Similarly, the use of the points recommended under options 3, 4, and 5 should be carefully evaluated according to the case being treated.

The points and accessory techniques we recommend using are listed below.

Clinical Notes

- Treatment of supraspinatus tendonitis and impingement and AC disorders usually ensures excellent outcomes.
- Effectiveness of treatment may be reduced if severely restricted range of motion is observed. In this specific case, pain may disappear with rest or movement leaving behind residual limited range of motion, which, however, does not prevent the patient from performing everyday activities.
- Improvement following treatment may turn intense pain to dull pain and then to a feeling of weakness. Should this be the case, the principle of treatment has to be changed as follows: it is no longer necessary to remove Qì stagnation and Blood stasis and expel EPFs, if any; instead, Qì and Blood should be tonified to strengthen tissues and avoid pain exacerbation from physical activities or invasion of EPFs.
- Sometimes, treatment may not achieve the expected results. An explanation for the poorer outcome could be the fact that the supraspinatus tendonitis may be caused not only by dysfunctions at SC, AC, and GH level but also by dysfunctions of the upper tract of the upper back. Further investigations are therefore mandatory.

Order of Needling

Option One: Distal Points

First Step: Small Intestine and Triple Energizer Muscle Channels

SI1 and TE1 These Jing-Well points activate the Small Intestine and Triple Energizer Muscle channels, and they remove Qì stagnation and Blood stasis with needling and bleeding techniques, respectively.

Second Step: Small Intestine and Triple Energizer Connecting Channels

SI7 and TE5 (Opposite Side) These Luo points activate the Small Intestine and Triple Energizer Connecting channels, and they remove Qì stagnation and Blood stasis in acute and chronic conditions from Excess.

HT5 and PC6 (Opposite Side) These Luo points activate the Heart and Pericardium Connecting channels. They are also used in chronic Deficiency conditions with dull pain to tonify Qì and Blood in the respective internally-externally related channels. In this case, we associate Yuan point SI4 with Luo point HT5 and Yuan point TE4 with Luo point PC6, which is the well-known Luo-Yuan point combination: first, as the main point, we needle the Yuan point on the affected side and then, as a secondary point, the Luo point on the internally-externally related channel on the opposite side.

Third Step: Empirical Points

There is no point that is classically recommended.

Fourth Step: Opposite Extremity (Upper/Lower)

BL53 and BL54 (Opposite Side) They are located in the posterior hip joint, which corresponds to the shoulder joint on the paired channel according to the Six Stages. Insertion of these needles requires the patient to be recumbent on the affected side.

BL40 (Opposite Side) Although located distal to the hip joint, it is used more often because it mobilizes more energy than the previous point.

GB30 (Opposite Side) It is located in the posterior hip joint, which corresponds to the shoulder joint on the paired channel according to the Six Stages. Insertion of this needle requires the patient to be recumbent on the affected side.

GB34 (Opposite Side) Although located distal to the hip joint, it is used more often because it mobilizes more energy than the previous point.

Our technique involves needling the opposite extremity (lower/upper) on the opposite side in acute and chronic conditions.

Alternatively, the most tender point on palpation is selected on the same or opposite side.

Fifth Step: Categories of Traditional Points

SI3 (Affected Side) and BL65 (Opposite Side), TE3 (Affected Side) and GB41 (Opposite Side) A good combination includes the Shu-Stream points on the paired channel according to the Six Stages.

First, we needle the Shu-Stream point on the channel involved on the affected side and then the Shu-Stream point on the coupled channel on the opposite side and opposite extremity (upper/lower). We use this technique in acute and chronic Excess conditions to treat pain and expel or prevent invasion of EPFs.

SI5 and TE6 The Jing-River points are used in acute or chronic Excess conditions due to the invasion of an EPF and they are needled to promote its expulsion from their respective channels. They are also useful to prevent pain exacerbation from seasonal changes or invasion of EPFs.

SI6 and TE7 The Xi-Cleft points are specifically used in acute conditions to treat Blood stasis in their respective channels. However, they are more effective in the *Yin* rather than in the Yang channels: that is why we would rather avoid using them to treat this condition.

SI4 and TE4 We recommend using these Yuan-Source points in chronic Deficiency conditions with dull pain, in case of weakness, or in the resolution phases of infraspinatus tendonitis, to tonify Qì and Blood in their respective channels.

In this situation, we can also associate the Yuan point SI4 with the Luo point HT5 and the Yuan point TE4 with the Luo point PC6, that is to say the well-known Luo-Yuan point combination. First, as the main point, we needle the Yuan point on the affected side and then, as a secondary point, the Luo point on the internally-externally related channel on the opposite side.

Sixth Step: Extraordinary Vessels

SI3 (Affected Side) and BL62 (Opposite Side) SI3 is the opening point of the Governing Vessel (Du Mai), while BL62 is the coupled point and opening point of the Yang Qiao Mai. The Governing Vessel is treated when cervical pain is observed and a concomitant irritation of the corresponding cervical roots is suspected.

In this case, we associate BL60 and BL10 with either the cervical Jiaji C3–C4–C5–C6 on the affected side or the most tender point on palpation.

First, as the main point, the opening point of the Governing Vessel is needled on the same side and then, as a secondary point, the coupled point on the opposite side. As cervical pain is rarely observed, treatment of the Governing Vessel is not often required and only the cervical Jiaji are to be needled if tender on palpation.

Option Two: Local Points

First Step: Painful Points (Ah Shi)

Ah Shi Point(s) Palpation of the posterior GH joint or scapula reveals either the most painful point(s) (Ah Shi) corresponding to Blood stasis and therefore to be bled or an area of widespread pain corresponding to Qì stagnation and requiring needling. Pain could radiate distally to the posterolateral aspect of the arm.

When the needle is inserted, its depth depends on the targeted area, the osteotendinous junction, the tendon, the musculotendinous junction, or the muscle belly. The needle is inserted perpendicularly to the required depth to reach the osteotendinous junction, the tendon sheath, the musculotendinous junction, or the muscle sheath.

Instead, if taut bands are found within the muscle belly, the 0.30 × 40 mm needles are inserted from oblique to transverse and into the muscle belly with a twisting and rotating manipulation. Alternatively, needles can be inserted deeply and perpendicularly until they reach the intermediate layers of the muscle. Electroacupuncture stimulation can be taken into consideration and used between two of these points.

TE14 In anatomical terms, it corresponds to the osteotendinous junction of the infraspinatus to the humerus.

SI10 It can be considered a local point to treat infraspinatus tendonitis since it is located very close to the osteotendinous junction of the infraspinatus to the humerus although, in anatomical terms, it corresponds to GH joint. We also use it because it is an insertion point of the Small Intestine Muscle channel, as we will see later.

Extra Point This Extraordinary point was suggested by W. Reaves.[1] It is located below SI10 and is one-quarter of the way along the line between SI10 and SI9; in anatomical terms, it corresponds to the musculotendinous junction.

To ensure the accuracy and precision of needle placement and manipulation, we prefer the sitting position, paying attention to the risk of fainting. Then, the patient is asked to lie supine except for treatment with electroacupuncture, which is administered with the patient side lying on the unaffected side.

Second Step: Anatomically Mirrored Points (Opposite Side)

The points to be needled are located on the opposite side and should correspond as precisely as possible to the anatomical mirror of the Ah Shi point(s) to be treated. The point(s) may or may not be tender on palpation.

To ensure accuracy and precision of needle placement, we prefer the sitting position, paying attention to the risk of fainting.

Option Three: Adjacent Points

First Step: Adjacent Points

LI15 It helps promote the horizontal flow of local Qì.

SI10 It is a very important point since it is the insertion point of the Small Intestine Muscle channel in the shoulder, and as such, it promotes the longitudinal flow of local Qì.

SI8 It is the insertion point of the Small Intestine Muscle channel in the elbow where shoulder pain can seldom radiate. In this specific case, it can be considered a local point. It is used to promote the longitudinal flow of local Qì and should be needled obliquely and distally to avoid hitting the underlying ulnar nerve.

Option Four: Etiological Points

First Step: Points According to Patterns
LI4 and LR3 (Bilaterally) They promote the flow of Qì and help remove Blood stasis. Since LR3 is the Yuan point of the Liver, it also helps nourish muscles and tendons.

ST36 (Bilaterally) It is used to tonify Qì and Blood in chronic Deficiency conditions or the phases of pain resolution that can turn into muscle weakness.

Second Step: General Points
GB34 (Bilaterally) It is the Hui-Gathering point of Sinews and is specifically used for infraspinatus tendonitis. In addition, it promotes the flow of Qì thus contributing to remove Blood stasis.

BL17 (Bilaterally) It is the Hui-Gathering point of Blood and is used to remove Blood stasis.

BL18 (Bilaterally) It treats all Excess and Deficiency conditions of the Liver that may favor the onset or duration of musculotendinous symptoms. It harmonizes the flow of Qì and Blood and enhances treatment of tendons and muscle.

Option Five: Microsystems

First Step: Wrist and Ankle Acupuncture
Upper 6. It roughly corresponds to the pathway of the Small Intestine channels (Fig. 2.32).

Upper 5 It controls upper limb mobility and the scapular region, the upper back, and the cervical paravertebral regions (Fig. 2.33).

Second Step: Ear Acupuncture
Local Point: Shoulder
Zang Fu Point: Liver
General Points: Subcortex and Shenmen (Fig. 2.34)

Acute or Chronic Pain from Excess.
Intense Pain or Range of Motion Reduced by Pain Principle of treatment: to remove Qì stagnation and Blood stasis and expel EPFs, if any (Box 2.3).

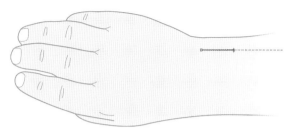

Fig. 2.32 Upper 6.

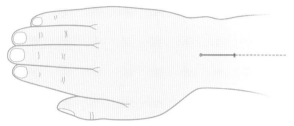

Fig. 2.33 Upper 5.

Chronic Pain from Deficiency.
Dull Pain or Muscle Weakness Principle of treatment: to tonify Qì and Blood, strengthen tissues, and avoid pain exacerbation from physical activities or invasion of EPFs (Box 2.4).

Therapeutic Program, Frequency of Sessions

The frequency of sessions depends on the clinical condition of the patient. If the condition is acute or chronic with intense pain, we recommend sessions twice a week for 2 weeks and then once a week for another 2 weeks. If improvement is observed, sessions are then scheduled once a week until complete pain relief or at least reduction by 80% to 90%. If not, the whole clinical picture should be reconsidered, and the patient should be referred to another specialist.

If the condition is chronic with dull pain, we recommend sessions once a week for 4 weeks. Afterward, and if the patient continues to improve, sessions are then scheduled once a week until complete pain relief or at least reduction by 80% to 90%.

Tendonitis of the Long Head of the Biceps

The Five Options and Selection of Acupoints
The approach we suggest is widely described in the section dedicated to the fundamentals of acupuncture for MSK pain in the limbs (see Chapter 1).

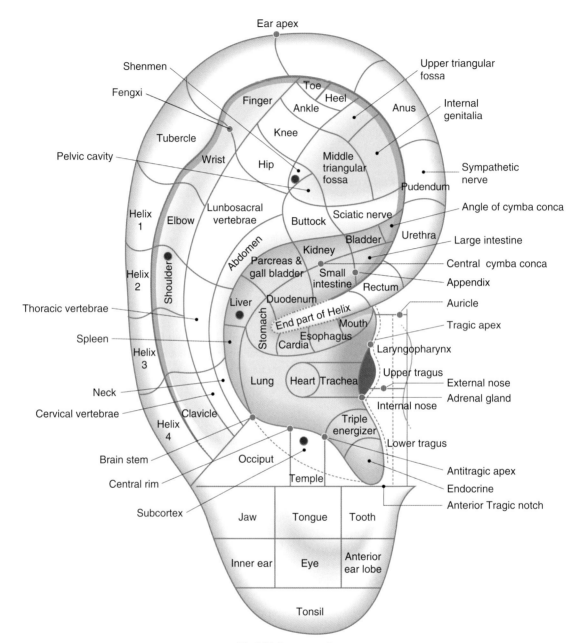

Fig. 2.34 Ear acupuncture.

The most important aspect is the identification of the Ah Shi point(s) to determine which channels are affected. In this specific case, the Lung Muscle and Connecting channels are involved.

It is worth reminding that the Lung Muscle channel runs in all of the portions of the biceps, except for its musculotendinous junction proximal to the upper arm that is covered by the Lung Main channel.

Since the Large Intestine Muscle and Connecting channels run along the intracapsular LHB and the Lung Main channel reaches point LI15, we can say that the Large Intestine channels may also be involved

BOX 2.3 ACUTE OR CHRONIC PAIN FROM EXCESS ACUPUNCTURE TREATMENT

Option 1 Distal points	• Jing-Well points SI1 and TE1 • Luo points SI7 and TE5 (opposite side) • Points according to the Six Stages BL53, BL54 or BL40 and GB30 or GB34 (opposite side) • Shu-Stream points SI3 and TE3 (affected side) and Shu-Stream points BL65 and GB41 (opposite side) • Jing-River points SI5 and TE6
Option 2 Local points	• Ah Shi • TE14 • SI10 • Extra point below SI10 • Anatomically mirrored point(s) (opposite side)
Option 3 Adjacent points	• LI15 • Insertion points SI10 and SI8
Option 4 Etiological and general points	• LI4 and LR3 (bilaterally) • GB34 (bilaterally) • BL17 (bilaterally) • BL18 (bilaterally)

Option 5 Microsystems	• W-A acupuncture
	  • Upper 6
	  • Upper 5
	• Ear acupuncture (opposite side)
	  • Shoulder
	  • Liver
	  • Subcortex and Shenmen

BOX 2.4 CHRONIC PAIN FROM DEFICIENCY ACUPUNCTURE TREATMENT

Option 1 Distal points	• Yuan points SI4 and TE4 • Luo points HT5 and PC6 (opposite side) • Points according to the 6 Stages BL53, BL54 or BL40 and GB30 or GB34 (opposite side) • Jing-River points SI5 and TE6
Option 2 Local points	• Ah Shi • TE14 • Extra point below SI10
Option 3 Adjacent points	• LI15 • Insertion points SI0 and SI8
Option 4 Etiological and general points	• ST36 (bilaterally) • GB34 (bilaterally) • LR3 (bilaterally) • BL18 (bilaterally)

Option 5 Microsystems	• W-A acupuncture
	  • Upper 6
	  • Upper 5
	• Ear acupuncture (opposite side)
	  • Shoulder
	  • Liver
	  • Subcortex and Shenmen

as widely demonstrated by clinical experience. The often-concomitant involvement of the Lung and Large Intestine channels may be explained by the fact that in anatomical terms the bicipital groove approximately lies between these two channels.

Therefore, when a combination of two points (LU and LI) is presented, the first point to be needled or bled is the LU point, whereas the LI point is the second option in case of results not satisfactory. Once the most effective channel is identified, selection of distal points continues along it.

Pricking pain localized on the tendon is a sign of Blood stasis to be treated with the bleeding technique, whereas widespread pain radiating distally along the bicipital groove is a sign of Qì stagnation to be treated with the needling technique.

It is worth reminding that the distal points should be needled one at a time and their effectiveness in terms of pain and range of motion tested after each insertion. The same applies to the local points.

Finally, since both options 1 and 2 consist of several steps, it is important to highlight how selection should be made. Specifically, the practitioner might wonder if all or some of the steps should be followed. The rule

Clinical Notes

- Treatment of infraspinatus tendonitis usually ensures excellent outcomes.
- Effectiveness of treatment may be reduced if severely restricted range of motion is observed. In this specific case, pain may disappear with rest or movement leaving behind residual limited range of motion, which, however, does not prevent the patient from performing everyday activities.
- Improvement following treatment may turn intense pain to dull pain and then to a feeling of weakness. Should this be the case, the principle of treatment has to be changed as follows: it is no longer necessary to remove Qì stagnation and Blood stasis and expel EPFs, if any; instead, Qì and Blood should be tonified to strengthen tissues and avoid pain exacerbation from physical activities or invasion of EPFs.

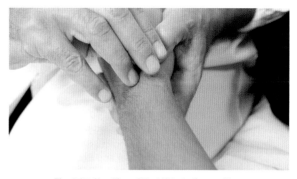

Fig. 2.35 Needling of the LU7: starting position.

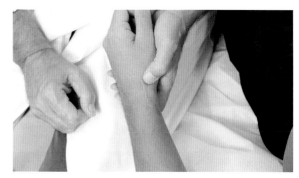

Fig. 2.36 Needling of the LU7: final position.

we follow is simple: when the result achieved is satisfactory, the remaining steps should be skipped, and the practitioner should move to the following option. Similarly, the use of the points recommended under options 3, 4, and 5 should be carefully evaluated according to the case being treated.

The points and accessory techniques we recommend using are listed below.

Order of Needling

Option One: Distal Points

First Step: Lung and Large Intestine Muscle Channels

LU11 and LI1 These Jing-Well points activate the Lung and Large Intestine Muscle channels, and they remove Qì stagnation and Blood stasis with needling and bleeding techniques, respectively.

Second Step: Lung and Large Intestine Connecting Channels

LU7 and LI6 (Opposite Side) These Luo points activate the Lung and Large Intestine Connecting channels, and they remove Qì stagnation and Blood stasis in acute or chronic conditions from Excess.

LU7 and LI6 are needled from oblique to transverse in proximal direction along the pathways of the Lung and Large Intestine Main channels, respectively.

The same Luo points are also used in chronic Deficiency conditions with dull pain to tonify Qì and

Blood in their respective internally-externally related channels. In this case, we associate Yuan point LI4 with Luo point LU7 and Yuan point LU9 with Luo point LI6, which is the well-known Luo-Yuan point combination: first, as the main point, we needle the Yuan point on the affected side and then, as a secondary point, the Luo point on the internally-externally related channel on the opposite side. (see Figs. 2.35–2.38; Videos 2.16 and 2.17).

Third step: Empirical Points

There is no point which is classically recommended.

Fourth step: Opposite Extremity (upper/lower)

SP12 (Opposite Side) It is located in the hip joint, which corresponds to the shoulder joint on the paired channel according to the Six Stages.

SP9 (Opposite Side) Although located distal to the hip joint, it is used more often because it mobilizes more energy than the previous point. Practitioners can also use a point that is tender on palpation and located about 1 or 2 cm distal to SP9 and along the Spleen Main channel.

Between these two points, we would suggest choosing the more tender one on palpation.

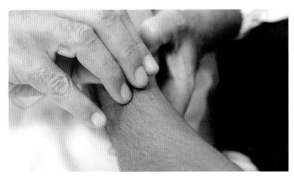

Fig. 2.37 Needling of the LI6: starting position.

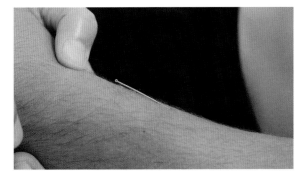

Fig. 2.38 Needling of the LI6: final position.

ST31 (Opposite Side) It is located in the hip joint, which corresponds to the shoulder joint on the paired channel according to the Six Stages.

Reaves[1] suggests also trying the point he refers to as the "medial" ST31, which is positioned medial to the sartorius muscle, whereas ST31 is on the lateral side.

ST36 (Opposite Side) Although located distal to the hip joint, it is used more often because it mobilizes more energy than the previous point.

Our technique consists of needling the opposite extremity (lower/upper) on the opposite side in acute and chronic conditions.

Alternatively, the most tender point on palpation is selected on the same or opposite side.

Fifth Step: Categories of Traditional Points

LU9 (Affected Side) and SP3 (Opposite Side), LI3 (Affected Side) and St43 (Opposite Side) A good combination includes the Shu-Stream points on the paired channel according to the Six Stages. First, we needle the Shu-Stream point on the channel involved on the affected side, and then the Shu-Stream point on the coupled channel on the opposite side and opposite extremity (upper/lower).

We use this technique in acute and chronic Excess conditions to treat pain and expel or prevent invasion of EPFs. It is worth reminding that in the Yin channels the Shu-Stream point corresponds to the Yuan-Source point. That is why LU9 could also be used in chronic Deficiency conditions, as we will see later.

LU8 and LI5 The Jing-River points are used in acute or chronic Excess conditions due to the invasion of an EPF, and they are needled to promote its expulsion from their respective channels. They are also useful to prevent pain exacerbation from seasonal changes or invasion of EPFs. However, they are more effective in the Yang rather than in the Yin channels; that is why we use LI5 to treat this condition and we would rather avoid using LU8.

LU6 and LI7 The Xi-Cleft points are used especially in acute conditions for the treatment of Blood stasis in their respective channels. However, they are more effective in the Yin rather than in the Yang channels; that is why we use LU6 to treat this condition and we would rather avoid using LI7.

LU9 and LI4 We recommend using these Yuan-Source point(s) in chronic Deficiency conditions with dull pain, in the case of weakness, or in the resolution phases of tendonitis of the LHB, to tonify Qi and Blood flow in their respective channels.

In this situation, we can also associate Yuan point LU9 with Luo point LI6 and Yuan point LI4 with Luo point LU7, which is the well-known Luo-Yuan point combination. First, as the main point, we needle the Yuan point on the affected side and then, as a secondary point, the Luo point on the internally-externally related channel on the opposite side.

Sixth Step: Extraordinary Vessels

In our opinion, no Extraordinary Vessel is effective to treat this disorder.

Option Two: Local Points

First Step: Painful Points (Ah Shi)

Ah Shi Point(s) Palpation of the anterior GH joint reveals either the most painful point(s) (Ah Shi) corresponding to Blood stasis and therefore to be bled or an area of widespread pain corresponding to Qi stagnation and requiring needling. Pain could radiate distally to the bicipital groove, 1 or 2 cm in length and about 0.5 cm in width (Figs. 2.39 and 2.40).

The cupping therapy should be used to bleed the Ah Shi point(s) (Video 2.18).

Needles are inserted perpendicularly to the required depth until the tendon sheath is reached; practitioners can choose two or three points that are about 1 cm apart.

We use a 0.25 × 25 mm or a 0.30 × 40 mm needle: the diameter and length of the needle to be used depending on the patient physique (Figs. 2.41 and 2.42). Electroacupuncture stimulation can be taken into consideration and used between two of these points (Video 2.19).

Jianqian

This point can be considered the local point for this disorder because it lies very proximal to the bicipital groove although not exactly in it.

In acute or chronic conditions, a moxa stick can be useful to promote the flow of Qì and Blood. We can also use it to treat the invasion of EPFs, Cold in particular.

However, attention should be paid, since too much heat can increase the ongoing inflammatory process.

To ensure the accuracy and precision of local needle placement and manipulation, we prefer the supine position.

Second Step: Anatomically Mirrored Points (Opposite Side)

The points to be needled are located on the opposite side, which means on the anterior side of the opposite shoulder, and should correspond as precisely as possible to the anatomical mirror of the Ah Shi point(s) to be treated. The point(s) may or may not be tender on palpation. To ensure the accuracy and precision of needle placement and manipulation, we prefer the supine position.

Option Three: Adjacent Points

First Step: Adjacent Points

LI15 It can be considered the most important adjacent point to treat this disorder as it is the meeting point of the Large Intestine and Lung Muscle channels. In anatomical terms, it is the closest acupoint, even if it does not correspond to the LHB, corresponding instead to the osteotendinous junction of the supraspinatus to the humerus. We also use it because it is the insertion point of the Large Intestine Muscle

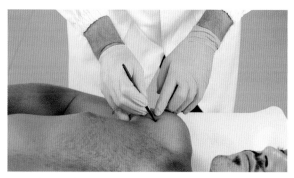

Fig. 2.39 Bleeding of the Ah Shi point(s): starting position.

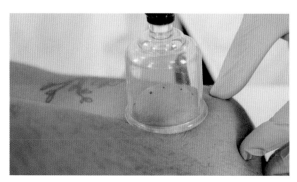

Fig. 2.40 Bleeding of the Ah Shi point(s): final position.

channel in the shoulder, and as such it promotes the longitudinal flow of local Qì.

LU1 and LU2 They help promote the longitudinal flow of local Qì.

SI11 and SI12 They help promote shoulder muscle balance since they represent the infraspinatus and supraspinatus, respectively.

LU3 It is the insertion point of the Lung Muscle channel located close to the shoulder, exactly where shoulder pain can radiate to. In this specific case, it can be considered a local point. It helps promote the longitudinal flow of local Qì.

LU5 It is the insertion point of the Lung Muscle channel in the elbow, where shoulder pain can seldom radiate to, and is located close to the osteotendinous junction of the biceps on the radius. In this specific case, it can be considered a local point. It is used to promote the longitudinal flow of local Qì.

LI11 It is the insertion point of the Large Intestine Muscle channel in the elbow, and it can help promote the longitudinal flow of Qì.

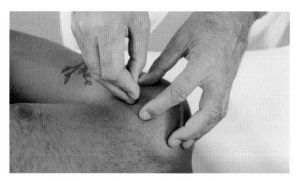

Fig. 2.41 Needling of the Ah Shi point(s): starting position.

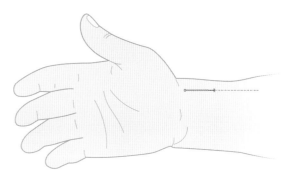

Fig. 2.43 Upper 3.

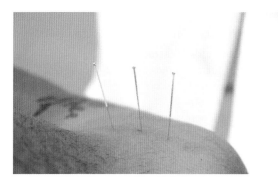

Fig. 2.42 Needling of the Ah Shi point(s): final position.

Option Four: Etiological Points

First Step: Points According to Patterns

LI4 and LR3 (Bilaterally) They promote the flow of Qì and help remove Blood stasis. Since LR3 is the Shu/Yuan point of the Liver, it also helps nourish muscles and tendons.

ST36 (Bilaterally) It is used to tonify Qì and Blood in chronic Deficiency conditions or the phases of pain resolution that can turn into muscle weakness.

Second Step: General Points

GB34 (Bilaterally) It is the Hui-Gathering point of Sinews and is specifically used for tendonitis of the LHB. In addition, it promotes the flow of Qì, thus contributing to remove Blood stasis.

BL17 (Bilaterally) It is the Hui-Gathering point of Blood and is used to remove Blood stasis.

BL18 (Bilaterally) It treats all Excess and Deficiency conditions of the Liver that may favor the onset or duration of musculotendinous symptoms. It harmonizes the flow of Qì and Blood and enhances treatment of tendons and muscle.

Option Five: Microsystems

First Step: Wrist and Ankle Acupuncture

Upper 3 It roughly corresponds to the pathway of the Lung channels (Fig. 2.43).

Upper 4 It roughly corresponds to the pathway of the Large Intestine channels (Fig. 2.44).

Upper 5 It controls upper limb mobility. Sometimes, it can help relieve pain and improve shoulder strength and range of motion (Fig. 2.45).

Second Step: Ear Acupuncture
Local Point: Shoulder
Zang Fu Point: Liver
General Points: Subcortex and Shenmen (Fig. 2.46)

The Order of Needling

Acute or Chronic Pain From Excess.

Intense Pain or Range of Motion Reduced by Pain Principle of treatment: to remove Qì stagnation and Blood stasis and expel EPFs, if any (Box 2.5).

Chronic Pain From Deficiency.

Dull Pain or Muscle Weakness Principle of treatment: to tonify Qì and Blood, strengthen tissues, and avoid pain exacerbation from physical activities or invasion of EPFs (Box 2.6).

Therapeutic Program, Frequency of Sessions

The frequency of sessions depends on the clinical condition of the patient. If the condition is acute or chronic with intense pain, we recommend sessions twice a week for 2 weeks and then once a week for another 2 weeks. If improvement is observed, sessions are then scheduled once a week until complete pain relief or at least reduction by 80% to 90%. If not, the

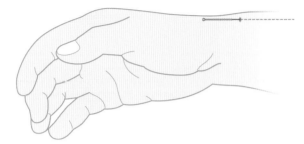

Fig. 2.44 Upper 4.

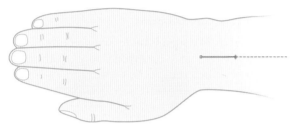

Fig. 2.45 Upper 5.

Clinical Notes

- Treatment usually ensures very good outcomes.
- Improvement following treatment may turn intense pain to dull pain and then to a feeling of weakness. Should this be the case, the principle of treatment has to be changed as follows: it is no longer necessary to remove Qì stagnation and Blood stasis and expel EPFs, if any; instead, Qì and Blood should be tonified to strengthen tissues and avoid pain exacerbation from physical activities or invasion of EPFs.

---

whole clinical picture should be reconsidered and the patient should be referred to another specialist.

If the condition is chronic with dull pain, we recommend sessions once a week for 4 weeks. Afterward, and if the patient continues to improve, sessions are then scheduled once a week until complete pain relief or at least reduction by 80% to 90%.

OSTEOPATHIC MANIPULATIVE TREATMENT

This section deals with osteopathic manipulations to treat shoulder joint dysfunctions. As already mentioned in the section dedicated to the fundamentals of osteopathy for MSK pain in the limbs (see Chapter 1), the key concept of the osteopathic therapeutic process is the treatment not only of the somatic dysfunctions of the shoulder but also of those functionally and anatomically related.

Consequently, the osteopathic manipulative approach to MSK shoulder pain is based on the identification of joint somatic dysfunctions not only of the shoulder but also of the elbow and wrist.

Regardless of the condition to be treated, be it supraspinatus or infraspinatus tendonitis, tendonitis of the LHB, AC joint disorders, arthritis of the shoulder, or surgical outcomes, all of the dysfunctions identified should be treated.

Somatic Dysfunctions of the Sternoclavicular Joint

Anterior Clavicle: Treatment

Anterior dysfunction: anterior sliding of the clavicular medial end is better than posterior sliding.

The patient sits.

The practitioner stands behind the patient with the thenar eminence of the right and left hand placed behind the right shoulder and on the clavicular medial end, respectively. The practitioner performs a combined movement: right hand forward and left hand backward.

After joint decoaptation and rebalancing, the thrust is performed at the beginning of inspiration (Fig. 2.47; Video 2.20).

Posterior Clavicle: Treatment

Posterior dysfunction: posterior sliding of the clavicular medial end is better than anterior sliding.

The patient sits.

The practitioner stands behind the patient with the right forearm under the axilla to lift the right arm to 90 degrees. The fingers of the left hand hold the sternal manubrium. The practitioner counterbalances the backward force with the chest while pulling the shoulder backward and laterally with the right hand.

After joint decoaptation and rebalancing, the thrust is performed by pulling with the right hand slightly backward and laterally and at the same time applying a gentle pressure forward with the chest at the beginning of inspiration (Fig. 2.48; Video 2.21).

Somatic Dysfunctions of the Acromioclavicular Joint

Anterior Rotation of the Clavicle: Treatment

Anterior rotation dysfunction: anterior rotation of the clavicular lateral end is better than posterior rotation.

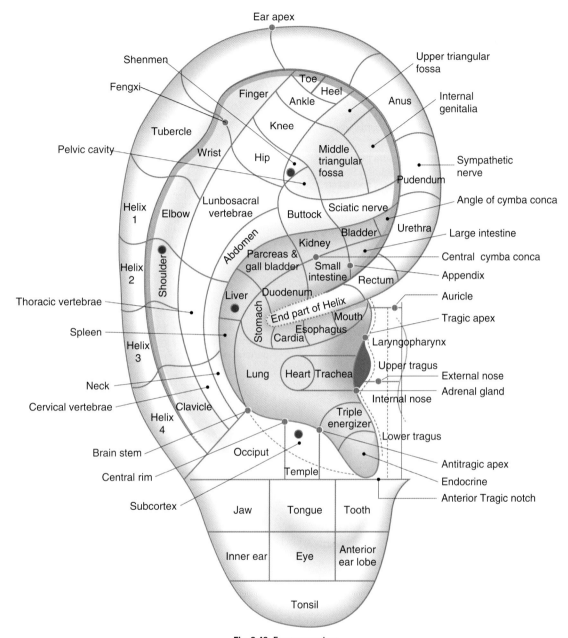

Fig. 2.46 Ear acupuncture.

The patient sits.

The practitioner stands behind the patient and holds the right clavicular lateral end with the second and third distal phalanges of the left hand fingers, while the right hand holds the elbow in a backward position.

The practitioner pulls the clavicle backward while pushing the elbow forward and then, while holding

BOX 2.5 ACUTE OR CHRONIC PAIN FROM EXCESS ACUPUNCTURE TREATMENT

Option 1 Distal points	• Jing-Well points LU11 and LI1 • Luo points LU7 and LI6 (opposite side) • Points according to the 6 stages SP12 or SP9, and ST31 or "medial" ST31, or ST36 (opposite site) • Shu-Stream points LU9 and LI3 (affected site) and Shu-Stream points SP3 and ST43 (opposite site) • Xi-Cleft point LU6 • Jing-River point LI5
Option 2 Local points	• Ah Shi • Jianqian • Anatomically mirrored point(s) (opposite side)
Option 3 Adjacent points	• LU1 • LU2 • LU3 • SI11 • SI12 • Insertion points LI15, LU5, and LI11
Option 4 Etiological and general points	• LI4 and LR3 (bilaterally) • GB34 (bilaterally) • BL17 (bilaterally) • BL18 (bilaterally)

Option 5
Microsystems
	• W-A acupuncture
	  • Upper 3
	  • Upper 4
	  • Upper 5
	• Ear acupuncture (opposite side)
	  • Shoulder
	  • Liver
	  • Subcortex and Shenmen

BOX 2.6 CHRONIC PAIN FROM DEFICIENCY ACUPUNCTURE TREATMENT

Option 1 Distal points	• Yuan points LU9 and LI4 • Luo points LI6 and LU7 (opposite side) • Points according to the 6 stages SP12 or SP9 and ST31, "medial" ST31, or ST36 (opposite side) • Jing-River point LI5
Option 2 Local points	• Ah Shi • Jianqian
Option 3 Adjacent points	• LU1 • LU2 • LU3 • SI11 • SI12 • Insertion points LI15, LU5, and LI11
Option 4 Etiological and general points	• ST36 (bilaterally) • GB34 (bilaterally) • LR3 (bilaterally) • BL18 (bilaterally)

Option 5
Microsystems
	• W-A acupuncture
	  • Upper 3
	  • Upper 4
	  • Upper 5
	• Ear acupuncture (opposite side)
	  • Shoulder
	  • Liver
	  • Subcortex and Shenmen

the clavicular end to prevent its anterior rotation, the elbow is pulled backward (Figs. 2.49 and 2.50).

The sequence should be repeated three times (Video 2.22).

Posterior Rotation of the Clavicle: Treatment

Posterior rotation dysfunction: posterior rotation of the clavicular lateral end is better than anterior rotation.

The patient sits.

The practitioner stands behind the patient and places the metacarpophalangeal joint of the left index finger behind the right clavicular lateral end while holding the elbow in a forward position with the right hand.

The practitioner pushes the clavicle forward while pulling the elbow backward and then, while holding the clavicular end to prevent its posterior rotation, the elbow is pushed forward (Figs. 2.51 and 2.52).

The sequence should be repeated three times (Video 2.23).

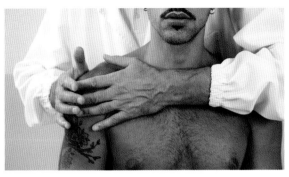
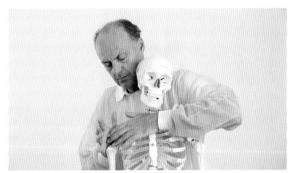

Fig. 2.47 Anterior clavicle: treatment.

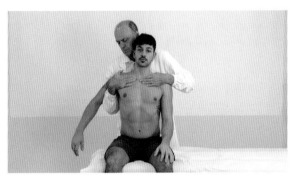
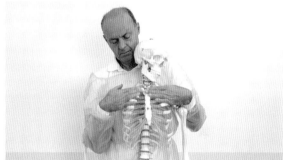

Fig. 2.48 Posterior clavicle: treatment.

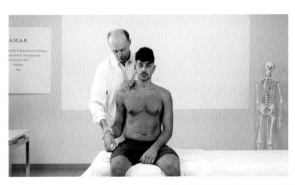
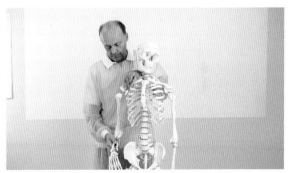

Fig. 2.49 Anterior rotation of the clavicle: treatment. Starting position.

Somatic Dysfunctions of the Glenohumeral Joint

Anterior Humeral Head: Treatment

Anterior dysfunction: anterior sliding of the humeral head is better than posterior sliding.

The patient is supine with the right shoulder on the bed edge. The practitioner stands close to the patient's right side.

The practitioner raises the patient's arm with the left hand, places the second metacarpophalangeal

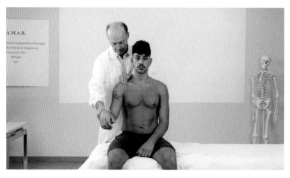

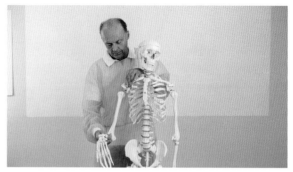

Fig. 2.50 Anterior rotation of the clavicle: treatment. Final position.

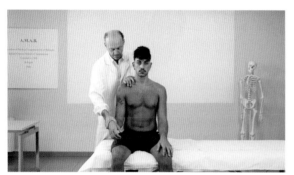

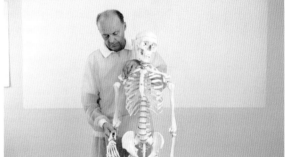

Fig. 2.51 Posterior rotation of the clavicle: treatment. Starting position.

joint of the right hand on the anterior side of the humeral head and, at the same time, holds the forearm in vertical position with the elbow extended (Fig. 2.53).

After joint decoaptation and rebalancing, the thrust is performed with the right hand from above downward and in an outward direction (Video 2.24).

Superior Humeral Head: Treatment

Superior dysfunction: upward sliding of the humeral head is better than downward sliding.

The patient sits on the bed edge.

The practitioner stands perpendicular to the patient's right side. The practitioner applies little lateral traction on the patient's right arm, which lies at 90 degrees on the practitioner's shoulder.

The practitioner's fingers are intertwined on the GH joint (Fig. 2.54).

After joint decoaptation and rebalancing, the thrust is performed vertically from above downward with the ulnar margin of the hands (Video 2.25).

Somatic Dysfunctions of the Long Head of the Biceps

Medial Malposition of the Long Head of the Biceps: Treatment

The patient sits on the bed edge.

The practitioner stands behind the patient. With the right hand the practitioner holds the patient's right wrist with the elbow held at 90 degrees.

The left hand is on the patient's shoulder, with the second and third fingers holding the LHB medially (Figs. 2.55 and 2.56).

Treatment consists of three steps:

1. During passive external rotation of the shoulder, the practitioner prevents the tendon from sliding medially.

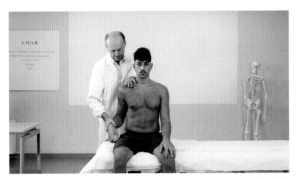
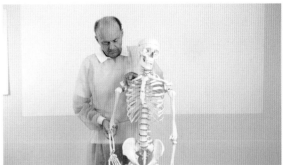

Fig. 2.52 Posterior rotation of the clavicle: treatment. Final position.

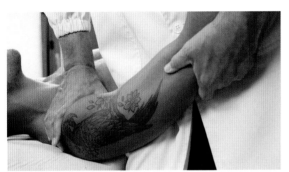
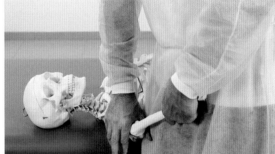

Fig. 2.53 Anterior humeral head: treatment.

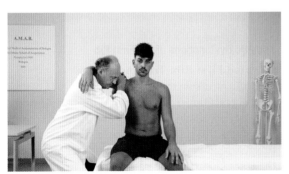
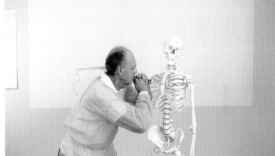

Fig. 2.54 Superior humeral head: treatment.

2. During passive internal rotation of the shoulder and while pushing the patient's arm downward, the practitioner holds the tendon medially and pulls it laterally to its physiological position.
3. During passive external rotation of the shoulder and while pulling the patient's arm upward, the fingers hold the tendon in its physiological position.

The sequence should be repeated three times (Video 2.26).

Lateral Malposition of the Long Head of the Biceps: Treatment

The patient sits on the bed edge.

The practitioner stands behind the patient. With the right hand the practitioner holds the patient's wrist with the elbow extended, shoulder in internal rotation, and forearm pronated.

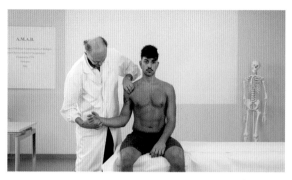
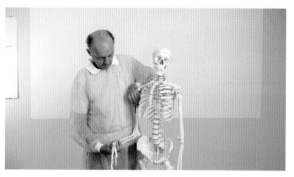

Fig. 2.55 Medial malposition of the long head of the biceps: treatment. Starting position.

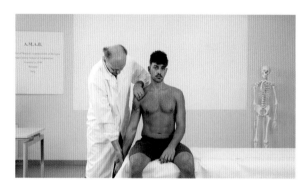
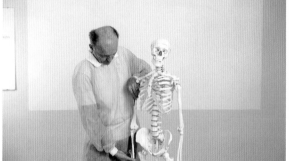

Fig. 2.56 Medial malposition of the long head of the biceps: treatment. Final position.

The left hand is on the patient's shoulder, with the second and third fingers placed lateral to the LHB (Figs. 2.57 and 2.58).

Treatment consists of three steps:

1. During passive external rotation of the shoulder and while pulling the patient's right arm upward, the practitioner prevents the tendon from sliding laterally.
2. During passive internal rotation of the shoulder and while pushing the patient's arm downward, the practitioner pushes the tendon medially toward its physiological position.
3. During passive external rotation of the shoulder and while pulling the patient's arm upward, the fingers hold the tendon in its physiological position.

The sequence should be repeated three times (Video 2.27).

Somatic Dysfunctions of the First Rib

Elevated First Rib: Treatment

The patient sits on the bed edge.

The practitioner stands behind the patient with the metacarpophalangeal joints of the right index finger placed on the superior surface of the first right rib tubercle in front of the trapezius anterior border, while the left hand bends the patient's head to the right and rotates it slightly to the left.

The practitioner pushes the tubercle of the rib in an inward, downward, and forward direction, while increasing right side bending (Fig. 2.59).

After joint decoaptation and rebalancing, the thrust is performed at the beginning of expiration (Video 2.28).

Therapeutic Program, Frequency of Sessions

The AcuOsteo Method of treatment combines acupuncture and osteopathic manipulations, and, in

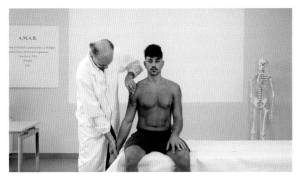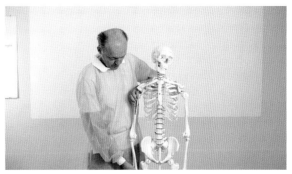

Fig. 2.57 Lateral malposition of the long head of the biceps: treatment. Starting position.

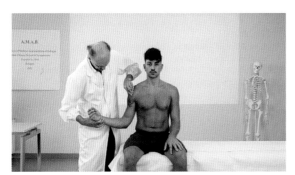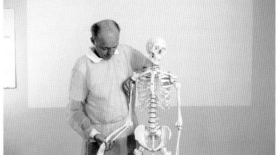

Fig. 2.58 Lateral malposition of the long head of the biceps: treatment. Final position.

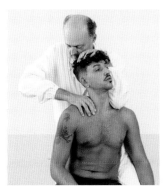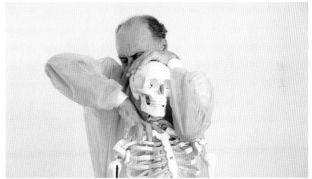

Fig. 2.59 Elevated first rib: treatment.

principle, both therapeutic techniques are used during each session and at the same time.

If the condition is acute or chronic with intense pain, we recommend sessions twice a week for 2 weeks and then once a week for another 2 weeks. If improvement is observed, sessions are then scheduled once a week until complete pain relief or at least reduction by 80% to 90%.

In practice, however, as the osteopathic approach differs from acupuncture in that it follows a mechanical principle and aims to restore proper joint mobility, we opt for a parsimonious use of osteopathic manipulations over acupuncture: there may be no need to repeat them in every session.

Osteopathic maneuvers are therefore performed in case of persistent somatic dysfunction. Hence the patient should always be reevaluated at the beginning of each session to assess joint conditions and compare them with preexisting dysfunction.

REFERENCE

1. Reaves W, Bong C. *The Acupuncture Handbook of Sports Injuries & Pain*. 3rd ed. Hidden Needle Press; 2013.

BIBLIOGRAPHY

Baldry PE. *Acupuncture, Trigger Points and Musculoskeletal Pain*. 3rd ed. Elsevier; 2005.
Buckup K. *Test ortopedici*. Verduci Editore; 1997.
Cipriano JJ. *Test Ortopedici e Neurologici*. Verduci Editore; 1998.
De Seze S, Ryckewaert A. *Malattie dell'osso e delle articolazioni*. Aulo Gaggi Editore; 1979.
Osteopatia Gay J. *l'Arto Superiore*. Editore Marrapese; 1989.
Giusti R. *Glossary of osteophatic terminology*. 3rd ed. American Association of Colleges of Osteophatic Medicine; 2017.
Greenman PE. *Principles of Manual Medicine*. 2nd ed. Williams & Wilkins; 1996.
Guolo F. *Atlante di Tecniche di Energia Muscolare*. Piccin; 2014.
Hoppenfeld S. *L'Esame Obiettivo dell'Apparato Locomotore*. Aulo Gaggi Editore; 1985.
Legge D. *Close to the bone*. Sydney College Press; 2010.
Maciocia G. *The Practice of Chinese Medicine*. 3rd ed. Elsevier; 2022.
Misulis KE, Head TC. *Neurologia di Netter*. Elsevier; 2008.
Nicholas AS, Nicholas EA. *Atlas of Osteophatic Thechniques*. Lippincott Williams & Wilkins; 2012.
Qiao W. (Association of Medical Acupuncturist of Bologna) Seminar *Wrist and Ankle and Balance Acupuncture*. Italian Chine School of Acupuncture-A.M.A.B; 2007.
Romoli M. *Auricular Acupuncture Diagnosis*. Churchill Livingstone Elsevier; 2009.
Tan RT. In: Besinger JW, ed. *Dr. Tan's Strategy of Twelve Magical Points*. 2003.
Tixa S. *Atlas d'Anatomie Palpatoire, tome 1, Cou, Tronc, Membre Superior*. 2é ed. Elsevier Masson; 2005.
Tixa S, Ebenegger B. *Atlas de Techniques articulaires ostéopathiques, tome 1, Les Membres*. 3é ed. Elsevier Masson; 2016.

Chapter 3

The Elbow

Lateral and Medial Epicondylitis

Lateral (tennis elbow) and medial (golfer's elbow) epicondylitis are two types of insertional tendinopathy affecting their respective humeral epicondyles. Mechanical overloading is a major cause of tendinopathy which often results from work- or sports-related repetitive microtrauma. Local pain can radiate to the forearm muscles.

Anatomy and Biomechanics According to Western Medicine

JOINTS AND MUSCLES

The elbow is characterized by stable bony architecture. Despite being intrinsically more stable, its peculiar joint architecture allows a wide range of motion. Additionally, its bone anatomy is involved in forearm rotation, regardless of the shoulder or flexion/extension of the elbow itself.

The elbow is a compound joint involving three articulations completely enclosed in a joint capsule and referred to as:

- The medial humeroulnar joint
- The lateral humeroradial joint
- The central, proximal radioulnar joint

These three articulations exist between the distal epiphysis of the humerus and the proximal epiphyses of the radius and ulna (Figs. 3.1 and 3.2).

In anatomy, the distal radioulnar joint is part of the wrist, although together with the proximal radioulnar joint, it allows supination and pronation of the forearm. The ulna articulates with the humerus in a stable way thanks to a tight conforming of the two joint surfaces. The radius articulates with the humerus in a stable way: stability mainly comes from the strong lateral ligament and the osseous articulation.

These two articulations form a uniaxial hinge joint allowing flexion-extension of the forearm. The radius also articulates with the ulna proximally and distally, thus allowing for pronation-supination of the forearm.

The radius and ulna, linked by the interosseous membrane, make up the functional unit of the forearm allowing hand and wrist rotation and they also act as a stable fulcrum to allow hand manipulation for gross and fine motor tasks.

The distal epiphysis of the humerus ends with a central portion, the humeral condyle, which is covered by hyaline cartilage, and two bony prominences, the lateral and medial epicondyles: the medial is the larger of the two.

Also distal to the humerus are three depressions, known as the coronoid and radial fossae located anteriorly, and the olecranon fossa posteriorly. They accommodate the ulnar and radial counterparts during flexion or extension at the elbow.

The medial epicondyle or epitrochlea serves as an attachment site for the flexor-pronator muscles and the ulnar collateral ligament; the lateral epicondyle or epicondyle serves as an attachment site for the extensor-supinator muscles and the radial collateral ligament.

The proximal end of the ulna is massive and posteriorly it is characterized by a large bony projection, the so-called olecranon, where the triceps attaches.

The proximal end or head of the radius is small, prism-shaped, and situated on the lateral side of the elbow. The distal end, which is larger, is the main component of the wrist.

Below the head, on the anterior aspect, there is the radial tuberosity, a bony prominence which serves as the distal place of attachment of the biceps. The elbow architecture is as complex as its joint structure. The muscles that attach to the ulna distally can flex or extend the elbow, but they can neither pronate nor supinate the forearm. The muscles with attach to the radius can flex or extend the elbow and can also pronate or supinate the forearm.

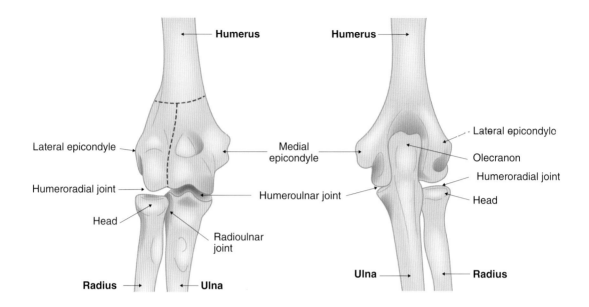

Fig. 3.1 The elbow anatomy: anterior and posterior view.

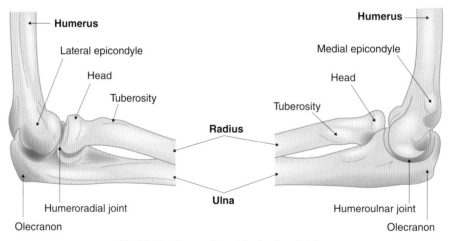

Fig. 3.2 The elbow anatomy: lateral and medial view.

When describing the muscles of the elbow, several criteria may be used to identify them, thus resulting in a functional (elbow flexors and extensors, forearm pronators and supinators) or topographical (anterior, posterior, medial and lateral) classification.

ANATOMICAL LANDMARKS

The most useful anatomical landmarks are listed in the following (Figs. 3.3 and 3.4):

- Lateral epicondyle: it is an eminence located on the lateral side of the elbow, at the distal end

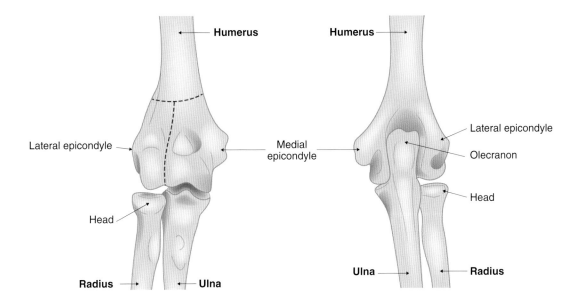

Fig. 3.3 Anatomical landmarks: anterior and posterior view.

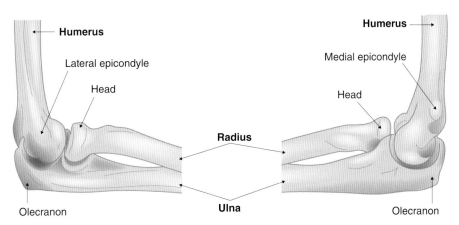

Fig. 3.4 Anatomical landmarks: lateral and medial view.

of the humerus and close to the humeroradial joint.
- Radial head: it is the proximal end of the radius located on the lateral side of the elbow. It is disk shaped with a flattened end that articulates with the distal end of the humerus.
- Medial epicondyle (epitrochlea): it is an eminence located on the medial side of the elbow,

at the distal end of the humerus and close to the humeroulnar joint.
- Olecranon process: it is a bony prominence characterizing the posterior and superior portions of the proximal ulna. It is nothing but the bony tip that can be palpated on the posterior aspect of the elbow.

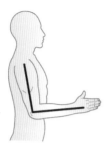

Fig. 3.5 Neutral position.

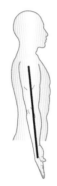

Fig. 3.6 Extension.

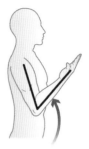

Fig. 3.7 Flexion.

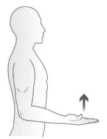

Fig. 3.8 Supination.

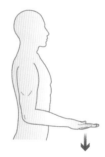

Fig. 3.9 Pronation.

JOINT MOVEMENTS

The Physiological Movements of the Proximal Radioulnar Joint

The radius pivots around the ulna to produce movement at the radioulnar joint. The neutral position of the elbow is with the upper limb close to the trunk. The starting positions to assess the physiological movements of the elbow are two:

- The forearm is in neutral position (Fig. 3.5), elbow at 90 degrees, the palm of the hand neither turned up nor turned down.
  - Extension: the forearm moves away from the arm (Fig. 3.6).
  - Flexion: the forearm moves towards the arm (Fig. 3.7).
  - Supination: the forearm rotates externally which means the hand is turned so the palm is upward (Fig. 3.8).
  - Pronation: the forearm rotates internally which means the hand is turned so the palm is downward (Fig. 3.9).

- The forearm is supinated with incomplete elbow extension; if it was complete, the following joint movements would be locked.
  - Adduction (passive): the forearm moves medially towards the patient (Fig. 3.10).
  - Abduction (passive): the forearm moves laterally away from the patient (Fig. 3.11).

The normal range of motion of the elbow:
- Full extension to full flexion is 0 degrees to about 150 degrees

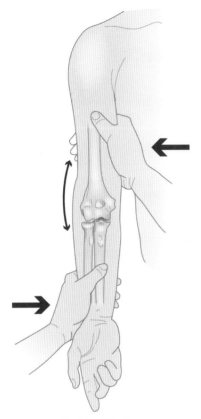

Fig. 3.10 Adduction.

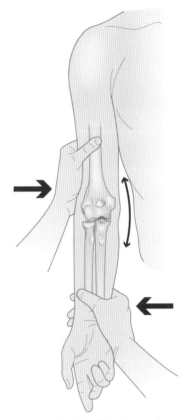

Fig. 3.11 Abduction.

- Full supination to full pronation 0 degrees to about 180 degrees

Range of motion required for most daily activities is:

- 30 degrees of flexion to 130 degrees of extension (with the elbow flexed to 90 degrees)
- 50 degrees of supination to 50 degrees of pronation (with the forearm in neutral position or thumb up)

Success of treatment may be defined as the achievement of at least these clinical outcomes.

Diagnosis in Western Medicine

LATERAL EPICONDYLITIS

Lateral epicondylitis is a tendinopathy injury, either inflammatory or degenerative (tendinosis), often involving the extensor digitorum communis and extensor carpi radialis brevis originating from the lateral epicondyle, i.e. the bony prominence on the lateral side of the elbow. In most cases, insertional tendinitis is diagnosed in the lateral epicondyle.

Lateral epicondylitis may be the result of gradual wear and tear to the tendon from overuse or work- or sport-related repetitive strain injury; however, pain may also be sudden and severe and occur after excessive muscular effort or local trauma.

The most common symptoms are the following:

- Lateral elbow pain, either well localized or radiating to the extensor muscles of the forearm
- Tenderness on palpation on the lateral epicondyle
- Pain when grasping small objects or performing certain tasks (e.g., screwing a lid to a container,

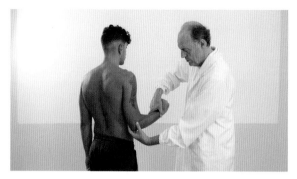

Fig. 3.12 Cozen test.

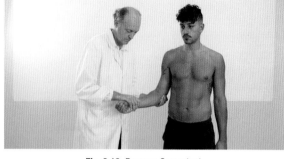

Fig. 3.13 Reverse Cozen test.

turning the key to lock the door, shaking hands or lifting objects with a pronated forearm)
- In chronic conditions, pain may be dull with a feeling of stiffness
- Positive Cozen test

Cozen Test

It is used to assess lateral epicondylitis (tennis elbow). The patient sits (Fig. 3.12; Video 3.1).

The practitioner stands opposite the patient. The right elbow is flexed at 90 degrees and the forearm is in pronation. The patient is asked to keep the wrist extended while the practitioner pulls the wrist into flexion with the right hand and palpates the lateral epicondyle with the left hand. The test is considered positive if the patient reports pain over the lateral epicondyle.

MEDIAL EPICONDYLITIS

Medial epicondylitis is a tendinopathy injury, either inflammatory or degenerative, involving the medial humeral epicondyle or epitrochlea, and more often the pronator teres, flexor carpi radialis and ulnaris, and palmaris longus muscles originating from the medial epicondyle, that is, the bony prominence on the medial side of the elbow. In most cases, insertional tendinitis is diagnosed in the medial epicondyle.

It is less common than lateral epicondylitis; in general, its onset is progressive and it results from overuse or work- or sports-related repetitive strain injury (golfer's elbow). However, pain may also be sudden and severe and occur after excessive muscular effort or local trauma.

The most common symptoms are the following:
- Medial elbow pain, either localized or radiating to the flexors and pronators of the forearm
- Tenderness on palpation on the medial epicondyle
- Pain when grasping small objects or performing certain tasks (e.g., unscrewing a lid to a container and turning the key to unlock the door)
- In chronic conditions, pain may be dull with a feeling of stiffness of the flexors and pronators
- Positive Reverse Cozen test

Reverse Cozen Test

It is used to assess medial epicondylitis (golfer's elbow). The patient sits (Fig. 3.13; Video 3.2).

The practitioner stands opposite the patient. The right elbow is flexed at 90 degrees and the forearm is in supination. The patient is asked to pronate the wrist while the practitioner holds the forearm with the right hand and palpates the medial epicondyle with the left hand. The test is considered positive if the patient reports pain over the medial epicondyle.

JOINT PAIN, ARTHRITIS, AND STIFFNESS

Patients with elbow arthritis and postsurgical outcomes usually complain of pain, weakness, and restricted range of motion. Among the most common causes of elbow arthritis are fractures, or rheumatoid arthritis, septic arthritis and primary osteoarthritis. Diagnosis is based on the patient's medical history, clinical findings, and radiographic examinations. The most common complications that may occur after surgery or as a result of fracture include:

- Elbow stiffness with possible loss of motion (flexion, extension, pronation and supination)
- Late-onset osteoarthritis
- Failed fusion
- Persistent pain

RED FLAGS IN WESTERN MEDICINE

The presence of heat (calor), redness (rubor), swelling (tumor), pain (dolor) and loss of function (function laesa) determines the need for diagnostic investigations.

Elbow trauma is a common occurrence. Among the signs and symptoms of fracture or dislocation are swelling and deformity of the limb. A fracture affects the continuity of a bone, whereas a dislocation involves a joint.

Patients with rheumatoid arthritis of the elbow usually complain of pain throughout the range of motion; the elbow is usually affected in the later stages the disease. Both fatigue and general discomfort can also be observed.

Special attention should be paid if concomitant symptoms are observed, such as numbness, tingling, paresthesia (abnormal sensation), muscle weakness, decreased tendon reflexes and pain, mainly at night.

Abnormalities uncovered on history taking or physical examination may require medical evaluation, laboratory tests, and imaging investigations, such as x-rays, US, CT, and MRI.

Diagnosis in Chinese Medicine

In Chinese Medicine, musculoskeletal pain results from the obstruction of Qì and Blood circulation or inadequate Qì and Blood for the nourishment of the secondary channels, especially the Muscle and Connecting channels.

The Muscle and Connecting channels more often involved in elbow disorders are listed below:

- Large Intestine
- Small Intestine
- Heart
- Triple Energizer
- Lung

The channels affected vary according to pain location:

- Large Intestine: pain is on the lateral epicondyle, the pathology is epicondylitis (tennis elbow)

Red Flags	Pain	Inspection	Other Signs	Neurological Signs	Recommendations
Inflammation	Pain	Redness, swelling, and heat		Functional deficit	Physician evaluation Imaging investigations
Fracture	Spontaneous pain	Deformity and swelling	Movement beyond normal range of motion	Functional deficit	Physician evaluation Imaging investigations
Dislocation	Pain with movement	Deformity and joint swelling	Hematoma	Functional deficit	Physician evaluation Imaging investigations
Rheumatoid arthritis	Pain with or without movement	Redness and swelling	Fatigue and general discomfort	Functional deficit	Physician evaluation Imaging investigations Laboratory tests
Herniated disc or cervical radiculopathy	Cervical pain radiating to the elbow			Paraesthesia, hypoesthesia, tingling and lack of deep tendon reflexes	Physician evaluation Imaging investigations

- Small Intestine: pain is on the medial epicondyle, the pathology is medial epicondylitis (golfer's elbow)
- Heart: pain is on the medial volar aspect of the proximal forearm (golfer's elbow)
- Triple Energizer: pain is in the olecranon, the pathology is olecranon bursitis
- Lung: pain is in the anterior crease, the pathology is joint pain or biceps insertional tendinitis

What matters most is to identify the affected channel where pain is located.

Sometimes, it is not so easy to determine it and consequently, the following data concerning the Muscle channels involved in elbow movements should be acquired for a better identification.

- Extension: LI, TE, and SI
- Flexion: PC, LU, and HT
- Supination: LI
- Pronation: LU

The information so acquired on the channel which is likely to be involved, that is, pain location and related movement restriction, can also be integrated with the results from Western medicine orthopedic tests in order to identify which muscle, tendon, and joint is affected in case of

- Lateral epicondylitis
- Medial epicondylitis
- Olecranon bursitis
- Joint pain or biceps insertional tendinitis

ETIOLOGY

Elbow pain is usually caused by:

- *Overuse, repetitive strain injury*. Through work (jackhammer) or sports (tennis or golfer's elbow); performing the same movement over and over again causes local Qì stagnation or Qì and Blood deficiency.
- *Trauma, sport injuries*. If mild, they cause local Qì stagnation; if severe, they cause local Blood stasis.
- *Cold*. Local invasion causes Qì stagnation or Blood stasis.

Previous accidents often predispose the elbow to more frequent invasions of external pathogenic factors, especially Cold.

PATHOLOGY

The Muscle and Connecting channels are often affected by Qì stagnation and Blood stasis:

- Qì stagnation manifests itself with widespread pain radiating proximally or distally along the pathway of the Muscle channels and could be associated with muscle contracture and stiffness of the forearm, also perceived upon palpation.
- Blood stasis, usually occurring in the Connecting channels, manifests itself with more intense pain localized in the joint or, more frequently, at the site of muscle insertion with consequent limited range of motion or joint stiffness.

As already mentioned in the Fundamentals of acupuncture for MSK pain in the limbs (see Chapter 1), the term Connecting channels includes not only the Connecting channel "proper" but also the Connecting channel "area" that covers the whole pathway of the Main channel.

LATERAL EPICONDYLITIS (TENNIS ELBOW)

To identify the Muscle and Connecting channels affected, we check location and characteristics of musculoskeletal pain, palpate the affected area, test the range of motion for each elbow movement and perform orthopaedic tests to elicit pain.

The Pathways of the Large Intestine Secondary Channels

In case of lateral epicondylitis the Large Intestine Muscle and Connecting channels are involved (Fig. 3.14).

The pathway of the Large Intestine Muscle and Connecting channels explains pain on the lateral side of the elbow, which could radiate distally to the radial forearm.

MEDIAL EPICONDYLITIS (GOLFER'S ELBOW)

To identify the Muscle and Connecting channels affected, we check location and characteristics of musculoskeletal pain, palpate the affected area, test the range of motion for each elbow movement and perform orthopaedic tests to elicit pain.

The Pathways of the Small Intestine Secondary Channels

In case of medial epicondylitis, the Small Intestine Muscle and Connecting channels are involved (Fig. 3.15).

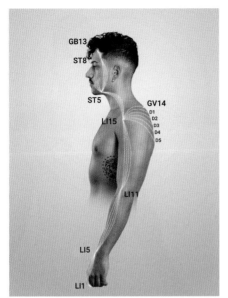 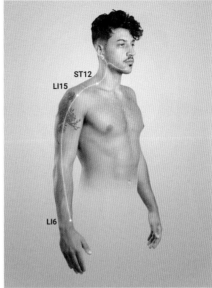

Fig. 3.14 The pathways of the Large Intestine Muscle and Connecting "proper" channels.

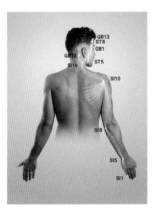 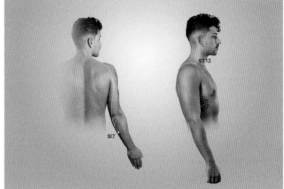

Fig. 3.15 The pathways of the Small Intestine Muscle and Connecting "proper" channels.

The pathway of the Small Intestine Muscle and Connecting channels explains pain on the posteromedial aspect of the elbow, which could radiate distally to the ulnar forearm.

The Pathways of the Heart Secondary Channels

In case of medial epicondylitis the Heart Muscle and Connecting channels may be involved (Fig. 3.16).

The pathway of the Heart Muscle and Connecting channels explains pain on the anteromedial aspect of the elbow, which could radiate distally to the anteromedial aspect of the proximal forearm.

Diagnosis in Osteopathic Medicine

The examination for "somatic dysfunction" is the central concept of the diagnostic process: palpation of

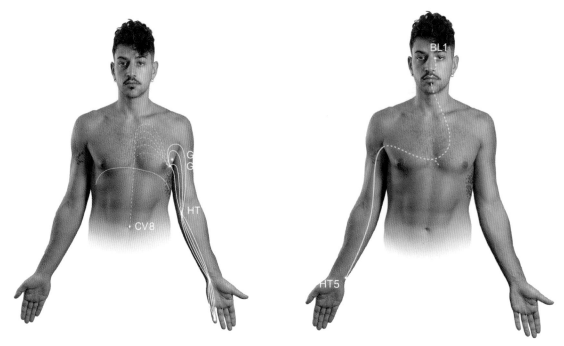

Fig. 3.16 The pathways of the Heart Muscle and Connecting "proper" channels.

the affected area and functionally/anatomically related components of the somatic system is the only way to assess it.

Consequently, the osteopathic diagnostic approach to musculoskeletal elbow pain is based on the identification of joint somatic dysfunctions not only of the elbow, but also of the shoulder and wrist.

Regardless of the condition to be treated, be it lateral or medial epicondylitis, arthritis of the elbow or surgical outcomes, all of the recommended tests should be performed to identify the dysfunctions that occur more frequently.

It is therefore evident that the osteopathic diagnosis is developed regardless of the condition to be treated and consequently, the osteopathic tests recommended for the shoulder, elbow, and wrist will not be repeated when the "injuries" are treated.

TESTS FOR THE MAIN SOMATIC DYSFUNCTIONS

The only way to diagnose somatic dysfunctions of a joint is to assess the passive movements of its articular ends in relation to one another and compare them

with the same movements of the joint on the healthy side. Testing of all elbow joints is required.

On the same plane of motion, there is passive mobility quantitatively and qualitatively equal on both sides of a theoretical neutral point that represents the reference point.

When the balance is lost and range and quality of motion are not the same in both directions, then there is somatic dysfunction.

Tests of the Humeroulnar Joint

Tests are performed to assess the most common ulnar dysfunctions:

1. Adduction of the ulna
2. Abduction of the ulna
3. Internal rotation of the ulna
4. External rotation of the ulna

Adduction Test of the Ulna

The patient is supine close to the bed edge with incomplete elbow extension. The practitioner stands close

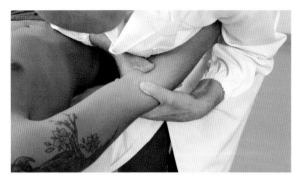 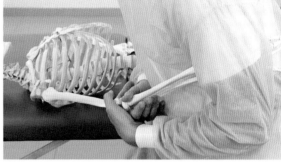

Fig. 3.17 Adduction test of the ulna.

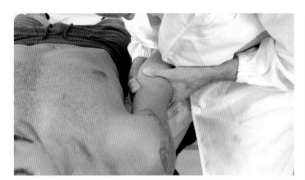 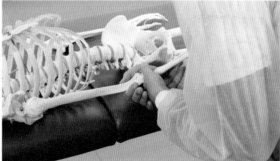

Fig. 3.18 Abduction test of the ulna.

to the patient's right side. The practitioner stabilizes the patient's wrist under the left axilla and the elbow by placing the left hand on the lateral aspect of the elbow.

The adduction test is then performed by pushing the elbow laterally with the margin of the first intermetacarpal space of the right hand placed on the medial joint line. The practitioner appreciates adduction range and quality of motion and then compares them with abduction. If the elbow slides more easily in adduction, then there is ulnar adduction dysfunction (Fig. 3.17; Video 3.3).

Abduction Test of the Ulna
The patient is supine close to the bed edge with incomplete elbow extension. The practitioner stands close to the patient's right side. The practitioner stabilizes the patient's wrist under the right axilla and the elbow by placing the right hand on the medial aspect of the elbow.

The abduction test is then performed by pushing the elbow medially with the margin of the first

intermetacarpal space of the left hand placed on the lateral joint line.

The practitioner appreciates abduction range and quality of motion and then compares them with adduction. If the elbow slides more easily in abduction, then there is ulnar abduction dysfunction (Fig. 3.18; Video 3.4).

Internal Rotation Test of the Ulna
The patient sits with elbow flexed at 90 degrees and forearm in neutral position. The practitioner stands opposite the patient. The practitioner holds the patient's elbow with the left hand and the wrist with the right hand: the internal rotation test is performed by rotating the forearm from supination to pronation with the right hand.

The practitioner appreciates range and quality of motion for internal rotation and compares them with external rotation. If the ulna slides more easily in internal rotation, then there is internal rotation dysfunction (Figs. 3.19 and 3.20; Video 3.5).

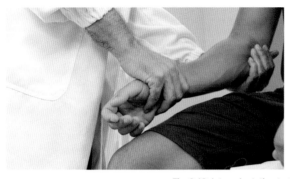 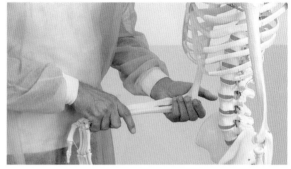

Fig. 3.19 Internal rotation test of the ulna: starting position.

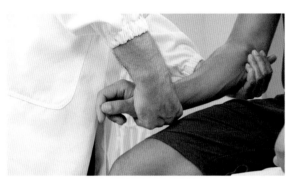 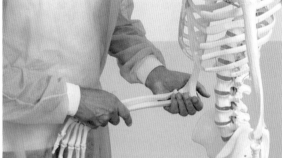

Fig. 3.20 Internal rotation test of the ulna: final position.

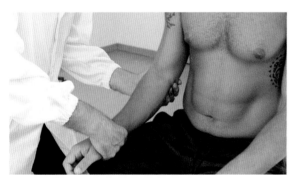 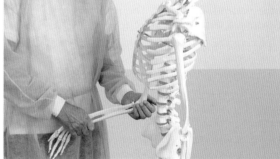

Fig. 3.21 External rotation test of the ulna: starting position.

External Rotation Test of the Ulna

The patient sits with elbow flexed at 90 degrees and forearm in neutral position. The practitioner stands opposite the patient. The practitioner holds the patient's elbow with the left hand and the wrist with the right hand. The external rotation test is performed by rotating the forearm from pronation to supination with the right hand. The practitioner appreciates range and quality of motion for external rotation and compares them with internal rotation. If the ulna slides more easily in external rotation, then there is external rotation dysfunction (Figs. 3.21 and 3.22; Video 3.6).

Test of the Proximal Radioulnar Joint

A test is performed to assess the most common radial dysfunctions:

- Anterior radial head
- Posterior radial head

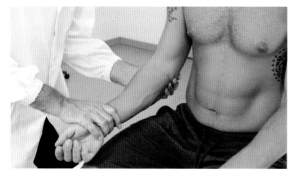
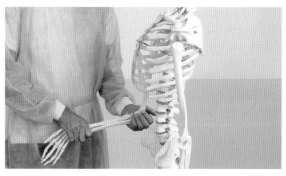

Fig. 3.22 External rotation test of the ulna: final position.

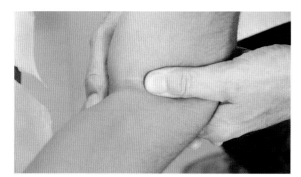
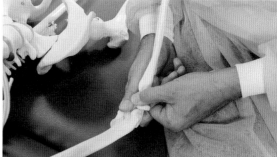

Fig. 3.23 Anteroposterior test of the radial head.

Anteroposterior Test of the Radial Head

The patient is supine close to the bed edge with incomplete elbow extension.

The practitioner stands close to the patient's right side with the patient's wrist under the right axilla and the right hand holding the ulna, while the left thumb and index finger are in front of and behind the radial head, respectively:

- The anterior test is performed by pushing the radial head forward with the index finger to assess anterior sliding.
- The posterior test is performed by pushing the radial head backward with the thumb to assess posterior sliding.

The practitioner appreciates range and quality of motion of anterior sliding and posterior sliding to compare them with posterior and anterior sliding, respectively.

If the radius slides more easily anteriorly, then there is anterior dysfunction, and vice versa (Fig. 3.23; Video 3.7).

Treatment With the AcuOsteo Method: The Choice of an Integrated Approach

The therapeutic approach of the AcuOsteo Method aims to treat those musculoskeletal injuries which do not require consultation with a surgeon or a physician.

Once this fundamental aspect has been defined, treatment envisages the use of acupuncture and osteopathy according to their diagnostic and therapeutic approaches.

We would like to stress that at this point in diagnostic assessment, we do not have to follow the rules of Western medicine, except for some specific cases, such as arthritis of the elbow, posttraumatic and postsurgical pain, and stiffness, which will be covered later.

In addition, we should not be misled by diagnostic imaging investigations and should rely only on the rules of Chinese and osteopathic medicine, which means selecting points according to symptoms and channel pathways and treating all of the somatic dysfunctions encountered.

For didactic purposes treatment with acupuncture will precede osteopathic treatment, whereas in clinical practice the order is reversed since it may be difficult to perform osteopathic manipulations once the needles have been inserted.

An exception to this methodology is represented by those morbidities where marked stiffness prevents joint mobilization as required by osteopathic manipulations. Specifically, we are referring to the outcomes after immobilization following surgery, fractures, and elbow dislocation.

In these cases, we suggest first using acupuncture, especially the bleeding techniques, and then, at the end of the session and after removing the needles, osteopathy.

In any case, it is always the practitioner's clinical experience that will guide them along the most appropriate pathway to treat each patient's condition.

Osteopathic manipulation in the treatment of "somatic dysfunction" is the central concept of the therapeutic process to treat the affected joints and functionally/anatomically related components of the somatic system.

Consequently, the osteopathic manipulative approach to musculoskeletal elbow pain focuses on the treatment of joint somatic dysfunctions not only of the elbow, but also of the shoulder and wrist.

Regardless of the condition to be treated, be it lateral or medial epicondylitis, arthritis of the elbow or postsurgical outcomes, all of the dysfunctions diagnosed should be treated.

It is therefore evident that the osteopathic therapeutic approach does not vary with the condition to be treated and thus the osteopathic manipulations described for the elbow, as well as those for the shoulder and wrist, will not be repeated under the paragraphs dedicated to the "injuries."

ACUPUNCTURE TREATMENT

Lateral Epicondylitis

The Five Options and Selection of Acupoints

The approach we suggest is widely described in the section dedicated to the Fundamentals of acupuncture for MSK pain in the limbs (see Chapter 1).

The most important aspect is the identification of the Ah Shi point(s) to determine which channels are affected. In this specific case, the Large Intestine Muscle and Connecting channels are involved.

Pricking pain localized on the lateral epicondyle is a sign of Blood Stasis to be treated with the bleeding technique, whereas widespread pain radiating along the forearm is a sign of Qì stagnation to be treated with the needling technique.

It is worth reminding that the distal points should be needled one at a time and their effectiveness in terms of pain and range of motion tested after each insertion. The same applies to the local points.

Finally, since both options 1 and 2 consist of several steps, it is important to highlight how selection should be made. Specifically, the practitioner might wonder if all or some of the steps should be followed. The rule we follow is simple: when the result achieved is satisfactory, the remaining steps should be skipped, and the practitioner should move to the following option. Similarly, the use of the points recommended under options 3, 4, and 5 should be carefully evaluated according to the case being treated.

The points and accessory techniques we recommend using are listed below.

Order of Needling

Option One: Distal Points
First Step: Large Intestine Muscle Channel
LI1. This Jing-Well point is used to activate the Large Intestine Muscle channel and remove Qì stagnation and Blood stasis with needling and bleeding techniques, respectively.

Second Step: Large Intestine Connecting Channels
LI6 (Opposite Side). This Luo point activates the Large Intestine Connecting channels and removes Qì stagnation and Blood stasis in acute and chronic conditions from Excess.

Our technique consists of needling from oblique to transverse in proximal direction along the pathway of the Large Intestine Main channel (Figs. 3.24 and 3.25; Video 3.8).

LU7 (Opposite Side). This Luo point activates the Lung Connecting channels and is also used in chronic Deficiency conditions with dull pain to tonify Qì and Blood in the internally-externally related Large Intestine channels. In the latter case, we associate the Yuan point LI4 with the Luo point LU7, that is to say the well-known Luo-Yuan point combination. First, as main point, we needle the Yuan point on the affected side and

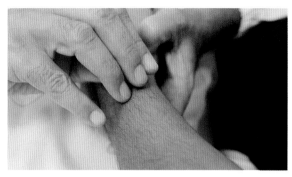

Fig. 3.24 Needling of the LI6: starting position.

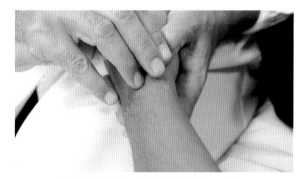

Fig. 3.26 Needling of the LU7: starting position.

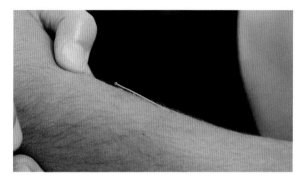

Fig. 3.25 Needling of the LI6: final position.

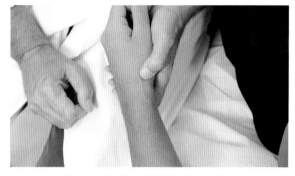

Fig. 3.27 Needling of the LU7: final position.

then, as secondary point, the Luo point on the internally-externally related channel on the opposite side.

Our technique consists of needling LU7 from oblique to transverse in proximal direction along the pathway of the Lung Main Channel (Figs. 3.26 and 3.27; Video 3.9).

Third step: Empirical Points

There is no point which is classically recommended. Richard Tan suggests the "anterior" GB33 which is located anterior to the ilio-tibial band on the same level as GB33. The point is needled on the opposite side.

Fourth Step: Opposite Extremity (Upper/ Lower)

ST35 (Opposite Side). It is located in the knee joint which corresponds to the elbow joint on the paired channel according to the Six Stages.

It is worth remembering that the lateral styloid is not exactly in the elbow joint; it is in fact slightly proximally located and this means we could palpate the leg in an upward direction along the Stomach Main channel to find another or more tender point(s).

In clinical practice, the anatomical mirror concept can lead us to select a point, which may be tender or not, on the area corresponding to the lateral femoral condyle which corresponds exactly to the lateral epicondyle, although it is not located on the Stomach Main channel.

In line with our principle of treatment, we first needle ST35 or a more proximal point and then test its effectiveness soon after insertion: if the result is not satisfactory, we remove the needle and move to another option.

ST36 (Opposite Side). It is used more often because it mobilizes more energy than the previous point, although it is located distal to the knee joint.

It would be more correct to use the first point when pain is on the lateral epicondyle and the second point when it radiates to the forearm. However, nothing prevents us from using both of them at the same time. Alternatively, the most tender on palpation is selected.

Our technique consists of needling the opposite extremity (lower/upper) on the opposite side in acute and chronic conditions.

Alternatively, the most tender point on palpation is selected on the same or opposite side.

Fifth Step: Categories of Traditional Points

LI3 (Affected Side) and ST43 (Opposite Side). A good combination includes the Shu-Stream points on the paired channel according to the Six Stages.

First, we needle the Shu-Stream point on the channel involved on the affected side and then the Shu-Stream point on the coupled channel on the opposite side and opposite extremity (upper/lower).

We use this technique in acute and chronic Excess conditions to treat pain and expel or prevent the invasion of external pathogenic factors.

LI5. The Jing-River points are used in acute or chronic Excess conditions due to the invasion of an external pathogenic factor and they are needled to promote its expulsion from their respective channels. They are also useful to prevent pain exacerbation from seasonal changes or invasion of external pathogenic factors.

LI7. The Xi-Cleft points are specifically used in acute conditions to treat Blood stasis in their respective channels. However, they are more effective in the Yin rather than in the Yang channels: that is why we would rather avoid using LI7 to treat this condition.

LI4. We recommend using this Yuan-Source point in chronic Deficiency conditions with dull pain, in case of weakness, or in the resolution phases of lateral epicondylitis, to tonify Qì and Blood in the Large Intestine channels.

In this situation, we can also associate the Yuan point LI4 with the Luo point LU7, that is to say the well-known Luo-Yuan point combination. First, as main point, we needle the Yuan point on the affected side and then, as secondary point the Luo point on the internally-externally related channel on the opposite side.

Sixth Step: Extraordinary Vessels

SI3 (Affected Side) and BL62 (Opposite Side). SI3 is the opening point of the Governing Vessel (Du Mai), while BL62 is the coupled point and opening point of the Yang Qiao Mai. The Governing Vessel is treated when cervical pain with concomitant irritation of the corresponding cervical roots is suspected. In this case, we associate BL60 and BL10 with either the cervical Jiaji C4-C5-C6-C7 on the affected side or the most tender cervical Jiaji on palpation.

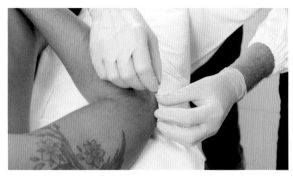

Fig. 3.28 Bleeding of the Ah Shi point(s): starting position.

First, as main point, the opening point of the Governing Vessel is needled on the same side and then, as secondary point, the coupled point on the opposite side. Cervical pain being rarely observed, treatment of the Governing Vessel is not often required and only the cervical Jiaji are to be needled if tender on palpation.

Option Two: Local Points

First Step: Painful Point(s) (Ah Shi)

Ah Shi Point(s). Palpation of the radial epicondyle reveals either the most painful point(s) (Ah Shi) corresponding to Blood stasis and therefore to be bled or an area of widespread pain corresponding to Qì stagnation and requiring needling. Pain could radiate distally to the lateral forearm.

When the bleeding technique is chosen and if the anatomical structure of the elbow allows us to, the cupping therapy should be used to bleed the most painful point(s) (Ah Shi) along with another 4 points around it, paying attention not to damage the tendinous tissue with the lancet or the soft tissues with a too strong cupping (Figs. 3.28 and 3.29; Video 3.10).

When needles are inserted, the first point to select is the most painful one (Ah Shi). The 0.25 × 25 mm needle is inserted perpendicularly to the required depth to reach the osteotendinous junction. Then, four needles are inserted from oblique to transverse, so as to create a circle at about 1 cun from the first needle, and their tips are directed towards the perpendicular needle (Figs. 3.30 and 3.31; Video 3.11).

One or two needles can also be inserted at 1 cun distal to the lateral epicondyle in the tendinous

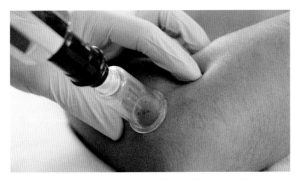

Fig. 3.29 Bleeding of the Ah Shi point(s): final position.

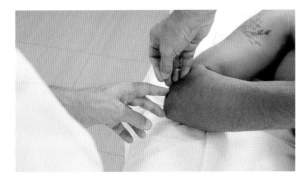

Fig. 3.30 Needling of the Ah Shi point(s): starting position.

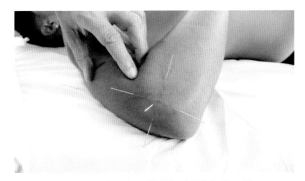

Fig. 3.31 Needling of the Ah Shi point(s): final position.

zone of the extensor muscles. The 0.30 × 40 mm needles are inserted obliquely to a depth of about 1 cun, trying to approach the tendon tissue as much as possible. Electroacupuncture stimulation can be taken into consideration and used between these two points.

Both in acute and chronic conditions a moxa stick can be useful to promote the flow of Qì and Blood. We can also use it to treat invasion of external pathogenic factors, Cold in particular. However, attention should be paid since too much heat can increase the ongoing inflammatory.

LI11. It can be considered a local point to treat lateral epicondylitis, although in reality it is only adjacent to the lateral epicondyle. The needle is inserted perpendicularly or from oblique to transverse directed towards the lateral epicondyle. We also use it because it is an insertion point of the Large Intestine Muscle channel in the elbow, as we will see later.

To ensure accuracy and precision of local needle placement and manipulation, we prefer the supine position.

Second Step: Anatomically Mirrored Point(s) (Opposite Side)

The point(s) to be needled is located on the opposite side and should correspond as precisely as possible to the anatomical mirror of the Ah Shi point(s) to be treated. The point(s) may or may not be tender on palpation.

To ensure accuracy and precision of needle placement and manipulation, we prefer supine position.

Option Three: Adjacent Points

First Step: Adjacent Points

They can be considered local and not adjacent points if pain is radiating or stiffness affects the extensor muscles of the forearm.

The needles are inserted perpendicularly into both points or only in the most painful one until they reach the muscle sheath. Alternatively, needles can be inserted deeply and perpendicularly until they reach the intermediate layers of the muscle. Electroacupuncture stimulation can be taken into consideration and used between these two points.

Instead, if taut bands are found within the muscle belly, the 0.30 × 40 mm needles are inserted from oblique to transverse along the taut bands and then a twisting-rotating manipulation is performed.

LI12. It is needled directing the tip towards the lateral epicondyle.

TE10 and LU5. They help promote the horizontal flow of local Qì.

"Outer" SI8. It is located in the crease between the lateral epicondyle and the olecranon process of the ulna. It helps promote the horizontal flow of local Qì. This point is suggested by W. Reaves.[1]

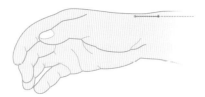

Fig. 3.32 Upper 4.

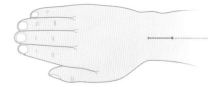

Fig. 3.33 Upper 5.

LI11. It is a very important point since it is the insertion point of the Large Intestine Muscle channel in the elbow and as such it promotes the longitudinal flow of local Qì.

Option Four: Etiological Points

First Step: According to Pattern

LI4 and LR3 (Bilaterally). They promote the flow of Qì and help remove Blood stasis. Since LR3 is the Shu/Yuan point of the Liver, it also helps nourish muscles and tendons.

ST36 (Bilaterally). It is used to tonify Qì and Blood in chronic Deficiency conditions or the phases of pain resolution that can turn into muscle weakness.

Second Step: General Points

GB34 (Bilaterally). It is the Hui-Gathering point of Sinews and is specifically used for lateral epicondylitis, which is often insertional tendinopathy or tendinitis. In addition, it promotes the flow of Qì thus contributing to remove Blood stasis.

BL17 (Bilaterally). It is the Hui-Gathering point of Blood to remove Blood stasis.

BL18 (Bilaterally). It treats all Excess and Deficiency conditions of the Liver that may favor the onset or duration of musculotendinous symptoms. It harmonizes the flow of Qì and Blood and enhances treatment of tendons and muscle.

Option Five: Microsystems

First Step: Wrist and Ankle Acupuncture

Upper 4. It roughly corresponds to the pathway of the Large Intestine channels (Fig. 3.32).

Upper 5. It controls upper limb mobility (Fig. 3.33).

Second Step: Ear Acupuncture (Opposite Side) (Fig. 3.34).

Local point: Elbow
Zang Fu point: Liver
General points: Subcortex and Shenmen

Acute or Chronic Pain From Excess

Intense Pain or Range of Motion Reduced by Pain. Principle of treatment: to remove Qì stagnation and Blood stasis and expel external or internal pathogenic factors, if any (Box 3.1).

Chronic Pain From Deficiency

Dull Pain or Muscle Weakness. Principle of treatment: to tonify Qì and Blood, strengthen tissues and avoid pain exacerbation from physical activities or invasion of external pathogenic factors (Box 3.2).

Therapeutic Program, Frequency of Sessions

The frequency of sessions depends on the clinical condition of the patient. If the condition is acute or chronic with intense pain, we recommend sessions twice a week for 2 weeks and then once a week for another 2 weeks. If improvement is observed, sessions are then scheduled once a week until complete pain relief or at least reduction by 80% to 90%. If not, the whole clinical picture should be reconsidered and the patient referred to another specialist.

If the condition is chronic with dull pain, we recommend sessions once a week for 4 weeks. Afterwards, and if the patient continues to improve, sessions are then scheduled once a week until complete pain relief or at least reduction by 80% to 90%.

Medial Epicondylitis

The Five Options and Selection of Acupoints

The approach we suggest is widely described in the section dedicated to the Fundamentals of acupuncture for MSK pain in the limbs (see Chapter 1).

The most important aspect is the identification of the Ah Shi point(s) to determine which channels are affected. In this specific case, the Small Intestine Muscle and Connecting channels are involved.

When treating medial epicondylitis, the challenge the practitioner faces is the presence of pain in two different regions: a Yang area—the Ah Shi point on

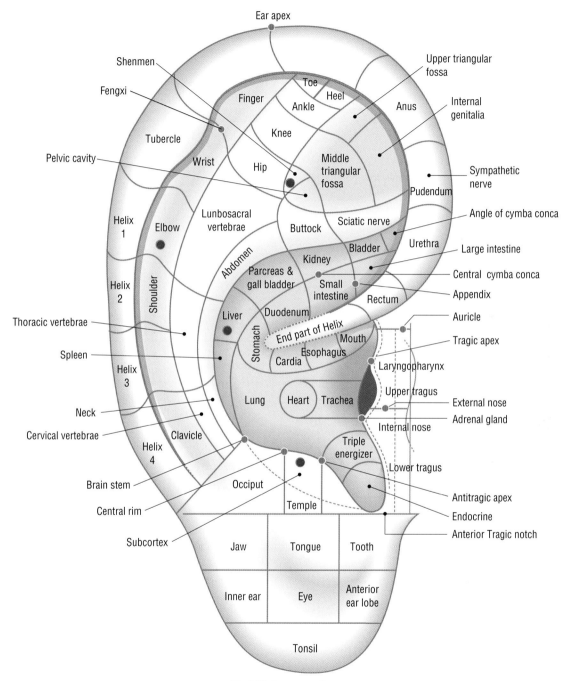

Fig. 3.34 Ear acupuncture.

BOX 3.1 ACUTE OR CHRONIC PAIN FROM EXCESS ACUPUNCTURE TREATMENT

Option 1 Distal points	• Jing-Well point LI1 • Luo point LI6 (opposite side) • Empirical point "anterior" GB33 (opposite side) • Point according to the Six Stages ST36 (opposite side) • Jing-River point LI5
Option 2 Local points	• Ah Shi • LI11 • Anatomically mirrored point(s) (opposite side)
Option 3 Adjacent points	• LI12 • LI10 • LI9 • TE10 • LU5 • Insertion point LI11 • "Outer" SI8
Option 4 Etiological and general points	• LI4 and LR3 (bilaterally) • GB34 (bilaterally) • BL17 (bilaterally) • BL18 (bilaterally) • Jiaji points C4-C5-C6-C7

Option 5 Microsystems	• W-A acupuncture
	  • Upper 4
	  • Upper 5
	• Ear acupuncture (opposite side)
	  • Elbow
	  • Liver
	  • Subcortex and Shenmen

BOX 3.2 CHRONIC PAIN FROM DEFICIENCY ACUPUNCTURE TREATMENT

Option 1 Distal points	• Yuan point LI4 • Luo point LU7 (opposite side) • Point according to the Six Stages ST36 (opposite side) • Jing-River point LI5
Option 2 Local points	• Ah Shi • LI11
Option 3 Adjacent points	• LI12 • LI10 • LI9 • TE10 • LU5 • Insertion point LI11 • "Outer" SI8
Option 4 Etiological and general points	• ST36 (bilaterally) • GB34 (bilaterally) • LR3 (bilaterally) • BL18 (bilaterally)

Option 5 Microsystems	• W-A acupuncture
	  • Upper 4
	  • Upper 5
	• Ear acupuncture (opposite side)
	  • Elbow
	  • Liver
	  • Subcortex and Shenmen

the posteromedial epicondyle—and a Yin area—pain radiating along the anteromedial forearm.

Though the latter is less frequently observed in medial epicondylitis, when pain affects these two regions, this peculiar condition requires treatment of both the Small Intestine (Yang) and the Heart (Yin) secondary channels.

Pricking pain localized on the medial epicondyle on the Small Intestine channels is a sign of Blood Stasis to be treated with the bleeding technique, whereas

pain radiating along the anteromedial forearm on the Heart channels is a sign of Qì to be treated with the needling technique.

It is worth reminding that the distal points should be needled one at a time and their effectiveness in terms of pain and range of motion tested after each insertion. The same applies to the local points.

Finally, since both options 1 and 2 consist of several steps, it is important to highlight how selection should be made. Specifically, the practitioner might wonder if

Clinical Notes

- Improvement following treatment may turn intense pain to dull pain and then to a feeling of weakness. Should this be the case, the principle of treatment has to be changed as follows; it is no longer necessary to remove Qì stagnation and Blood stasis and expel external pathogenic factors, if any; instead, Qì and Blood should be tonified to strengthen tissues and avoid pain exacerbation from physical activities or invasion of external pathogenic factors.
- When the anatomically mirrored point is used as local point, precise identification of its correspondence to the Ah Shi point(s) to be treated is mandatory.
- Treatment of lateral epicondylitis may not achieve the expected results.
- An explanation for the poorer outcome could be the fact that the lateral epicondyle is not located precisely on the pathway of the Large Intestine Main, Muscle, and Connecting channels. Since it is located more laterally, the epicondyle is directly covered only by the Connecting "area."

all or some of the steps should be followed. The rule we follow is simple: when the result achieved is satisfactory, the remaining steps should be skipped, and the practitioner should move to the following option. Similarly, the use of the points recommended under options 3, 4, and 5 should be carefully evaluated according to the case being treated

The points and accessory techniques we recommend using are listed below.

Order of Needling

Option One: Distal Points

First Step: Small Intestine and Heart Muscle Channels

SI1 and HT9. These Jing-Well points are used to activate the Small Intestine and Heart Muscle channels and they remove Qì stagnation and Blood stasis with needling and bleeding techniques, respectively.

Second Step: Small Intestine and Heart Connecting Channels

SI7 and HT5 (Opposite Side). These Luo points activate the Small Intestine and Heart Connecting

channels and they remove Qì stagnation and Blood stasis in acute or chronic conditions from Excess.

The same Luo points are also used in chronic Deficiency conditions with dull pain to tonify Qì and Blood in their respective internally-externally related channels. In this case, we associate the Yuan point HT7 with the Luo point SI7 and the Yuan point SI4 with the Luo point HT5, that is to say the well-known Luo-Yuan point combination. First, as main point, we needle the Yuan point on the affected side and then, as secondary point, the Luo point on the internally-externally related channel on the opposite side.

Third Step: Empirical Points

There is no point that is classically recommended.

Fourth Step: Opposite Extremity (Upper/ Lower)

BL40 and KI10 (Opposite Side). They are located in the knee joint which corresponds to the elbow joint on the paired channel according to the Six Stages.

BL40 should be used when pain is on the medial epicondyle on the Small Intestine Main channel, whereas KI10 when pain radiates along the anteromedial forearm on the Heart Main channel.

It is worth remembering that the medial epicondyle is not exactly in the elbow joint; it is in fact slightly proximally located and this means we should palpate the leg in an upward direction, starting from the knee joint line, along the Bladder or Kidney Main channel to find another or more tender points.

In clinical practice, the anatomical mirror concept can lead us to select a point, which may be tender or not, on the area corresponding to the medial femoral condyle which corresponds exactly to the medial epicondyle, although it is not located on the Bladder or Kidney Main channels.

In line with our principle of treatment, we first needle BL40 and KI10 or some other more proximal point(s) and then test their effectiveness soon after insertion: if the result is not satisfactory, we remove the needles and move to the subsequent option.

Our technique consists of needling the opposite extremity (lower/upper) on the opposite side if pain is intense in acute and chronic conditions.

Alternatively, the most tender point on palpation is selected on the same or opposite side.

Fifth Step: Categories of Traditional Points

SI3 (Affected Side) and BL65 (Opposite Side); HT7 (Affected Side) and KI3 (Opposite Side). A good combination includes the Shu-Stream points on the paired channel according to the Six Stages.

First, we needle the Shu-Stream point on the channel involved on the affected side and then the Shu-Stream point on the coupled channel on the opposite side and opposite extremity (upper/lower).

We use this technique in acute and chronic Excess conditions to treat pain and expel or prevent the invasion of external pathogenic factors.

It is worth reminding that in the Yin channels the Shu-Stream point corresponds to the Yuan-Source point. That is why HT7 could also be used in chronic Deficiency conditions, as we will see later.

SI5 and HT4. The Jing-River points are used in acute or chronic Excess conditions due to the invasion of an external pathogenic factor and they are needled to promote its expulsion from their respective channels. It is also useful to prevent pain exacerbation from seasonal changes or invasion of external pathogenic factors. However, they are more effective in the Yang rather than in the Yin channels: that is why we would rather avoid using HT4 to treat this condition.

SI6 and HT6. The Xi-Cleft points are specifically used in acute conditions to treat Blood stasis in their respective channels. However, they are more effective in the *Yin* rather than in the *Yang* channels: that is why we would rather avoid using SI6 to treat this condition; not even HT6 has proved to be effective in the treatment of musculoskeletal diseases.

SI4 and HT7. We recommend using these Yuan-Source point(s) in chronic Deficiency conditions with dull pain, in case of weakness, or in the resolution phases of medial epicondylitis, to tonify Qì and Blood in their respective channels.

In this situation, we can also associate the Yuan point SI4 with the Luo point HT5 and the Yuan point HT7 with the Luo point SI7, that is to say the well-known Luo-Yuan point combination. First, as main point, we needle the Yuan point on the affected side and then, as secondary point, the Luo point on the internally-externally related channel on the opposite side.

Sixth Step: Extraordinary Vessels

No extraordinary vessel is to be regarded as involved under these circumstances.

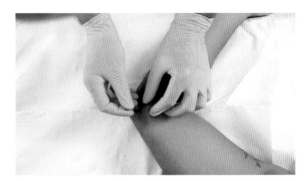

Fig. 3.35 Bleeding of the Ah Shi point(s): starting position.

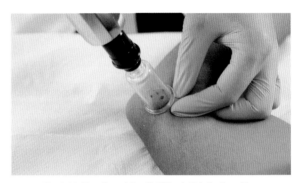

Fig. 3.36 Bleeding of the Ah Shi point(s): final position.

Option Two: Local Points

First Step: Painful Point(s) (Ah Shi)

Ah Shi Point(s). Palpation of the medial epicondyle reveals either the most painful point(s) (Ah Shi) corresponding to Blood stasis and therefore to be bled or an area of widespread pain corresponding to Qì stagnation and requiring needling. Pain could radiate distally to the to the anteromedial forearm.

When the bleeding technique is chosen and if the anatomical structure of the elbow allows us to, the cupping therapy should be used to bleed the most painful point (Ah Shi) along with another 4 points around it, paying attention not to damage the tendinous tissue with the lancet or the soft tissues with a too strong cupping (Figs. 3.35 and 3.36; Video 3.12).

When needles are inserted, the first point to select is the most painful one (Ah Shi). The needle is inserted perpendicularly to the required depth to reach the osteotendinous junction. Then, 4 needles are inserted

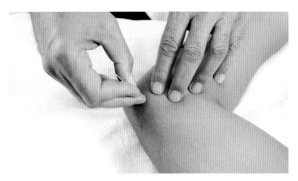

Fig. 3.37 Needling of the Ah Shi point(s): starting position.

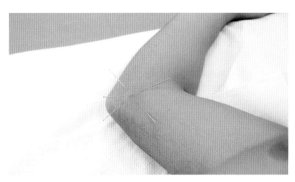

Fig. 3.38 Needling of the Ah Shi point(s): final position.

from oblique to transverse, so as to create a circle at about 1 cun from the first needle, and their tips are directed towards the perpendicular needle (Figs. 3.37 and 3.38; Video 3.13).

One or two needles can also be inserted at 1 cun distal to the medial epicondyle in the tendinous zone of the pronators and flexors.

The 0.30 × 40 mm needles are inserted obliquely to a depth of about 1 cun, trying to approach the tendon tissue as much as possible. Electroacupuncture stimulation can be taken into consideration and used between these two points.

Both in acute and chronic conditions a moxa stick can be useful to promote the flow of Qì and Blood. However, attention should be paid since too much heat can increase the ongoing inflammatory.

SI8. It can be considered a local point to treat medial epicondylitis, although in reality it is only adjacent to the medial epicondyle. We also use it because it is an

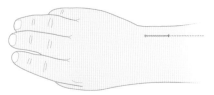

Fig. 3.39 Upper 6.

insertion point of the Small Intestine Muscle channel, as we will see later. S.I.-8 should be needled obliquely and distally to avoid hitting the underlying ulnar nerve.

To ensure accuracy and precision of local needle placement and manipulation, we prefer the supine position.

Second Step: Anatomically Mirrored Point(s) (Opposite Side)

The point(s) to be needled is located on the opposite side and should correspond as precisely as possible to the anatomical mirror of the Ah Shi point(s) to be treated. The point(s) may or may not be tender on palpation.

To ensure accuracy and precision of needle placement and manipulation, we prefer the supine position.

Option Three: Adjacent Points

First Step: Adjacent Points

SI8 and HT3. They are very important points since they are the insertion points of their respective Muscle channels in the elbow and as such, they promote the longitudinal flow of local Qì.

SI8 and HT3 can also be considered simple adjacent points and as such they help promote the horizontal flow of local Qì.

Option Four: Etiological Points

First Step: According to Patterns

LI4 and LR3 (Bilaterally). They promote the flow of Qì and help remove Blood stasis. Since LR3 is the Shu/Yuan point of the Liver, it also helps nourish muscles and tendons.

ST36 (Bilaterally). It is used to tonify Qì and Blood in chronic Deficiency conditions or the phases of pain resolution that can turn into muscle weakness.

Second Step: General Points

GB34 (Bilaterally). It is the Hui-Gathering point of Sinews and is specifically used for lateral epicondylitis, which is often insertional tendinopathy or tendinitis.

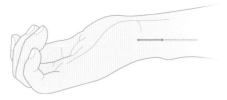

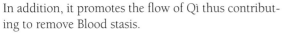

Fig. 3.40 Upper 1.

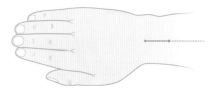

Fig. 3.41 Upper 5.

In addition, it promotes the flow of Qì thus contributing to remove Blood stasis.

BL17 (Bilaterally). It is the Hui-Gathering point of Blood and is used to remove Blood stasis.

BL18 (Bilaterally). It treats all Excess and Deficiency conditions of the Liver that may favor the onset or duration of musculotendinous symptoms. It harmonizes the flow of Qì and Blood and enhances treatment of tendons and muscle.

Option Five: Microsystems

First Step: Wrist and Ankle Acupuncture

Upper 6. It roughly corresponds to the pathway of the Small Intestine channels (Fig. 3.39).

Upper 1. It roughly corresponds to the pathway of the Heart channels (Fig. 3.40).

Upper 5. It controls upper limb mobility (Fig. 3.41).

Second step: Ear Acupuncture (Opposite Side)

(Fig. 3.42)

Local Point: Elbow

Zang Fu Point: Liver

General Points: Subcortex and Shenmen

Acute or Chronic Pain From Excess

I*ntense Pain or Range of Motion Reduced by Pain.* Principle of treatment: to remove Qì stagnation and Blood stasis and expel external or internal pathogenic factors, if any (Box 3.3).

Chronic Pain From Deficiency

Dull Pain or Muscle Weakness. Principle of treatment: to tonify Qì and Blood, strengthen tissues and avoid pain exacerbation from physical activities or invasion of external pathogenic factors (Box 3.4).

Therapeutic Program, Frequency of Sessions

The frequency of sessions depends on the clinical condition of the patient. If the condition is acute or

Clinical Notes

- When the anatomically mirrored point is used as local point, precise identification of its correspondence to the Ah Shi point(s) to be treated is mandatory.
- Treatment of medial epicondylitis may not achieve the expected results, even more than lateral epicondylitis.
- An explanation for the poorer outcome could be the fact that the medial epicondyle is not located precisely on the pathway of the Small Intestine Main, Muscle, and Connecting channels. Since it is located more medially, the epicondyle is directly covered only by the Connecting area. The Heart Main, Muscle, and Connecting channels correspond instead more precisely to the flexors and pronators of the forearm.

with intense pain, we recommend sessions twice a week for 2 weeks and then once a week for another 2 weeks. If improvement is observed, sessions are then scheduled once a week until complete pain relief or at least reduction by 80% to 90%. If not, the whole clinical picture should be reconsidered and the patient referred to another specialist.

If the condition is chronic or with dull pain, we recommend sessions once a week for 4 weeks. Afterwards, and if the patient continues to improve, sessions are then scheduled once a week until complete pain relief or at least reduction by 80% to 90%.

OSTEOPATHIC MANIPULATIVE TREATMENT

This paragraph will deal with osteopathic manipulations to treat elbow joint dysfunctions.

As already mentioned in the section dedicated to the Fundamentals of osteopathy for MSK pain in the limbs (see Chapter 1), the key point of the osteopathic

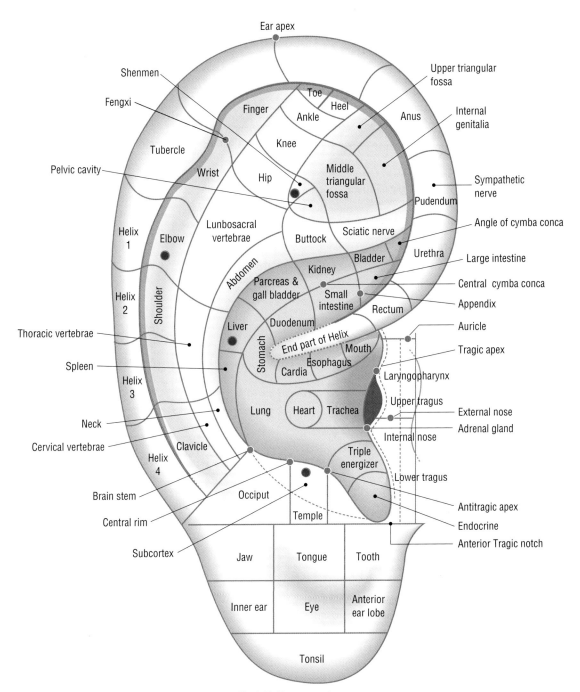

Fig. 3.42 Ear acupuncture.

BOX 3.3 ACUTE OR CHRONIC PAIN FROM EXCESS ACUPUNCTURE TREATMENT

Option 1 Distal points	• Jing-Well points SI1 and HT9 • Luo points SI7 and HT5 (opposite side) • Point according to the Six Stages BL40 and KI10 (opposite side) • Jing-River points SI5 and HT4
Option 2 Local points	• Ah Shi • SI8 • Anatomically mirrored point(s) (opposite side)
Option 3 Adjacent points	• Insertion points SI8 and HT3
Option 4 Etiological points	• LI4 and LR3 (bilaterally) • GB34 (bilaterally) • BL17 (bilaterally) • BL18 (bilaterally)

Option 5
Microsystems
	• W-A acupuncture
	  • Upper 6
	  • Upper 1
	  • Upper 5
	• Ear acupuncture (opposite side)
	  • Elbow
	  • Liver
	  • Subcortex and Shenmen

BOX 3.4 CHRONIC PAIN FROM DEFICIENCY ACUPUNCTURE TREATMENT

Option 1 Distal points	• Yuan point SI4 and HT7 • Luo points HT5 and SI7 (opposite side) • Point according to the Six Stages BL40 and KI10 (opposite side) • Jing-River point SI5 and HT4
Option 2 Local points	• Ah Shi • SI8
Option 3 Adjacent points	• Insertion points SI8 and HT3
Option 4 Etiological points and general points	• ST36 (bilaterally) • GB34 (bilaterally) • LR3 (bilaterally) • BL18 (bilaterally)

Option 5
Microsystems
	• W-A acupuncture
	  • Upper 6
	  • Upper 1
	  • Upper 5
	• Ear acupuncture (opposite side)
	  • Elbow
	  • Liver
	  • Subcortex and Shenmen

therapeutic process is the treatment not only of the somatic dysfunctions of the elbow but also of those which are functionally and anatomically related.

Consequently, the osteopathic manipulative approach to musculoskeletal elbow pain is based on the identification of joint somatic dysfunctions not only of the elbow, but also of the shoulder and wrist.

Regardless of the condition to be treated, be it lateral or medial epicondylitis, arthritis of the elbow or surgical outcomes, all of the dysfunctions identified should be treated.

Somatic Dysfunctions of the Humeroulnar Joint
Adduction of the Ulna: Treatment

Adduction dysfunction: elbow adduction is better than abduction.

The patient is supine close to bed edge with incomplete elbow extension (Fig. 3.43; Video 3.14).

The practitioner stands close to the patient's right side with the patient's wrist under the right axilla; the practitioner's right hand is placed on the medial aspect of the elbow to hold it, while the margin of the first intermetacarpal space of the left hand is placed on the lateral joint line of the elbow.

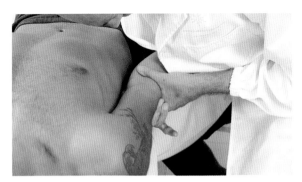 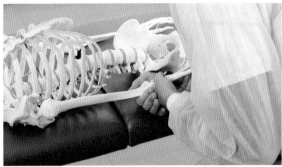

Fig. 3.43 Adduction of the ulna treatment.

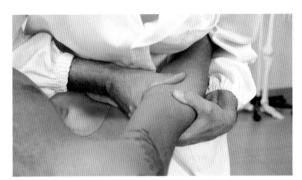 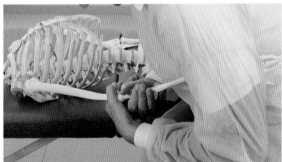

Fig. 3.44 Abduction of the ulna treatment.

After joint decoaptation and rebalancing, the thrust is performed by pushing the elbow internally with the left hand.

Abduction of the Ulna: Treatment

Abduction dysfunction: elbow abduction is better than adduction.

The patient is supine close to bed edge with incomplete elbow extension (Fig. 3.44; Video 3.15).

The practitioner stands close to the patient's right side with the patient's wrist under the left axilla; the practitioner's left hand is placed on the lateral aspect of the elbow to hold it, while the margin of the first intermetacarpal space of the right hand is placed on the medial joint line of the elbow.

After joint decoaptation and rebalancing, the thrust is performed by pushing the elbow externally with the right hand.

Internal Rotation of the Ulna: Treatment

Internal rotation dysfunction: elbow internal rotation is better than external rotation.

The patient sits with elbow flexed at 90 degrees (Figs. 3.45 and 3.46; Video 3.16).

The practitioner stands opposite the patient.

The practitioner holds the bottom of the patient's elbow with the left hand and the wrist with the right hand; the forearm is in neutral position.

After providing the medial side of the elbow with a counterpoint, the thrust is performed by increasing forearm supination with the right hand while holding the elbow flexed at 90 degrees.

External Rotation of the Ulna: Treatment

External rotation dysfunction: elbow external rotation is better than internal rotation.

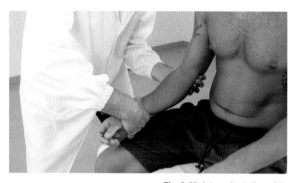 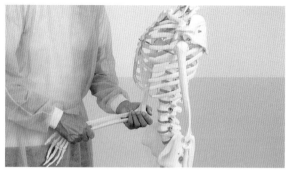

Fig. 3.45 Internal rotation of the ulna treatment: starting position.

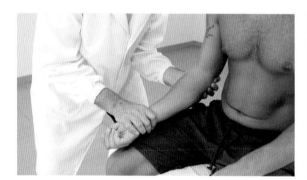 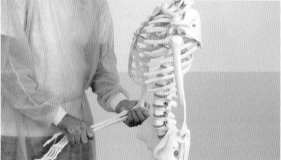

Fig. 3.46 Internal rotation of the ulna treatment: final position.

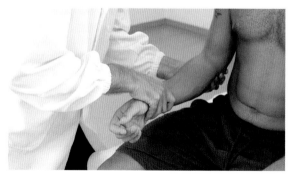 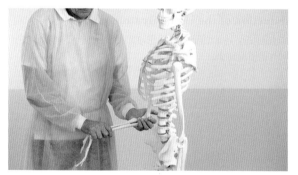

Fig. 3.47 External rotation of the ulna treatment: starting position.

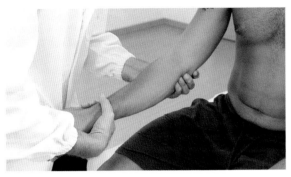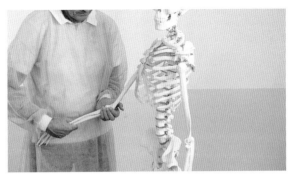

Fig. 3.48 External rotation of the ulna treatment: final position.

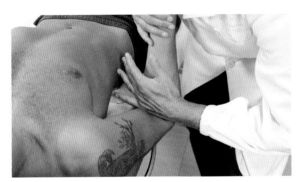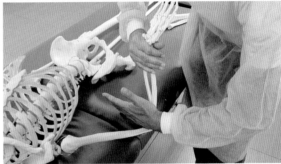

Fig. 3.49 Anterior radial head treatment: starting position.

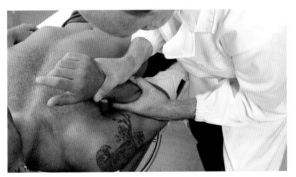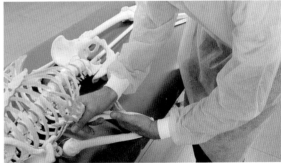

Fig. 3.50 Anterior radial head treatment: final position.

The patient sits with elbow flexed at 90 degrees (Figs. 3.47 and 3.48; Video 3.17).

The practitioner stands opposite the patient.

The practitioner holds the bottom of the patient's elbow by placing the left thenar eminence on the lateral side of the humeroulnar joint while the wrist is held with the right hand; the forearm is in neutral position.

After providing the lateral side of the elbow with a counterpoint, the thrust is performed by increasing

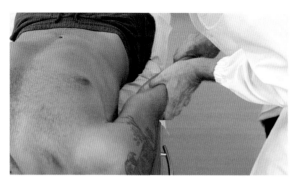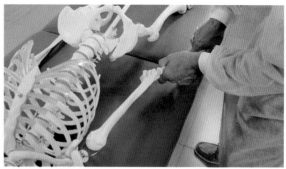

Fig. 3.51 Posterior radial head treatment.

forearm pronation while extending the elbow with the right hand.

Somatic Dysfunctions of the Radioulnar Joint

Anterior Radial Head: Treatment

Anterior dysfunction: anterior sliding of the radial head is better than posterior sliding.

The patient is supine close to bed edge (Figs. 3.49 and 3.50; Video 3.18).

The practitioner stands close to the patient's right side; the right hand holds the patient's wrist in supination while the left hand holds the forearm with the pisiform placed on the anterior side of the radial head.

The practitioner brings the patient's elbow into flexion and the forearm into pronation, while a wedge is created in the elbow crease by the left hand and the pisiform is tucked under the radial head.

After joint decoaptation and rebalancing, the thrust is performed by increasing flexion and pronation with the right hand.

Posterior Radial Head: Treatment

Posterior dysfunction: posterior sliding of the radial head is better than anterior sliding.

The patient is supine close to bed edge (Fig. 3.51; Video 3.19).

The practitioner stands close to the patient's right side; the right hand holds the patient's wrist in supination while the metacarpophalangeal joint of the

left index finger is placed on the posterior side of the radial head.

After joint decoaptation and rebalancing, the thrust is performed with the left hand in a forward direction while increasing extension and supination of the forearm with the right hand.

Therapeutic Program, Frequency of Sessions

The AcuOsteo Method of treatment combines acupuncture and osteopathic manipulations and, in principle, both therapeutic techniques are used during each session and at the same time.

If the condition is acute or chronic with intense pain, we recommend sessions twice a week for 2 weeks and then once a week for another 2 weeks. If improvement is observed, sessions are then scheduled once a week until complete pain relief or at least reduction by 80% to 90%.

In practice, however, since the osteopathic approach differs from acupuncture in that it follows a mechanical principle and aims to restore proper joint mobility, we opt for a *parsimonious* use of osteopathic manipulations over acupuncture: there may be no need to repeat them in every session.

Osteopathic manoeuvres are therefore performed in case of persistent somatic dysfunction. That is why the patient should always be reevaluated at the beginning of each session to assess joint conditions and compare them with preexisting dysfunction.

REFERENCE

1. Reaves W, Bong C. *The Acupuncture Handbook of Sports Injuries & Pain*. 3rd ed. Hidden Needle Press; 2013.

BIBLIOGRAPHY

Baldry PE. *Acupuncture, Trigger Points and Musculoskeletal Pain*. 3rd ed. Elsevier; 2005.

Buckup K. *Test Ortopedici*. Verduci Editore; 1997.

Cipriano JJ. *Test Ortopedici e Neurologici*. Verduci Editore; 1998.

De Seze S, Ryckewaert A. *Malattie dell'osso e delle articolazioni*. Aulo Gaggi Editore; 1979.

Gay J. *Osteopatia, l'Arto Superiore*. Editore Marrapese; 1989.

Giusti R. *Glossary of Osteophatic Terminology*. 3rd ed. American Association of Colleges of Osteophatic Medicine; 2017.

Greenman PE. *Principles of Manual Medicine*. 2nd ed. Williams & Wilkins; 1996.

Guolo F. *Atlante di Tecniche di Energia Muscolare*. Piccin; 2014.

Hoppenfeld S. *L'Esame Obiettivo dell'Apparato Locomotore*. Aulo Gaggi Editore; 1985.

Legge D. *Close to the Bone*. Sydney College Press; 2010.

Maciocia G. *The Practice of Chinese Medicine*. 3rd ed. Elsevier; 2022.

Misulis KE, Head TC. *Neurologia di Netter*. Elsevier; 2008.

Nicholas AS, Nicholas EA. *Atlas of Osteophatic Thechniques*. Lippincott Williams & Wilkins; 2012.

Qiao W. (Association of Medical Acupuncturist of Bologna) Seminar *Wrist and Ankle and Balance Acupuncture*. Italian Chine School of Acupuncture-A.M.A.B; 2007.

Romoli M. *Auricular Acupuncture Diagnosis*. Churchill Livingstone Elsevier; 2009.

Tan R.T., Dr. Tan's Strategy of Twelve Magical Points. Edited by Besinger J.W., San Diego, California, 2003

Tixa S. *Atlas d'Anatomie Palpatoire, tome 1, Cou, Tronc, Membre Superior*. 2e édition. Elsevier Masson; 2005.

Tixa S, Ebenegger B. *Atlas de Techniques articulaires ostéopathiques, tome 1, Les Membres*. 3e édition. Elsevier Masson; 2016.

Chapter 4

The Wrist

Radial (De Quervain tenosynovitis) and ulnar (ulnar wrist pain) styloiditis and extensor tenosynovitis

Radial and ulnar styloiditis are two types of inflammatory tendinopathy affecting their respective styloid processes.

They are of mechanical origin and occur as the consequence of work- or sports-related repetitive wrist movements, which cause the tendons to rub against underlying bony surfaces.

Extensor tenosynovitis is a condition that affects tendons and their protective synovium sheathing with inflammation. It results from work- or sports-related repetitive wrist movements or from distracting injury to the wrist.

Local pain can radiate to the fingers.

Anatomy and Biomechanics According to Western Medicine

JOINTS AND MUSCLES

The wrist is a complex joint marking the area of transition between the forearm and the hand. It connects the two bones in the forearm to the carpals in the hand allowing extension and flexion. It is made up of bones held together by tough bands of connective tissue called ligaments. Muscles and nerves are attached to bones with tendons and allow movement.

Specifically, the bones of the wrist are the two of the forearm (ulna and radius) and the eight carpal bones. The carpus can be divided into two rows of four bones. The proximal row (closer to wrist) is composed of (running from thumb to little finger) the scaphoid, lunate, triquetrum, and pisiform. The distal row is composed of the trapezium, trapezoid, capitate, and hamate.

The proximal row articulates with the radius and is known as the radiocarpal joint, whereas the distal row articulates with the five metacarpal bones and is known as the carpometacarpal joint (Fig. 4.1).

A series of ligaments that extend transversely across the dorsal surface of the wrist connect the carpal bones to one another and the carpal bones to the radius, ulna, and metacarpal bones.

The wrist and hand muscles are located primarily in the forearm and work synergistically to allow for the movement of wrist. They are the following:

- Extensors carpi radialis and ulnaris, digitorum, and pollicis communis
- Flexors carpi radialis and ulnaris, digitorum superficialis, and pollicis longus

ANATOMICAL LANDMARKS

The most useful anatomical landmarks are listed in the following (Fig. 4.2):

- Radial styloid process: an eminence located on the lateral side of the wrist at the distal end of the radius and close to the radiocarpal joint
- Ulnar styloid process: an eminence located on the medial side of the wrist at the distal end of the ulna and close to the radiocarpal joint
- Carpal bones: the anatomical region of the wrist is made up of the carpal bones that are arranged in two rows
- Metacarpal bones: articulate proximally with the carpal bones.

JOINT MOVEMENTS

The Physiological Movements of the Radiocarpal Joint

The neutral position of the wrist is with the patient supine, the upper limb extended.

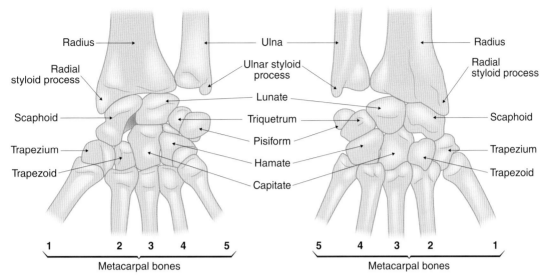

Fig. 4.1 The wrist anatomy: anterior and posterior view.

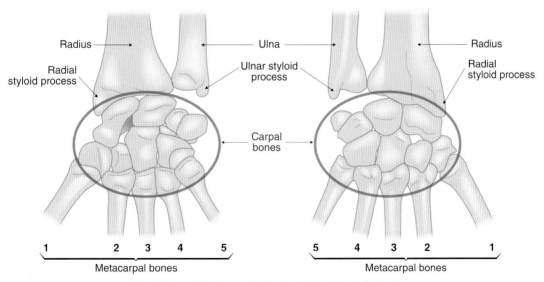

Fig. 4.2 The wrist anatomical landmarks: anterior and posterior view.

There are two starting positions to assess the physiological movements of the wrist:

1. The forearm is supinated with the palm up:
   - Adduction (ulnar flexion): the wrist moves medially toward the patient (Fig. 4.3).
   - Abduction (radial flexion): the wrist moves laterally away from the patient (Fig. 4.4).
2. The forearm is pronated with the palm down:
   - Flexion: the hand moves toward the anterior forearm (Fig. 4.5).
   - Extension: the hand moves away from the anterior forearm (Fig. 4.6).

The normal range of motion of the wrist from a neutral position:

- To full flexion is 0 to about 80 degrees
- To full extension is 0 to about 70 degrees
- To adduction (ulnar flexion) is 0 to about 30 degrees
- To abduction (radial flexion) is 0 to about 20 degrees

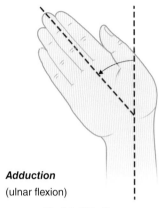

Adduction
(ulnar flexion)

Fig. 4.3 Adduction.

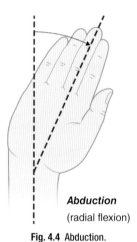

Abduction
(radial flexion)

Fig. 4.4 Abduction.

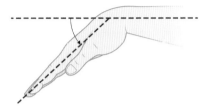

Fig. 4.5 Flexion.

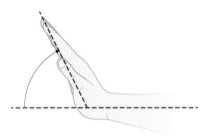

Fig. 4.6 Extension.

Diagnosis in Western Medicine

RADIAL STYLOIDITIS (DE QUERVAIN DISEASE)

Radial styloiditis is a form of stenosing tenosynovitis affecting tendons on the side of the wrist at the base of the thumb. These tendons include the abductor pollicis longus and extensor pollicis brevis, which are compressed by the fibers of the extensor retinaculum at the level of the radial styloid process. Most often, it is of mechanical origin and occurs as the consequence of repetitive wrist movements, which cause the tendons to rub against the underlying bony surfaces of the radial styloid.

Local swelling is usually observed. The onset of symptoms is usually gradual and results from overuse or work- and sports-related repetitive strain injury; however, the onset may also be acute and result from excessive physical effort or local distracting injury.

The most common symptoms are the following:
- Pain on the side of the wrist, either localized on the radial styloid or widespread: it radiates proximally to the forearm along its radial aspect and rarely to the thumb thus making a differential diagnosis of arthritis of the thumb (rhizarthrosis) mandatory.
- Tenderness on palpation on the radial styloid process and swelling of the tendon sheaths are frequently observed (a typical crunching sound is heard on palpation during radial or ulnar flexion of the wrist, similar to the sound you hear when you walk on new snow).
- Pain when grasping small objects or performing certain tasks (e.g., screwing/unscrewing a lid to a container, turning the key to lock/unlock the door, shaking hands or flexing the wrist with radial deviation against resistance).

- Dull pain with a feeling of stiffness in chronic conditions.
- Positive Finkelstein test.

Finkelstein Test

It is used to assess De Quervain disease (styloiditis or tenosynovitis). The patient sits. The practitioner is opposite the patient and holds the patient's right wrist with the left hand. The forearm is in a neutral position. The patient is asked to make a fist around the thumb. The practitioner slightly brings the wrist into ulnar flexion with the right hand. The test is considered positive if the patient reports pain over the radial styloid process (Fig. 4.7; Video 4.1).

ULNAR STYLOIDITIS (ULNAR WRIST PAIN)

Ulnar styloiditis is usually a form of tenosynovitis affecting the tendon of the extensor carpi ulnaris at the level of the ulnar styloid process. Most often, it is of mechanical origin and occurs as the consequence of repetitive wrist movements, which cause the tendons to rub against the underlying bony surfaces of the ulnar styloid.

Local swelling is usually observed. Less frequently observed than radial styloiditis, it is usually characterized by a gradual onset of symptoms from overuse or work- and sports-related repetitive strain injury; however, onset may also be acute and result from excessive physical effort, local distracting injury, or an accidental fall on the hand.

The most common symptoms are the following:
- Pain on the medial side of the wrist: it can be localized, but more often it radiates to the fifth metacarpal, sometimes to the fifth finger. In such cases, a differential diagnosis is mandatory to exclude pain from irritation (entrapment) of the ulnar nerve radiating to the wrist and sometimes proximally to the forearm along its ulnar aspect.
- Tenderness on palpation on the ulnar styloid process and possible swelling of the tendon sheaths.
- Pain when grasping small objects or performing certain tasks (e.g., screwing/unscrewing a lid to a container, turning the key to lock/unlock the door, shaking hands, or flexing the wrist with ulnar deviation against resistance).
- In chronic conditions, pain may be dull with a feeling of stiffness.
- Positive ulnocarpal stress test.

Ulnocarpal Stress Test

It is used to assess ulnar styloiditis. The patient is supine with the right elbow flexed at 90 degrees and the forearm in a neutral position. The practitioner stands close to the patient and holds the right wrist with the left hand while placing it in maximal ulnar deviation with the right hand. The test is performed by applying stress through passive supination and pronation while the wrist remains in maximal ulnar deviation. The test is considered positive if the patient reports pain over the ulnar styloid process. It is a very sensitive provocative test, however little specific, as it can often be positive and therefore can suggest the presence of many ulnar-sided wrist disorders (Fig. 4.8; Video 4.2).

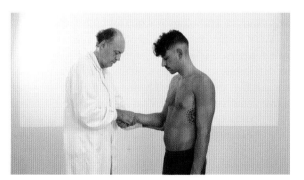

Fig. 4.7 Finkelstein test.

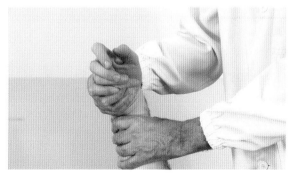

Fig. 4.8 Ulnocarpal stress test.

EXTENSOR TENOSYNOVITIS

Dorsal wrist pain is usually a form of tenosynovitis affecting the tendons of the extensor digitorum on the dorsal side of the wrist and resulting from repetitive wrist movements or inflammation due to a distracting injury to the wrist.

Local swelling is usually observed. It is usually characterized by a gradual onset of symptoms from overuse or work- and sports-related repetitive strain injury; however, the onset may also be acute and result from excessive physical effort or local distracting injury.

The most common symptoms are the following:

- Pain on the dorsal side of the wrist: it can be localized; more often it radiates to the dorsum of the hand, sometimes proximally to the forearm along its dorsal aspect.
- Tenderness on palpation on the extensor digitorum communis with swelling of its tendon sheaths is frequently observed.
- Pain and tenderness with hand extension or wrist flexion.

JOINT PAIN, ARTHRITIS, AND STIFFNESS

Patients with wrist arthritis and postsurgical outcomes usually complain of pain, weakness, and restricted range of motion. Among the most common causes of wrist arthritis are fractures, rheumatoid arthritis, septic arthritis, and primary osteoarthritis. Diagnosis is based on the patient's medical history, clinical findings, and radiographic examinations.

The most common complications that may occur after surgery or as a result of fracture include:

- Wrist stiffness with possible loss of motion (flexion, extension, adduction, and abduction)
- Late-onset osteoarthritis
- Failed fusion
- Persistent pain

RED FLAGS IN WESTERN MEDICINE

The presence of heat (calor), redness (rubor), swelling (tumor), pain (dolor), and loss of function (function laesa) determines the need for diagnostic investigations.

Wrist trauma is a common occurrence. Among the signs and symptoms of fracture or dislocation are swelling and deformity of the limb. A fracture affects the continuity of a bone, whereas a dislocation involves a joint.

Patients with rheumatoid arthritis of the wrist usually complain of pain throughout the range of motion; the wrist is usually affected in the later stages in the disease. Both fatigue and general discomfort can also be observed.

Special attention should be paid if concomitant symptoms are observed, such as numbness, tingling, paresthesia (abnormal sensation), muscle weakness, decreased tendon reflexes and pain, mainly at night.

Abnormalities uncovered on history taking or physical examination may require medical evaluation, laboratory tests, and imaging investigations, such as x-rays, US, CT, and MRI.

Diagnosis in Chinese Medicine

In Chinese Medicine, musculoskeletal pain results from the obstruction of Qì and Blood circulation or inadequate Qì and Blood for the nourishment of the secondary channels, especially the Muscle and Connecting channels.

The Muscle and Connecting channels more often involved in wrist disorders are listed below:

- Large Intestine
- Small Intestine
- Triple Energizer

The channels affected vary according to the pain location:

- Large Intestine: pain is on the radial side, and the pathology is radial styloiditis.
- Small Intestine: pain is on the ulnar side, and the pathology is ulnar styloiditis.
- Triple Energizer: pain is on the posterior side, and the pathology is extensor tenosynovitis.

What matters most is to identify the affected channel where the pain is located. Sometimes it is not so easy to determine it, and consequently, the following data concerning the Muscle channels involved in wrist movements should be acquired for better identification.

- Extension: TE, SI, and LI
- Flexion: LU, PC, and HT
- Abduction: LI and LU
- Adduction: SI, TE, and HT

Red Flags	Pain	Inspection	Other Signs	Neurological Signs	Recommendations
Inflammation	Pain	Redness, swelling, and heat	–	Functional deficit	Physician evaluation Imaging investigations
Fracture	Spontaneous pain	Deformity and swelling	Movement beyond normal range of motion	Functional deficit	Physician evaluation Imaging investigations
Rheumatoid arthritis	Pain with or without movement	Redness and swelling	Fatigue and general discomfort	Functional deficit	Physician evaluation Imaging investigations Laboratory tests
Herniated disc or cervical radiculopathy	Cervical pain radiating to the wrist	–	–	Paresthesia, hypoesthesia, tingling and lack of deep tendon reflexes	Physician evaluation Imaging investigations
Dorsal cyst	Pain	Visible lump with hard-elastic consistency	–	Paresthesia, hypoesthesia	Physician evaluation Imaging investigations
Cubital tunnel syndrome	Pain in the elbow and in the most severe cases spreading to the ulnar side of the forearm, wrist, little finger, and ring finger	–	–	Paresthesia, hypoesthesia, tingling and hyposthenia in the little and ring fingers, positive Tinel sign	Physician evaluation Imaging investigations
Carpal tunnel syndrome	Pain in the wrist spreading to the first three fingers	–	–	Paresthesia, hypoesthesia, and tingling in the first three fingers, positive Tinel sign, weakness and loss of pinch strength	Physician evaluation Imaging investigations

The information so acquired on the channel that is likely to be involved, that is, pain location and related movement restriction, can also be integrated with the results from Western medicine orthopedic tests in order to identify which muscle, tendon, and joint is affected in the case of:

- Radial styloiditis
- Ulnar styloiditis
- Extensor tenosynovitis

ETIOLOGY

Wrist pain is usually caused by:

- *Overuse, repetitive strain injury.* Through work (hair-dresser) or sports (tennis or rowing); performing the same movement over and over again causes local Qì stagnation or Qì and Blood deficiency.
- *Trauma, sport injuries.* If mild, they cause local Qì stagnation. If severe, they cause local Blood stasis.
- *Cold and Dampness.* Local invasion causes Qì stagnation or Blood stasis. Dampness also causes local swelling.

Previous accidents often predispose the wrist to more frequent invasions of external pathogenic factors (EPFs), especially Cold.

PATHOLOGY

The Muscle and Connecting channels are often affected by Qì stagnation and Blood stasis:

- Qì stagnation manifests itself with widespread pain radiating proximally or distally along the pathway of the Muscle channels.
- Blood stasis, usually occurring in the Connecting channels, manifests itself with more intense pain over the radial and ulnar styloid process, over the tendons or in the joint, with a consequent limited range of motion or joint stiffness.

As already mentioned in the fundamentals of acupuncture for MSK pain in the limbs (see Chapter 1), the term Connecting channels includes not only the Connecting channel "proper" but also the Connecting channel "area" that covers the whole pathway of the Main channel.

RADIAL STYLOIDITIS (DE QUERVAIN DISEASE)

To identify the Muscle and Connecting channels affected, we check the location and characteristics of musculoskeletal pain, palpate the affected area, test

the range of motion for each wrist movement, and perform orthopedic tests to elicit pain.

The Pathways of the Large Intestine Secondary Channels

In case of radial styloiditis the Large Intestine Muscle and Connecting channels are involved (Fig. 4.9).

The pathway of the Large Intestine Muscle channel explains pain on the radial side of the wrist, which could radiate proximally to the radial side of the forearm, whereas the pathway of the Large Intestine Connecting channel "proper" does not because it does not descend to the wrist and hand.

Since we are now referring to the Large Intestine Connecting channel "area", we regard the Large Intestine Connecting channels as channels involved.

ULNAR STYLOIDITIS (ULNAR WRIST PAIN)

To identify the Muscle and Connecting channels affected, we check the location and characteristics of musculoskeletal pain, palpate the affected area, test the range of motion for each wrist movement, and perform orthopedic tests to elicit pain.

The Pathways of the Small Intestine Secondary Channels

In case of ulnar styloiditis, the Small Intestine Muscle and Connecting channels are involved (Fig. 4.10).

The pathway of the Small Intestine Muscle channel explains pain on the ulnar side of the wrist, which could radiate distally to the fifth finger and proximally to the ulnar side of the forearm, whereas the pathway of the Small Intestine Connecting channel "proper" does not because it does not descend to the wrist and hand.

Since we are now referring to the Small Intestine Connecting channel "area," we regard the Small Intestine Connecting channels as channels involved.

EXTENSOR TENOSYNOVITIS

To identify the Muscle and Connecting channels affected, we check the location and characteristics of musculoskeletal pain, palpate the affected area, test the range of motion for each wrist movement, and perform orthopedic tests to elicit pain.

The Pathways of the Triple Energizer Secondary Channels

In the case of extensor tenosynovitis the Triple Energizer Muscle and Connecting channels are involved (Fig. 4.11).

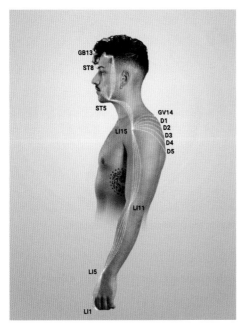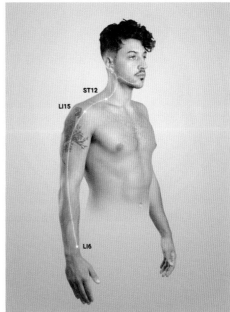

Fig. 4.9 The pathways of the Large Intestine Muscle and Connecting "proper" channels.

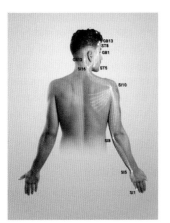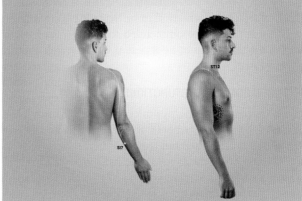

Fig. 4.10 The pathways of the Small Intestine Muscle and Connecting "proper" channels.

The pathway of the Triple Energizer Muscle channel explains pain on the dorsal aspect of the wrist, which could radiate distally to the dorsum of the hand and proximally to the posterior forearm, whereas the pathway of the Triple Energizer Connecting channel "proper" does not because it does not descend to the wrist and hand.

Since we are now referring to the Triple Energizer Connecting channel "area", we regard the Triple Energizer Connecting channels as channels involved.

Diagnosis in Osteopathic Medicine

The examination for "somatic dysfunction" is the central concept of the diagnostic process; palpation of the affected area and functionally/anatomically related components of the somatic system is the only way to assess it.

Consequently, the osteopathic diagnostic approach to musculoskeletal wrist pain is based on the identification of joint somatic dysfunctions not only of the wrist but also of the shoulder and elbow.

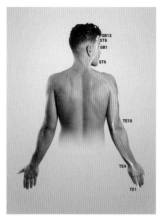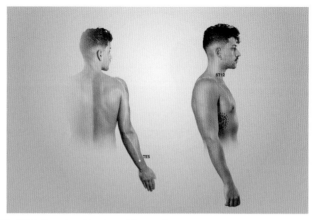

Fig. 4.11 The pathways of the Triple Energizer Muscle and Connecting "proper" channels.

Regardless of the condition to be treated, be it radial or ulnar styloiditis, extensor tenosynovitis, arthritis of the wrist, or surgical outcomes, all of the recommended tests should be performed to identify the dysfunctions that occur more frequently.

It is therefore evident that the osteopathic diagnosis is developed regardless of the condition to be treated; therefore the osteopathic tests recommended for the wrist, shoulder, and elbow will not be repeated when the "injuries" are treated.

TESTS FOR THE MAIN SOMATIC DYSFUNCTIONS

The only way to diagnose somatic dysfunctions of a joint is to assess the passive movements of its articular ends in relation to one another and compare them with the same movements of the joint on the healthy side. Testing of all wrist joints is required.

On the same plane of motion, there is passive mobility quantitatively and qualitatively equally on both sides of a theoretical neutral point that represents the reference point.

When the balance is lost and the range and quality of motion are not the same in both directions, then there is somatic dysfunction.

Test of the Distal Radioulnar Joint

A test is performed to assess the most common ulnar dysfunctions:

1. Posterior ulna
2. Anterior ulna

Anteroposterior Test of the Ulna

The patient is supine with incomplete elbow extension and wrist in a neutral position. The practitioner stands close to the patient's right side with the right thumb and index finger holding the patient's radius. The posterior test is performed by pulling the ulna backward with the left index finger to assess posterior sliding. The anterior test is performed by pushing the ulna forward with the left thumb to assess anterior sliding. The practitioner appreciates the range and quality of motion of anterior and posterior sliding and compares them with posterior and anterior sliding, respectively. If the ulna slides more easily posteriorly, then there is posterior dysfunction, and vice versa (Fig. 4.12; Video 4.3).

Tests of the Radiocarpal Joint

Tests are performed to assess the most common carpal dysfunctions:

1. Anterior carpus
2. Posterior carpus

Anterior Test of the Carpus

The patient is supine with incomplete elbow extension and wrist in pronation. The practitioner stands on the patient's right side and holds the wrist. The anterior test is performed with the thumbs on the carpal bones posteriorly and the index fingers on the radius anteriorly.

The practitioner applies gentle traction and makes the carpal bones slide anteriorly to appreciate the

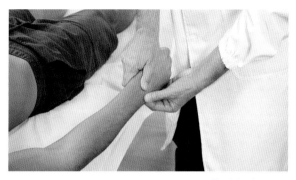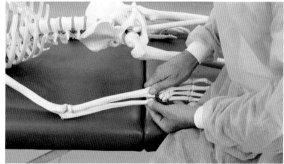

Fig. 4.12 Anteroposterior test of the ulna.

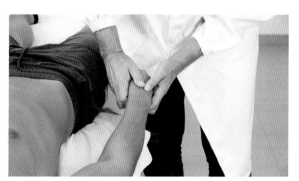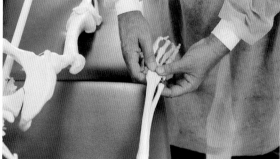

Fig. 4.13 Anterior test of the carpus: starting position.

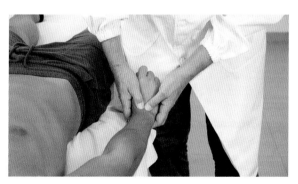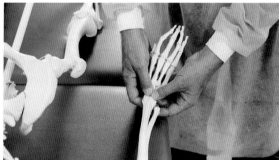

Fig. 4.14 Anterior test of the carpus: final position.

range and quality of motion with the thumbs and compare them with the posterior test.

If the carpal bones slide more easily anteriorly than posteriorly, then there is anterior dysfunction (Figs. 4.13 and 4.14; Video 4.4).

Posterior Test of the Carpus

The patient is supine with incomplete elbow extension and wrist in pronation. The practitioner stands on the patient's right side and holds the wrist. The posterior

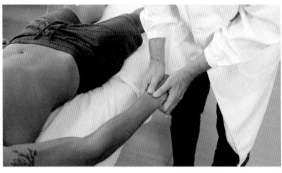
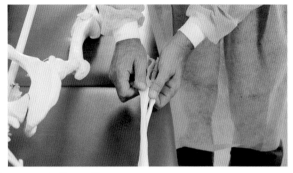

Fig. 4.15 Posterior test of the carpus: starting position.

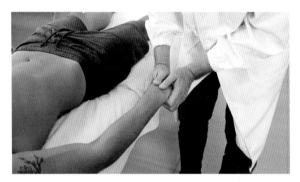
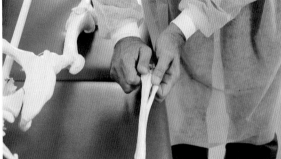

Fig. 4.16 Posterior test of the carpus: final position.

test is performed with the index fingers on the carpal bones anteriorly and the thumbs on the radius posteriorly.

The practitioner applies gentle traction and makes the carpal bones slide posteriorly to appreciate the range and quality of motion with the index fingers and compare them with the anterior test. If the carpal bones slide more easily posteriorly than anteriorly, then there is posterior dysfunction (Figs. 4.15 and 4.16; Video 4.5).

Treatment With the AcuOsteo Method: The Choice of an Integrated Approach

The therapeutic approach of the AcuOsteo Method aims to treat those musculoskeletal injuries that do not require consultation with a surgeon or a physician. Once this fundamental aspect has been defined, the treatment envisages the use of acupuncture and osteopathy according to their diagnostic and therapeutic approaches.

We would like to stress that at this point in diagnostic assessment, we do not have to follow the rules of Western medicine, except for some specific cases, such as wrist arthritis, posttraumatic and postsurgical pain, and stiffness, which will be covered later.

In addition, we should not be misled by diagnostic imaging investigations and should rely only on the rules of Chinese and Osteopathic medicine, which means selecting points according to symptoms and channel pathways and treating all of the somatic dysfunctions encountered.

For didactic purposes, acupuncture treatment will precede osteopathic treatment, whereas in clinical practice the order is reversed since it may be difficult to perform osteopathic manipulations once the needles have been inserted.

An exception to this methodology is represented by those morbidities where marked stiffness prevents joint mobilization as required by osteopathic manipulations. Specifically, we are referring to the outcomes after immobilization following surgery, fractures, and wrist dislocation.

In these cases, we suggest first using acupuncture, especially the bleeding techniques, and then, at the end of the session and after removing the needles, osteopathy. In any case, it is always the practitioner's clinical experience that will guide them along the most appropriate pathway to treat each patient's condition.

Osteopathic manipulation in the treatment of "somatic dysfunction" is the central concept of the therapeutic process to treat the affected joints and functionally/anatomically related components of the somatic system.

Consequently, the osteopathic manipulative approach to musculoskeletal wrist pain focuses on the treatment of joint somatic dysfunctions not only of the wrist but also of the shoulder and elbow.

Regardless of the condition to be treated, be it radial or ulnar styloiditis, extensor tenosynovitis, arthritis of the wrist, or surgical outcomes, all of the dysfunctions diagnosed should be treated.

It is therefore evident that the osteopathic therapeutic approach does not vary with the condition to be treated and thus the osteopathic manipulations described for the wrist, as well as those for the shoulder and elbow, will not be repeated under the paragraphs dedicated to the "injuries."

ACUPUNCTURE TREATMENT
Radial Styloiditis

The Five Options and Selection of Acupoints

The approach we suggest is widely described in the section dedicated to the fundamentals of acupuncture for MSK pain in the limbs (see Chapter 1).

The most important aspect is the identification of the Ah Shi point(s) to determine which channels are affected. In this specific case, the Large Intestine Muscle and Connecting channels are involved.

Pricking pain localized on the radial styloid process is a sign of Blood stasis to be treated with the bleeding technique, whereas widespread pain radiating proximally to the forearm is a sign of Qì stagnation to be treated with the needling technique.

Pain radiating distally to the thumb, which is a rarer occurrence, usually indicates involvement of the Lung secondary channels: in this case treatment should follow the principles of the Five Options;

alternatively, their Jing-Well and Luo points should at least be needled.

It is worth reminding that the distal points should be needled one at a time and their effectiveness in terms of pain and range of motion tested after each insertion. The same applies to the local points.

Finally, since both options 1 and 2 consist of several steps, it is important to highlight how selection should be made. Specifically, the practitioner might wonder if all or some of the steps should be followed. The rule we follow is simple: when the result achieved is satisfactory, the remaining steps should be skipped, and the practitioner should move to the following option. Similarly, the use of the points recommended under options 3, 4, and 5 should be carefully evaluated according to the case being treated.

The points and accessory techniques we recommend using are listed below.

Order of Needling
Option One: Distal Points
First Step: Large Intestine Muscle Channel
LI1. This Jing-Well point activates the Large Intestine Muscle channel and removes Qì stagnation and Blood stasis with needling and bleeding techniques, respectively.

Second Step: Large Intestine Connecting Channels
LI6 (Opposite Side). This Luo point activates the Large Intestine Connecting channels and removes Qì stagnation and Blood stasis in acute and chronic conditions from Excess.

Our technique consists of needling LI6 from oblique to transverse in a proximal direction along the pathway of the Large Intestine Main channel (Figs. 4.17 and 4.18; Video 4.6).

LU7 (Opposite Side). This Luo point activates the Lung Connecting channels and is also used in chronic Deficiency conditions with dull pain to tonify Qì and Blood in the internally-externally related Large Intestine channels. In the latter case, we associate Yuan point LI4 with Luo Point LU7, which is the well-known Luo-Yuan combination. First, as the main point, we needle the Yuan point on the affected side and then, as a secondary point, the Luo point on the internally-externally related channel on the opposite side.

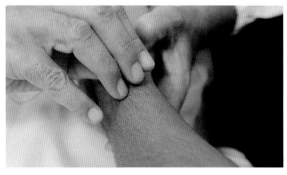

Fig. 4.17 Needling of the LI6: starting position.

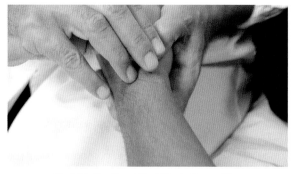

Fig. 4.19 Needling of the LU7: starting position.

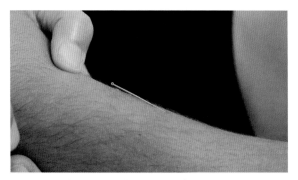

Fig. 4.18 Needling of the LI6: final position.

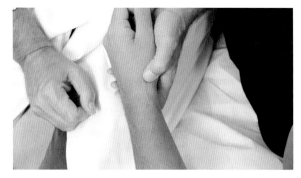

Fig. 4.20 Needling of the LU7: final position.

Our technique consists of needling LU7 from oblique to transverse in a proximal direction along the pathway of the Lung Main channel (Figs. 4.19 and 4.20; Video 4.7).

Third step: Empirical Points

There is no point that is classically recommended.

Fourth Step: Opposite Extremity (Upper/Lower)

ST41 (Opposite Side). It is located in the ankle joint, which corresponds to the wrist joint on the paired channel according to the Six Stages.

It is worth remembering that the radial styloid is not exactly in the wrist joint; it is in fact slightly proximally located, and this means we could palpate the leg in an upward direction along the Stomach Main channel to possibly find a tender point(s).

In clinical practice, the mirror concept can lead us to select a point, which may be tender or not, on the area corresponding to the medial malleolus, which corresponds exactly to the radial styloid, although it is not located on the Stomach Main channel.

In line with our principle of treatment, we first needle ST41 or a more proximal point and then test its effectiveness soon after insertion; if the result is not satisfactory, we remove the needle and move to the second option.

Our technique consists of needling the opposite extremity (lower/upper) on the opposite side in acute and chronic conditions.

Alternatively, the most tender point on palpation is selected on the same or opposite side.

Fifth Step: Categories of Traditional Points

LI3 (Affected Side) and ST43 (Opposite Side). A good combination includes the Shu-Stream points on the paired channel according to the Six Stages. First, we needle the Shu-Stream point on the channel involved on the affected side and then the Shu-Stream point on the coupled channel on the opposite side and opposite extremity (upper/lower). We use this technique in acute and chronic Excess conditions to treat pain and expel or prevent invasion of EPFs.

LI5. The Jing-River points are used in acute or chronic Excess conditions due to the invasion of an EPF, and they are needled to promote its expulsion from their respective channels. They are also useful to prevent pain exacerbation from seasonal changes or invasion of EPFs. We also use LI5 because it is a local point of the wrist and an insertion point of the Large Intestine Muscle channel, as we will see later.

LI7. The Xi-Cleft points are specifically used in acute conditions to treat Blood stasis in their respective channels. However, they are more effective in the Yin rather than in the Yang channels: that is why we would rather avoid using LI7 to treat this condition.

LI4. We recommend using this Yuan-Source point in chronic Deficiency conditions with dull pain, in case of weakness, or in the resolution phases of radial styloiditis, to tonify Qì and Blood in the Large Intestine channels.

In this situation, we can also associate Yuan point LI4 with Luo point LU7, which is the well-known Luo-Yuan point combination. First, as the main point, we needle the Yuan point on the affected side and then, as a secondary point, the Luo point on the internally-externally related channel on the opposite side.

Sixth Step: Extraordinary Vessels

In our opinion, no Extraordinary Vessel is effective to treat this inflammation.

Option Two: Local Points

First Step: Painful Point(s) (Ah Shi)

Ah Shi Point(s). Palpation of the radial styloid reveals either the most painful point(s) (Ah Shi) corresponding to Blood stasis and therefore to be bled or an area of widespread pain corresponding to Qì stagnation and requiring needling. The pain could radiate proximally to the lateral forearm or distally to the thumb.

When the anatomical structure of the wrist allows us to, the cupping therapy should be used to bleed this point(s) paying attention not to damage the tendinous tissue with the lancet or the soft tissues with a too strong cupping (Figs. 4.21 and 4.22; Video 4.8).

The needle should be inserted superficially, from oblique to transverse, lateral to the involved tendons. We use four needles, two inserted from the medial side and two from the lateral side, at a distance of about half a cun one from the other.

The 0.25 × 25 mm needles are inserted tangentially to a depth of about half a centimeter until the tendon sheath is reached (Figs. 4.23 and 4.24; Video 4.9).

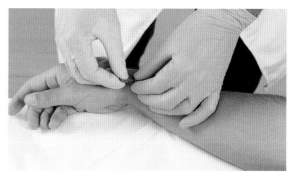

Fig. 4.21 Bleeding of the Ah Shi point(s): starting position.

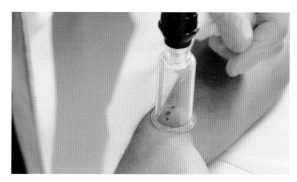

Fig. 4.22 Bleeding of the Ah Shi point(s): final position.

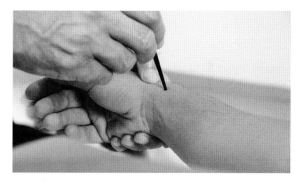

Fig. 4.23 Needling of the Ah Shi point(s): starting position.

Electroacupuncture stimulation can be taken into consideration and used between these two points. Both in acute and chronic conditions a moxa stick can be useful to promote the flow of Qì and Blood. However, attention should be paid since too much heat can increase the ongoing inflammatory process.

LI5. It can be considered a local point to treat radial styloiditis, although in reality it is only adjacent to the

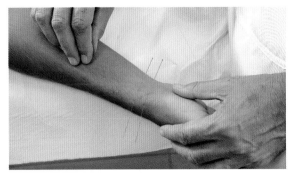

Fig. 4.24 Needling of the Ah Shi point(s): final position.

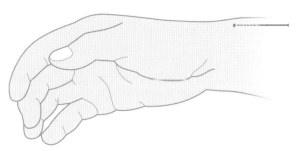

Fig. 4.25 Upper 4.

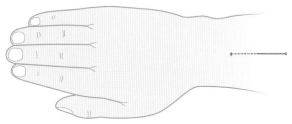

Fig. 4.26 Upper 5.

radial styloid process. We also use it because it is an insertion point of the Large Intestine Muscle channel in the wrist, as we will see later.

To ensure the accuracy and precision of local needle placement and manipulation, we prefer the supine position.

Second Step: Anatomically Mirrored Point(s) (Opposite Side)

The points to be needled are located on the opposite side and should correspond as precisely as possible to the anatomical mirror of the Ah Shi point(s) to be treated. The point(s) may or may not be tender on palpation. To ensure the accuracy and precision of needle placement and manipulation, we prefer the supine position.

Option Three: Adjacent Points

First Step: Adjacent Points

TE4 and LU9. They help promote the horizontal flow of local Qì.

LI5. It is a very important point since it is the insertion point of the Large Intestine Muscle channel in the wrist and as such it promotes the longitudinal flow of local Qì.

Option Four: Etiological Points

First Step: According to Patterns

LI4 and LR3 (Bilaterally). They promote the flow of Qì and help remove Blood stasis. Since LR3 is the Shu/Yuan point of the Liver, it also helps nourish muscles and tendons.

ST36 (Bilaterally). It is used to tonify Qì and Blood in chronic Deficiency conditions or the phases of pain resolution that can turn into muscle weakness.

Second Step: General Points

GB34 (Bilaterally). It is the Hui-Gathering point of Sinews and is specifically used for radial styloiditis, which is a type of tenosynovitis. In addition, it promotes the flow of Qì thus contributing to remove Blood stasis.

BL17 (Bilaterally). It is the Hui-Gathering point of Blood to remove Blood stasis.

BL18 (Bilaterally). It treats all Excess and Deficiency conditions of the Liver that may favor the onset or duration of musculotendinous symptoms. It harmonizes the flow of Qì and Blood and enhances the treatment of tendons and muscle.

Option Five: Microsystems

First Step: Wrist and Ankle Acupuncture

Upper 4. It roughly corresponds to the pathway of the Large Intestine channels, which is directed toward the radial styloid (Fig. 4.25).

Upper 5. It controls upper limb mobility. In this specific case, we recommend directing the needle toward the hand (Fig. 4.26).

Second Step: Ear Acupuncture (Fig. 4.27)

Local point: Wrist
Zang Fu point: Liver
General points: Subcortex and Shenmen

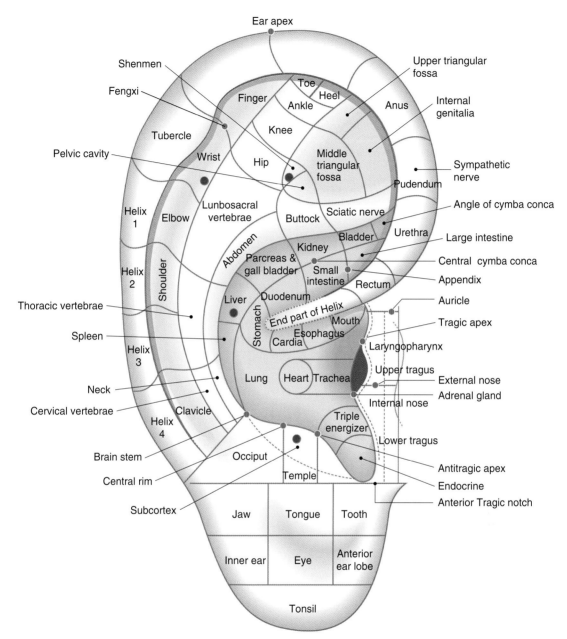

Fig. 4.27 Ear acupuncture.

Acute or Chronic Pain From Excess

Intense Pain or Range of Motion Reduced by Pain. The principle of treatment is to remove Qì stagnation and Blood stasis and expel EPFs or internal pathogenic factors (IPFs), if any (Box 4.1).

Chronic Pain From Deficiency

Dull Pain or Muscle Weakness. The principle of treatment is to tonify Qì and Blood, strengthen tissues, and avoid pain exacerbation from physical activities or invasion of EPFs (Box 4.2).

BOX 4.1 ACUTE OR CHRONIC PAIN FROM EXCESS ACUPUNCTURE TREATMENT

Option 1 Distal points	• Jing-Well point LI1 • Luo point LI6 (opposite side) • Point according to the Six Stages ST41 (opposite side) • Jing-River point LI5
Option 2 Local points	• Ah Shi • LI5 • Anatomically mirrored point(s) (opposite side)
Option 3 Adjacent points	• TE4 • LU9 • Insertion point LI5
Option 4 Etiological and general points	• LI4 and LR3 (bilaterally) • GB34 (bilaterally) • BL17 (bilaterally) • BL18 (bilaterally)

Option 5
Microsystems
	• W-A acupuncture
	  • Upper 4
	  • Upper 5
	• Ear acupuncture (opposite side)
	  • Wrist
	  • Liver
	  • Subcortex and Shenmen

BOX 4.2 CHRONIC PAIN FROM DEFICIENCY ACUPUNCTURE TREATMENT

Option 1 Distal points	• Yuan point LI4 • Luo point LU7 (opposite side) • Point according to the Six Stages ST41 (opposite side) • Jing-River point LI5
Option 2 Local points	• Ah Shi • LI5
Option 3 Adjacent points	• TE4 • LU9 • Insertion point LI5
Option 4 Etiological and general points	• ST36 (bilaterally) • GB34 (bilaterally) • LR3 (bilaterally) • BL18 (bilaterally)

Option 5
Microsystems
	• W-A acupuncture
	  • Upper 4
	  • Upper 5
	• Ear acupuncture (opposite side)
	  • Wrist
	  • Liver
	  • Subcortex and Shenmen

Therapeutic Program, Frequency of Sessions

The frequency of sessions depends on the clinical condition of the patient. If the condition is acute or chronic with intense pain, we recommend sessions twice a week for 2 weeks and then once a week for another 2 weeks. If improvement is observed, sessions are then scheduled once a week until complete pain relief or at least a reduction by 80% to 90%. If not, the whole clinical picture should be reconsidered, and the patient should be referred to another specialist.

If the condition is chronic with dull pain, we recommend sessions once a week for 4 weeks. Afterward,

Clinical Notes

• Improvement following treatment may turn intense pain into dull pain and then into a feeling of weakness. Should this be the case, the principle of treatment has to be changed as follows: it is no longer necessary to remove Qì stagnation and Blood stasis and expel EPF, if any; instead, Qì and Blood should be tonified to strengthen tissues and avoid pain exacerbation from physical activities or invasion of EPFs.

and if the patient continues to improve, sessions are then scheduled once a week until complete pain relief or at least a reduction by 80% to 90%.

Ulnar Styloiditis (Ulnar Wrist Pain)

The Five Options and Selection of Acupoints

The approach we suggest is widely described in the section dedicated to the fundamentals of acupuncture for MSK pain in the limbs (see Chapter 1).

The most important aspect is the identification of the Ah Shi point(s) to determine which channels are affected. In this specific case, the Small Intestine Muscle and Connecting channels are involved.

Pricking pain localized on the ulnar styloid process is a sign of Blood stasis to be treated with the bleeding technique, whereas widespread pain radiating along the forearm and to the hand and little finger is a sign of Qì stagnation to be treated with the needling technique.

It is worth reminding that the distal points should be needled one at a time and their effectiveness in terms of pain and range of motion tested after each insertion. The same applies to the local points.

Finally, since both options 1 and 2 consist of several steps, it is important to highlight how selection should be made. Specifically, the practitioner might wonder if all or some of the steps should be followed. The rule we follow is simple: when the result achieved is satisfactory, the remaining steps should be skipped, and the practitioner should move to the following option. Similarly, the use of the points recommended under options 3, 4, and 5 should be carefully evaluated according to the case being treated.

The points and accessory techniques we recommend using are listed below.

The Order of Needling

Option One: Distal Points

First Step: Small Intestine Muscle Channel

SI1. This Jing-Well point activates the Small Intestine Muscle channel and removes Qì stagnation and Blood stasis with needling and bleeding techniques, respectively.

Second Step: Small Intestine Connecting Channels

SI7 (Opposite Side). This Luo point activates the Small Intestine Connecting channels and removes Qì stagnation and Blood stasis in acute or chronic conditions from Excess.

HT5 (Opposite Side). This Luo point activates the Heart Connecting channels and is also used in chronic Deficiency conditions with dull pain to tonify Qì and Blood in the internally-externally related Small Intestine channels. In the latter case, we associate Yuan point SI4 with Luo point HT5, which is the well-known Luo-Yuan point combination. First, as the main point, we needle the Yuan point on the affected side and then, as a secondary point, the Luo point on the internally-externally related channel on the opposite side.

Third Step: Empirical Points

There is no point that is classically recommended.

Fourth Step: Opposite Extremity (Upper/Lower)

BL60 (Opposite Side). It is located in the ankle joint, which corresponds to the wrist joint on the paired channel according to the Six Stages.

It is worth remembering that the ulnar styloid is not exactly in the wrist joint; it is in fact slightly proximally located, and this means we could palpate the leg in an upward direction along the Bladder Main channel to possibly find a tender point(s).

In clinical practice, the mirror concept can lead us to select the point, which may be tender or not, on the area corresponding to the apex of the lateral malleolus, which corresponds exactly to the ulnar styloid, although it is not located on the Bladder Main channel.

In line with our principle of treatment, we first needle BL60 or a more proximal point and then test its effectiveness soon after insertion; if the result is not satisfactory, we remove the needle and move to the second option.

Our technique consists of needling the opposite extremity (lower/upper) on the opposite side in acute and chronic conditions. Alternatively, the most tender point on palpation is selected on the same or opposite side.

Fifth Step: Categories of Traditional Points

SI3 (Affected Side) and BL65 (Opposite Side). A good combination includes the Shu-Stream points on the paired channel according to the Six Stages. We first needle the Shu-Stream point on the channel involved on the affected side and then the Shu-Stream point on the coupled channel on the opposite side and opposite extremity (upper/lower). We use this technique in acute and chronic Excess conditions to treat pain and expel or prevent invasion of EPFs.

SI5. The Jing-River points are used in acute or chronic Excess conditions due to the invasion of an

EPF, and they are needled to promote its expulsion from their respective channels. They are also useful to prevent pain exacerbation from seasonal changes or invasion of EPFs. We also use SI5 because it is a local point of the wrist and an insertion point of the Small Intestine Muscle channel, as we will see later.

SI6. The Xi-Cleft points are specially used in acute conditions to treat Blood stasis in their respective channels. However, they are more effective in the Yin rather than in the Yang channels: that is why we would rather avoid using SI6 to treat this condition.

SI4. We recommend using this Yuan-Source point in chronic Deficiency conditions with dull pain, in case of weakness, or in the resolution phases of ulnar styloiditis, to tonify Qì and Blood in the Small Intestine channels.

In this situation, we can also associate Yuan point SI4 with Luo point HT5, which is the well-known Luo-Yuan point combination. First, as the main point, we needle the Yuan point on the affected side and then, as a secondary point, the Luo point on the internally-externally related channel on the opposite side.

Sixth Step: Extraordinary Vessels

In our opinion, no Extraordinary Vessel is effective to treat this disorder.

Option Two: Local Points

First Step: Painful Point(s) (Ah Shi)

Ah Shi Point(s). Palpation of the ulnar styloid reveals either the most painful point(s) (Ah Shi) corresponding to Blood stasis and therefore to be bled or an area of widespread pain corresponding to Qì stagnation and requiring needling. Pain could radiate distally to the ulnar side of the hand.

When the anatomical structure of the wrist allows us to, the cupping therapy should be used to bleed this point(s) paying attention not to damage the tendinous tissue with the lancet or the soft tissues with a too strong cupping. The needle should be inserted perpendicularly until the tendon sheath is reached.

Both in acute and chronic conditions, a moxa stick can be useful to promote the flow of Qì and Blood. However, attention should be paid since too much heat can increase the ongoing inflammatory process.

SI5. It can be considered a local point to treat ulnar styloiditis, although in reality it is only adjacent to the ulnar styloid process. We also use it because it is an insertion point of the Small Intestine Muscle

channel in the wrist, as we will see later. To ensure the accuracy and precision of local needle placement and manipulation, we prefer the supine position.

Second Step: Anatomically Mirrored Point(s) (Opposite Side)

The points to be needled are located on the opposite side and should correspond as precisely as possible to the anatomical mirror of the Ah Shi point(s) to be treated. The point(s) may or may not be tender on palpation. To ensure the accuracy and precision of needle placement and manipulation, we prefer the supine position.

Option Three: Adjacent Points

First Step: Adjacent Points

TE4 and HT7. They help promote the horizontal flow of local Qì.

SI5. It is a very important point since it is the insertion point of the Small Intestine Muscle channel in the wrist and as such it promotes the longitudinal flow of local Qì.

Option Four: Etiological Points

First Step: According to Patterns

LI4 and LR3 (Bilaterally). They promote the flow of Qì and help remove Blood stasis. Since LR3 is the Shu/Yuan point of the liver, it also helps nourish muscles and tendons.

ST36 (Bilaterally). It is used to tonify Qì and Blood in chronic Deficiency conditions or the phases of pain resolution that can turn into muscle weakness.

Second Step: General Points

GB34 (Bilaterally). It is the Hui-Gathering point of Sinews and is specifically used for ulnar styloiditis, which is a type of tenosynovitis. In addition, it promotes the flow of Qì thus contributing to remove Blood stasis.

BL17 (Bilaterally). It is the Hui-Gathering point of Blood to remove Blood stasis.

BL18 (bilaterally). It treats all Excess and Deficiency conditions of the Liver that may favor the onset or duration of musculotendinous symptoms. It harmonizes the flow of Qì and Blood and enhances the treatment of tendons and muscle.

Option Five: Microsystems

First Step: Wrist and Ankle Acupuncture

Upper 6. It roughly corresponds to the pathway of the Small Intestine channels, which is directed toward the ulnar styloid (Fig. 4.28).

BOX 4.3 ACUTE OR CHRONIC PAIN FROM EXCESS ACUPUNCTURE TREATMENT

Option 1 Distal points	• Jing-Well points SI1 • Luo points SI7 (opposite side) • Point according to the Six Stages BL-60 (opposite side) • Shu-Stream points SI3 (affected side) and Shu-Stream points BL65 (opposite side) • Jing-River points SI5
Option 2 Local points	• Ah Shi • SI5 • Anatomically mirrored point(s) (opposite side)
Option 3 Adjacent points	• TE4 • HT7 • Insertion points SI5
Option 4 Etiological points	• LI4 and LR3 (bilaterally) • GB34 (bilaterally) • BL17 (bilaterally) • BL18 (bilaterally)

Option 5
Microsystems
	• W-A acupuncture
	  • Upper 6
	  • Upper 5
	• Ear acupuncture (opposite side)
	  • Wrist
	  • Liver
	  • Subcortex and Shenmen

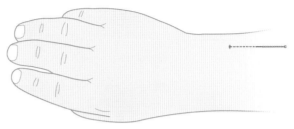

Fig. 4.28 Upper 6.

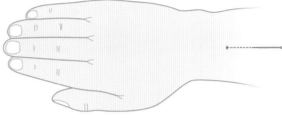

Fig. 4.29 Upper 5.

Upper 5. It controls upper limb mobility. In this specific case, we recommend directing the needle toward the hand (Fig. 4.29).

Second Step: Ear Acupuncture (Fig. 4.30)
Local point: Wrist
Zang Fu point: Liver
General points: Subcortex and Shenmen
Acute or Chronic Pain From Excess
Intense Pain or Range of Motion Reduced by Pain. The principle of treatment is to remove Qì stagnation and Blood stasis and expel EPFs or IPFs, if any (Box 4.3).
Chronic Pain From Deficiency
Dull Pain or Muscle Weakness. The principle of treatment is to tonify Qì and Blood, strengthen tissues,

and avoid pain exacerbation from physical activities or invasion of EPFs (Box 4.4).

Therapeutic Program, Frequency of Sessions

The frequency of sessions depends on the clinical condition of the patient. If the condition is acute or chronic with intense pain, we recommend sessions twice a week for 2 weeks and then once a week for another weeks. If improvement is observed, sessions are then scheduled once a week until complete pain relief or at least a reduction by 80% to 90%. If not, the whole clinical picture should be reconsidered, and the patient should be referred to another specialist.

If the condition is chronic with dull pain, we recommend sessions once a week for 4 weeks. Afterward, if the patient continues to improve, sessions are then scheduled once a week until complete pain relief or at a least reduction by 80% to 90%.

Clinical Notes

• Treatment of ulnar styloiditis results in better outcomes for patients than treatment of radial styloiditis.

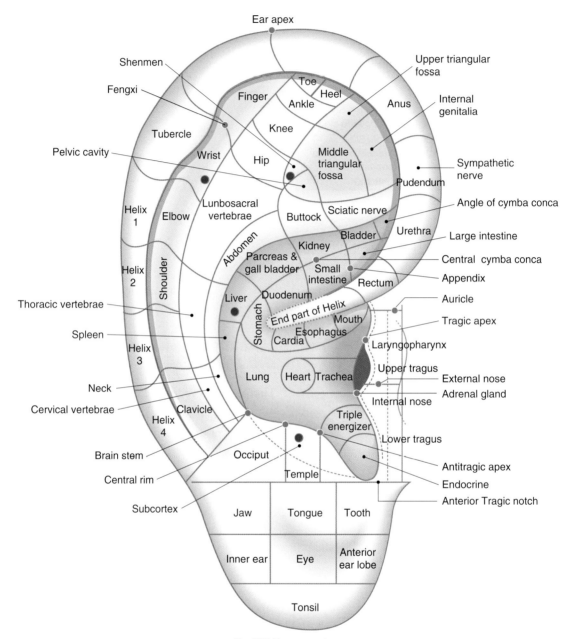

Fig. 4.30 Ear acupuncture.

Extensor Tenosynovitis

The Five Options and Selection of Acupoints

The approach we suggest is widely described in the section dedicated to the Fundamentals of acupuncture for MSK pain in the limbs (see Chapter 1).

The most important aspect is the identification of the Ah Shi point(s) to determine which channels are affected. In this specific case, the Triple Energizer Muscle and Connecting channels are involved.

BOX 4.4 CHRONIC PAIN FROM DEFICIENCY ACUPUNCTURE TREATMENT

Option 1 Distal points	• Yuan point SI4 • Luo points HT5 (opposite side) • Point according to the Six Stages BL60 (opposite side) • Jing-River point SI5
Option 2 Local points	• Ah Shi • SI5
Option 3 Adjacent points	• TE4 • HT7 • Insertion points SI5
Option 4 Etiological points and general points	• ST36 (bilaterally) • GB34 (bilaterally) • LR3 (bilaterally) • BL18 (bilaterally)

Option 5
Microsystems
	• W-A acupuncture
	  • Upper 6
	  • Upper 5
	• Ear acupuncture (opposite side)
	  • Wrist
	  • Liver
	  • Subcortex and Shenmen

Pricking pain localized on the tendon is a sign of Blood stasis to be treated with the bleeding technique, whereas pain radiating along the dorsum of the hand is a sign of Qì stagnation to be treated with the needling technique.

It is worth reminding that the distal points should be needled one at a time and their effectiveness in terms of pain and range of motion tested after each insertion. The same applies to the local points.

Finally, since both options 1 and 2 consist of several steps, it is important to highlight how selection should be made. Specifically, the practitioner might wonder if all or some of the steps should be followed. The rule we follow is simple: when the result achieved is satisfactory, the remaining steps should be skipped, and the practitioner should move to the following

option. Similarly, the use of the points recommended under options 3, 4, and 5 should be carefully evaluated according to the case being treated.

The points and accessory techniques we recommend using are listed below.

The Order of Needling

Option One: Distal Points

First Step: Triple Energizer Muscle Channel

TE1. This Jing-Well point activates the Triple Energizer Muscle channel and removes Qì stagnation and Blood stasis with needling and bleeding techniques, respectively.

Second Step: Triple Energizer Connecting Channels

TE5 (Opposite Side). This Luo point activates the Triple Energizer Connecting channels and removes Qì stagnation and Blood stasis in acute and chronic conditions from Excess.

PC6 (Opposite Side). This Luo point activates the Pericardium Connecting channels and is also used in chronic Deficiency conditions with dull pain to tonify Qì and Blood in the internally-externally related Triple Energizer channels. In the latter case, we associate Yuan point TE4 with Luo point PC6, which is the well-known Luo-Yuan point combination: first, as the main point, we needle the Yuan point on the affected side and then, as a secondary point, the Luo point on the internally-externally related channel on the opposite side.

Third Step: Empirical Points

There is no point that is classically recommended.

Fourth Step: Opposite Extremity (Upper/ Lower)

GB40 (Opposite Side). It is located in the ankle joint, which corresponds to the wrist joint on the paired channel according to the Six Stages.

It is worth remembering that the extensor synovitis of the wrist can radiate to the dorsum of the hand; this means we can palpate the lateral dorsum of the foot along the Gall Bladder Main channel to possibly find a tender point(s).

In clinical practice, the mirror concept can lead us to select the point, which may be tender or not, in the center and on the anterior side of the ankle, at the level of ST41, or on the dorsum of the foot, the area that in practice corresponds to the extensor muscles of the hand, although this area is not located on the Gall Bladder Main channel.

In line with our principle of treatment, we first needle GB40 and then test its effectiveness soon after insertion; if the result is not satisfactory, we remove the needle and move to the second option.

Our technique consists of needling the opposite extremity (lower/upper) on the opposite side in acute and chronic conditions. Alternatively, the most tender point on palpation is selected on the same or opposite side.

Fifth Step: Categories of Traditional Points

TE3 (Affected Side) and GB41 (Opposite Side). A good combination includes the Shu-Stream points on the paired channel according to the Six Stages. First, we needle the Shu-Stream point on the channel involved on the affected side and then the Shu-Stream point on the coupled channel on the opposite side and opposite extremity (upper/lower). We use this technique in acute and chronic Excess conditions to treat pain and expel or prevent invasion of EPFs.

TE6. The Jing-River points are used in acute or chronic Excess conditions due to the invasion of an EPF, and they are needled to promote its expulsion from their respective channels. They are also useful to prevent pain exacerbation from seasonal changes or invasion of EPFs.

TE7. The Xi-Cleft points are specifically used in acute conditions to treat Blood stasis in their respective channels. However, they are more effective in the Yin rather than in the Yang channels; hence, we would rather avoid using TE7 to treat this condition.

TE4. We recommend using this Yuan-Source point in chronic Deficiency conditions with dull pain, in case of weakness, or in the resolution phases of extensor tenosynovitis, to tonify Qì and Blood in the Triple Energizer channels.

In this situation, we can also associate Yuan point TE4 with Luo point PC6, which is the well-known Luo-Yuan point combination. First, as the main point, we needle the Yuan point on the affected side and then, as a secondary point, the Luo point on the internally-externally related channel on the opposite side.

We also use TE4 because it is a local point of the wrist and an insertion point in the Triple Energizer Muscle channel, as we will see later.

Sixth Step: Extraordinary Vessels

In our opinion, no Extraordinary Vessel is effective to treat this disorder.

Option Two: Local Points

First Step: Painful Point(s) (Ah Shi)

Ah Shi Point(s). Palpation of the dorsal aspect of the wrist and hand reveals either the most painful point(s) (Ah Shi) corresponding to Blood stasis and therefore to be bled or an area of widespread pain corresponding to Qì stagnation and requiring needling.

When the anatomical structure of the wrist allows us to, the cupping therapy should be used to bleed this point(s) paying attention not to damage the tendinous tissue with the lancet or the soft tissues with too strong cupping. The needle should be inserted perpendicularly until the tendon sheath is reached.

Both in acute and chronic conditions, a moxa stick can be useful to promote the flow of Qì and Blood. However, attention should be paid since too much heat can increase the ongoing inflammatory process.

TE4. It can be considered a local point to treat extensor tenosynovitis. We also use it because it is an insertion point of the Triple Energizer Muscle channel, as we will see later. To ensure the accuracy and precision of local needle placement and manipulation, we prefer the supine position.

Second Step: Anatomically Mirrored Point(s) (Opposite Side)

The points to be needled are located on the opposite side and should correspond as precisely as possible to the anatomical mirror of the Ah Shi point(s) to be treated. The point(s) may or may not be tender on palpation. To ensure the accuracy and precision of needle placement and manipulation, we prefer the supine position.

Option Three: Adjacent Points

First Step: Adjacent Points

TE5. It is a very important point since its classical target is the wrist, and furthermore, it is located on the affected channel.

LI5 and SI5. They help promote the horizontal flow of local Qì.

Option Four: Etiological Points

First Step: According to Patterns

LI4 and LR3 (Bilaterally). They promote the flow of Qì and help remove Blood stasis. Since LR3 is the Shu/Yuan point of the liver, it also helps nourish muscles and tendons.

ST36 (Bilaterally). It is used to tonify Qì and Blood in chronic Deficiency conditions or the phases of pain resolution that can turn into muscle weakness. In addition, it could be useful to apply moxa on the needle.

Second Step: General Points

GB34 (Bilaterally). It is the Hui-Gathering point of Sinews and is specifically used for extensor tenosynovitis. In addition, it promotes the flow of Qì thus contributing to remove Blood stasis.

BL17 (Bilaterally). It is the Hui-Gathering point of Blood to remove Blood stasis.

BL18 (Bilaterally). It treats all Excess and Deficiency conditions of the Liver that may favor the onset or duration of musculotendinous symptoms. It harmonizes the flow of Qì and Blood and enhances the treatment of tendons and muscle.

Option Five: Microsystems

First Step: Wrist and Ankle Acupuncture

Upper Five. It roughly corresponds to the pathway of the Triple Energizer channels and controls upper limb mobility. In this specific case, we recommend directing the needle toward the hand (Fig. 4.31).

Second Step: Ear Acupuncture (Fig. 4.32)

Local point: Wrist

Zang Fu point: Liver

General points: Subcortex and Shenmen

Acute or Chronic Pain From Excess

Intense Pain or Range of Motion Reduced by Pain. The principle of treatment is to remove Qì stagnation and Blood stasis and expel EPFs or IPFs, if any (Box 4.5).

Chronic pain from Deficiency

Dull pain or muscle weakness. The principle of treatment is to tonify Qì and Blood, strengthen tissues, and avoid pain exacerbation from physical activities or invasion of EPFs (Box 4.6).

Therapeutic Program, Frequency of Sessions

The frequency of sessions depends on the clinical condition of the patient. If the condition is acute or chronic with intense pain, we recommend sessions twice a week for 2 weeks and then once a week for another 2 weeks. If improvement is observed, sessions are then scheduled once a week until complete pain relief or at least a reduction by 80%–90%. If not, the whole clinical picture should be reconsidered and the patient referred to another specialist.

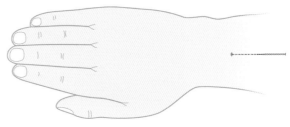

Fig. 4.31 Upper 5.

If the condition is chronic or with dull pain, we recommend sessions once a week for 4 weeks. Afterward, and if the patient continues to improve, sessions are then scheduled once a week until complete pain relief or at least a reduction by 80%–90%.

OSTEOPATHIC MANIPULATIVE TREATMENT

This section deals with osteopathic manipulations to treat wrist joint dysfunctions.

As already mentioned in the section dedicated to the fundamentals of osteopathy for MSK pain in the limbs (see Chapter 1), the key point of the osteopathic therapeutic process is the treatment not only of the somatic dysfunctions of the wrist but also of those which are functionally and anatomically related.

Consequently, the osteopathic manipulative approach to MSK wrist pain is based on the identification of joint somatic dysfunctions not only of the wrist, but also of the shoulder and elbow. Regardless of the condition to be treated, be it radial or ulnar styloiditis, extensor tenosynovitis, arthritis of the wrist, or surgical outcomes, all of the dysfunctions identified should be treated.

Somatic Dysfunctions of the Distal Radioulnar Joint

Posterior Ulna: Treatment

Posterior dysfunction: posterior sliding is better than anterior sliding. The patient is supine with incomplete elbow extension and forearm in pronation. The practitioner stands on the patient's right side with the thumbs placed posteriorly on the ulna and the index fingers anteriorly on the radius.

After joint decoaptation and rebalancing, first the wrist is slightly flexed, then the thrust is performed on the ulna in a forward direction by combining extension and supination of the hand (Figs. 4.33 and 4.34; Video 4.10).

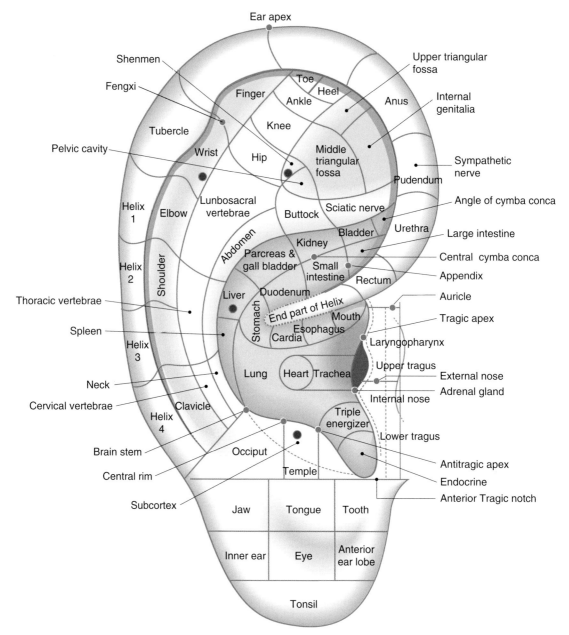

Fig. 4.32 Ear acupuncture.

ANTERIOR ULNA: TREATMENT

Anterior dysfunction: anterior sliding is better than posterior sliding. The patient is supine with incomplete elbow extension and forearm in supination. The practitioner stands on the patient's right side with the

BOX 4.5 ACUTE OR CHRONIC PAIN FROM EXCESS ACUPUNCTURE TREATMENT

Option 1 Distal points	• Jing-Well points TE1 • Luo points TE5 (opposite side) • Point according to the Six Stages GB40 (opposite side) • Shu-Stream points TE3 (affected side) and Shu-Stream points GB41 (opposite side) • Jing-River points TE6
Option 2 Local points	• Ah Shi • TE4 • Anatomically mirrored point(s) (opposite side)
Option 3 Adjacent points	• LI5 • SI5 • Insertion points TE4
Option 4 Etiological points	• LI4 and LR3 (bilaterally) • GB34 (bilaterally) • BL17 (bilaterally) • BL18 (bilaterally)

Option 5
Microsystems
	• W-A acupuncture
	  • Upper 5
	• Ear acupuncture (opposite side)
	  • Wrist
	  • Liver
	  • Subcortex and Shenmen

BOX 4.6 CHRONIC PAIN FROM DEFICIENCY ACUPUNCTURE TREATMENT

Option 1 Distal points	• Yuan point TE4 • Luo points PC6 (opposite side) • Point according to the Six Stages BL40 (opposite side) • Jing-River point TE6
Option 2 Local points	• Ah Shi • SI4
Option 3 Adjacent points	• LI5 • SI5 • Insertion points TE4
Option 4 Etiological points and general points	• ST36 (bilaterally) • GB34 (bilaterally) • LR3 (bilaterally) • BL18 (bilaterally)

Option 5
Microsystems
	• W-A acupuncture
	  • Upper 5
	• Ear acupuncture (opposite side)
	  • Wrist
	  • Liver
	  • Subcortex and Shenmen

thumbs placed anteriorly on the ulna and the index fingers posteriorly on the radius.

After joint decoaptation and rebalancing, first the wrist is slightly extended, then the thrust is performed on the ulna in a backward direction by combining flexion and pronation of the hand (Figs. 4.35 and 4.36; Video 4.11).

Somatic Dysfunctions of the Radiocarpal Joint

Posterior Carpus: Treatment

Posterior dysfunction: posterior sliding is better than anterior sliding. The patient is supine with incomplete elbow extension and forearm in pronation. The

practitioner stands on the patient's right side and holds the wrist by placing the thumbs posteriorly on the carpal bones and the index fingers anteriorly on the radius.

After joint decoaptation and rebalancing, slight wrist traction and extension, the thrust is performed with the thumbs in a downward direction while extending the wrist (Figs. 4.37 and 4.38; Video 4.12).

Anterior Carpus: Treatment

Anterior dysfunction: anterior sliding is better than posterior sliding. The patient is supine with incomplete elbow extension and forearm in pronation. The practitioner stands on the patient's right side and holds the wrist by placing the thumbs posteriorly on the radius and the index fingers anteriorly on the carpal bones.

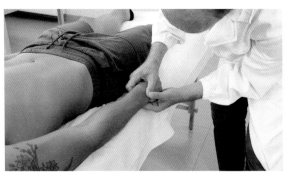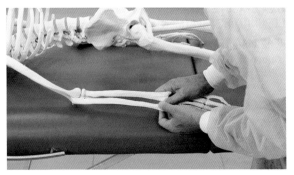

Fig. 4.33 Posterior ulna: treatment. Starting position.

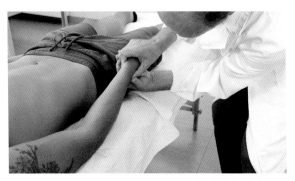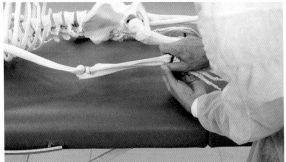

Fig. 4.34 Posterior ulna: treatment. Final position.

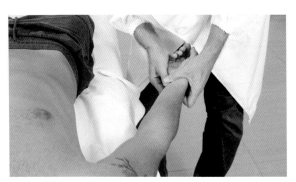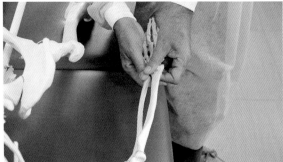

Fig. 4.35 Anterior ulna: treatment. Starting position.

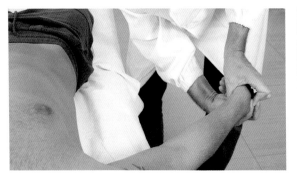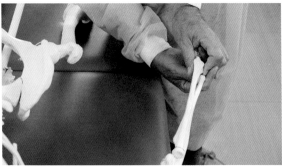

Fig. 4.36 Anterior ulna: treatment. Final position.

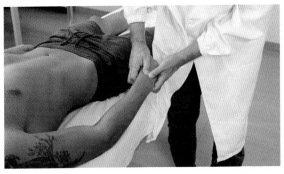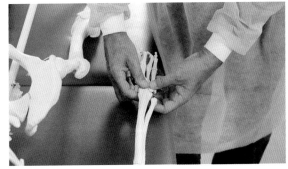

Fig. 4.37 Posterior carpus: treatment. Starting position.

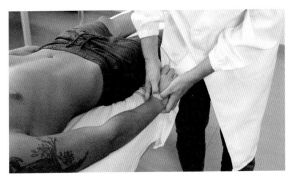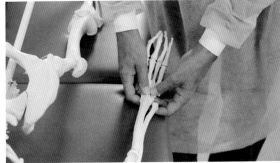

Fig. 4.38 Posterior carpus: treatment. Final position.

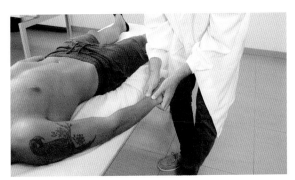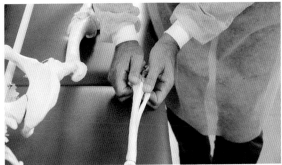

Fig. 4.39 Anterior carpus: treatment. Starting position.

After joint decoaptation and rebalancing, slight wrist traction and flexion, the thrust is performed with the index fingers in an upward direction while flexing the wrist (Figs. 4.39 and 4.40; Video 4.13).

Compression of the Carpus: Decompression Treatment

Carpal Dysfunction: Movements of the Carpal Bones are Restricted

The treatment consists of four steps. The patient is supine with the elbow flexed at 90 degrees and the

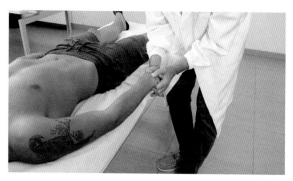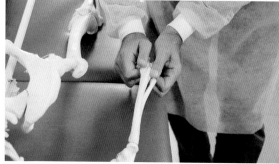

Fig. 4.40 Anterior carpus: treatment. Final position.

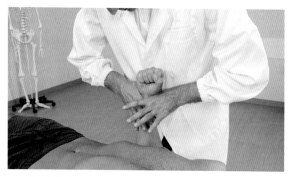

Fig. 4.41 Decompression treatment of the carpus: first step.

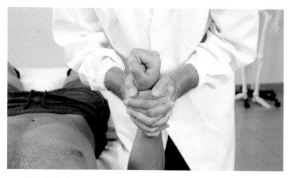

Fig. 4.43 Decompression treatment of the carpus: third step.

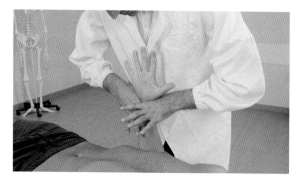

Fig. 4.42 Decompression treatment of the carpus: second step.

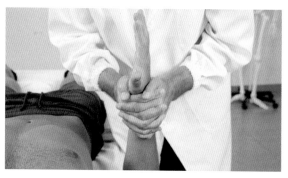

Fig. 4.44 Decompression treatment of the carpus: fourth step.

wrist in a neutral position. The practitioner stands close to the patient's right side. The practitioner stands close to the patient's right side and places the distal margins of the first intermetacarpal space on the sides of the radiocarpal joint to compress and decompress it. Then, the patient is asked to clench their fist and release it wide while compression is increased. The sequence is repeated three times, each

time increasing the force applied (Figs. 4.41 and 4.42; Video 4.14).

The practitioner places the thenar eminences posteriorly and anteriorly on the carpal bones to compress and decompress them. Then, the patient is asked to clench their fist and release it wide while compression is increased. The sequence is repeated three times, each time increasing the force applied (Figs. 4.43 and 4.44).

Therapeutic Program, Frequency of Sessions

The AcuOsteo Method of treatment combines acupuncture and osteopathic manipulations and, in principle, both therapeutic techniques are used during each session and at the same time.

If the condition is acute or chronic with intense pain, we recommend sessions twice a week for 2 weeks and then once a week for another 2 weeks. If improvement is observed, sessions are then scheduled once a week until complete pain relief or at least a reduction by 80%–90%.

In practice, however, as the osteopathic approach differs from acupuncture in that it follows a mechanical principle and aims to restore proper joint mobility, we opt for a parsimonious use of osteopathic manipulations over acupuncture; there may be no need to repeat them in every session.

Osteopathic maneuvres are therefore performed in case of persistent somatic dysfunction. That is why the patient should always be reevaluated at the beginning of each session to assess joint conditions and compare them with preexisting dysfunction.

Clinical Notes

- Treatment of extensor tenosynovis usually meet both patient's and practitioner's expectations.

BIBLIOGRAPHY

Baldry PE. *Acupuncture, Trigger Points and Musculoskeletal Pain.* 3rd ed. Elsevier; 2005.

Buckup K. *Test Ortopedici.* Verduci Editore; 1997.

Cipriano JJ. *Test Ortopedici e Neurologici.* Verduci Editore; 1998.

De Seze S, Ryckewaert A. *Malattie dell'osso e delle articolazioni.* Aulo Gaggi Editore; 1979.

Gay J. *Osteopatia, l'Arto Superiore.* Editore Marrapese; 1989.

Giusti R. *Glossary of Osteophatic Terminology.* 3rd ed. American Association of Colleges of Osteophatic Medicine; 2017.

Greenman PE. *Principles of Manual Medicine.* 2nd ed. Williams & Wilkins; 1996.

Guolo F. *Atlante di Tecniche di Energia Muscolare.* Piccin; 2014.

Hoppenfeld S. *L'Esame Obiettivo dell'Apparato Locomotore.* Aulo Gaggi Editore; 1985.

Legge D. *Close to the Bone.* Sydney College Press; 2010.

Maciocia G. *The Practice of Chinese Medicine.* 3rd ed. Elsevier; 2022.

Misulis KE, Head TC. *Neurologia di Netter.* Elsevier, Masson; 2008.

Nicholas AS, Nicholas EA. *Atlas of Osteophatic Thechniques.* Lippincott Williams & Wilkins; 2012.

Qiao W. *Wrist and Ankle and Balance Acupuncture, Italian Chine School of Acupuncture-A.M.A.B. (Association of Medical Acupuncturist of Bologna).* Seminar; 2007.

Romoli M. *Auricular Acupuncture Diagnosis.* Churchill Livingstone Elsevier; 2009.

Tan RT. *Dr. Tan's Strategy of Twelve Magical Points.* Edited by Besinger J.W., San Diego, California, 2003.

Tixa S. *Atlas d'Anatomie Palpatoire, tome 1, Cou, Tronc, Membre Superior.* 2é edition. Elsevier Masson; 2005.

Tixa S, Ebenegger B. *Atlas de Techniques articulaires ostéopathiques, tome 1, Les Membres.* 3é edition. Elsevier Masson; 2016.

Chapter 5

The Hip

Hip Pain and Trochanteric Bursitis

Hip pain is a common complaint. It is usually located in the groin and can be due to a variety of causes, such as femoroacetabular impingement (FAI), repetitive strain injuries, sports injuries, and arthritis.

Lateral hip pain is often due to trochanteric bursitis, which is inflammation of the superficial trochanteric bursa lying between the tensor fasciae latae and the greater trochanter.

Anatomy and Biomechanics According to Western Medicine

JOINTS AND MUSCLES

The Pelvic Girdle

The pelvic girdle is a bony ring consisting of the sacrum, the coccyx, and two hip bones. There are four articulations within the pelvis (Figs. 5.1 and 5.2):
- One sacrococcygeal joint
- Two sacroiliac joints
- One pubic symphysis

The sacrum is a triangle-shaped bone made up of five fused vertebrae, concave anteriorly and convex posteriorly. Its superior aspect articulates superiorly with the L5 vertebral body, whereas its inferior aspects articulate with the coccyx. The wings of the sacrum articulate bilaterally with the ilium thus forming the two sacroiliac joints.

The coccyx is a triangular bone consisting of three to five segments, concave anteriorly and convex posteriorly. It is the terminal part of the spine. The two hip bones are symmetrical and flat. Each hip bone consists of three fused bones: ilium, ischium, and pubis.

The upper portion of the hip bone is the ilium. The body of the ilium forms the acetabular roof, where the head of the femur articulates with the acetabulum itself to form the hip joint. The wing of the ilium is above the body and articulates posteriorly with the sacrum. The wing forms the iliac crest, which extends from the anterior superior iliac spine (ASIS) to the posterior superior iliac spine (PSIS).

The posteroinferior portion of the hip bone is the ischium, which is composed of a body, an inferior ramus, and a superior ramus. The body of the ischium joins the inferior and superior ramus. The inferior ischial ramus combines with the inferior pubic ramus forming the ischiopubic ramus. The ischiopubic ramus and the superior pubic ramus form the obturator foramen, which is covered by the homonymous membrane. The superior ischial ramus includes the posterior portion of the acetabulum and a bony prominence, the ischial tuberosity, which provides support when sitting.

The anterior portion of the hip bone is the pubis and consists of a body, a superior ramus, and an inferior ramus. The body joins the superior and inferior rami and articulates with the opposite pubic body to form the pubic symphysis. The superior pubic ramus extends laterally from the body and forms the anterior part of the acetabulum. The ischiopubic ramus results from the joining of the inferior pubic ramus with the inferior ischial ramus.

As already mentioned, the ischiopubic ramus with the superior pubic ramus form the obturator foramen, which is covered by the homonymous membrane.

The muscles attaching to and acting on the three joints of the pelvic girdle complex can be divided into:
- Muscles of the pelvis, strictly connected with the essential bodily functions of the organs they enclose (e.g., the pelvic floor muscles: elevator ani and urethral sphincter muscles).
- Muscles of the back, which stabilize and orientate the pelvis, and provide support to the spine (e.g., quadratus lumborum and multifidus).

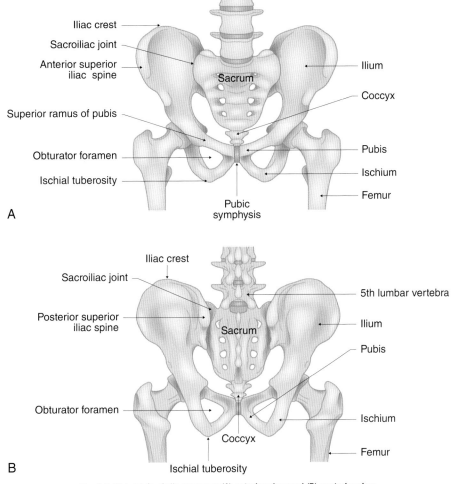

Fig. 5.1 The pelvic girdle anatomy: (A) anterior view and (B) posterior view.

- Muscles of the abdomen, which stabilize and orientate the pelvis through connection with the trunk (rectus abdominis, external and internal oblique muscles, and transversus abdominis).
- Muscles of the hip, to be divided into two groups for didactic purposes: those attaching to the femur and those to the pelvis (see below for an in-depth analysis).

The Hip

The hip joint, or coxofemoral joint, is made up of the femoral head and the acetabulum of the hip bone (Fig. 5.3).

The hip joint is commonly known as a ball and socket joint, where the ball is the head of the femur and the socket is the acetabulum of the hip bone. The ball fits perfectly inside the socket and ensures good mobility through its inherent stability.

As already mentioned, the acetabulum of the hip bone is made up of fused portions of the ilium, ischium, and pubis. The femur is a long bone, made up of a head, a shaft, and the femoral condyles.

- Head: it articulates with the acetabulum of the hip bone. The neck connects the head with the shaft. The neck projects in a superior and medial direction. Above and lateral to the neck-shaft

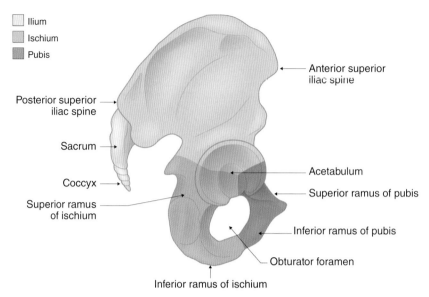

Ilium
Ischium
Pubis

Anterior superior iliac spine

Posterior superior iliac spine

Sacrum

Coccyx

Superior ramus of ischium

Acetabulum

Superior ramus of pubis

Inferior ramus of pubis

Obturator foramen

Inferior ramus of ischium

Fig. 5.2 The pelvic girdle anatomy lateral view.

junction, the greater trochanter projects from the anterior aspect, whereas medial and inferior to the neck-shaft junction, the lesser trochanter projects from the posteromedial side of the femur.

- Shaft: it is the long, straight part of the femur. Roughened ridges of bone (the linea aspera) are visible on the posterior surface of the shaft.
- Condyles: they articulate with the tibial plateau to form the knee joint.

The hip muscles that attach to the femur and pelvis can be grouped based on their functions:

- When they make a fixed point to the femur, they assist with pelvic stabilization and orientation.
- When they make a fixed point to the pelvis, they assist with hip movements and orientation.

Gluteus maximus, medius, and minimus; piriformis; iliopsoas; obturator externus and internus; superior and inferior gemellus; and quadratus femoris belong to the first group and are known as the muscles of the hip.

Tensor fasciae latae (TFL); quadriceps; sartorius; adductors longus, brevis, and magnus; hamstrings; gracilis; and pectineus belong to the second group and are known as the muscles of the thigh. Without getting into too many details, we can mention the following.

First Group

The gluteus maximus arises from the sacrum, coccyx, ilium, and sacrotuberous ligament. It attaches to the linea aspera on the proximal third of the femur and the iliotibial band (ITB) of the TFL. This muscle allows the hip to abduct, extend, and extrarotate.

The gluteus medius and minimus arise from the ilium and attach to the greater trochanter. These muscles allow the hip to abduct.

The obturator externus arises from the external bony margin of the obturator foramen and attaches to the posterior portion of the greater trochanter. This muscle allows the hip to extrarotate.

Second Group

The TFL is a muscle that arises from the ASIS, whose belly usually ends before the greater trochanter. Then, it runs as a fascia superficially to the greater trochanter and inserts distally to the ITB. Finally, the ITB attaches to the lateral condyle of the tibia. This muscle allows the hip to abduct.

The quadriceps femoris consists of four muscles: the vastus lateralis, medialis, and intermedius, which arise from the linea aspera of the femur, and the rectus femoris, which arises from the ASIS and the superior part of the acetabulum. These four muscles unite and

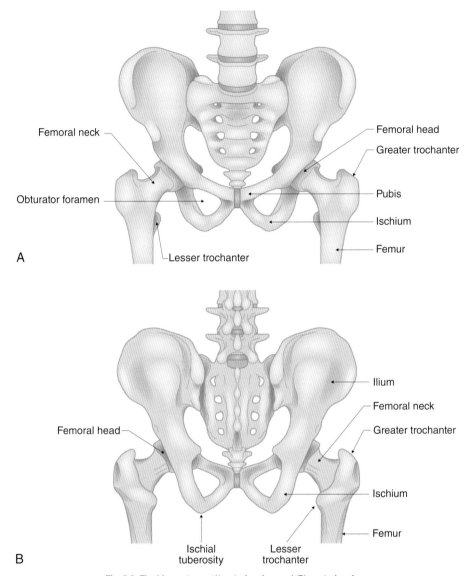

Fig. 5.3 The hip anatomy: (A) anterior view and (B) posterior view.

attach to the patella through the quadriceps tendon. In turn, the patellar tendon arises from the patella and attaches to the anterior tuberosity of the tibia. This muscle allows the hip to flex.

The sartorius arises from the ASIS and attaches to the medial condyle of the tibia where it joins with the tendons of the gracilis and semitendinosus in the pes anserinus (PA). This muscle allows the hip to flex.

The adductor longus arises from the superior pubic ramus lateral to the pubic symphysis and attaches to the linea aspera on the middle third of femur. This muscle allows the hip to adduct, extrarotate, and flex.

The hamstrings are a group of three muscles: the semitendinosus, semimembranosus, and biceps femoris. The semitendinosus arises from the ischial tuberosity and attaches to the medial condyle of the tibia,

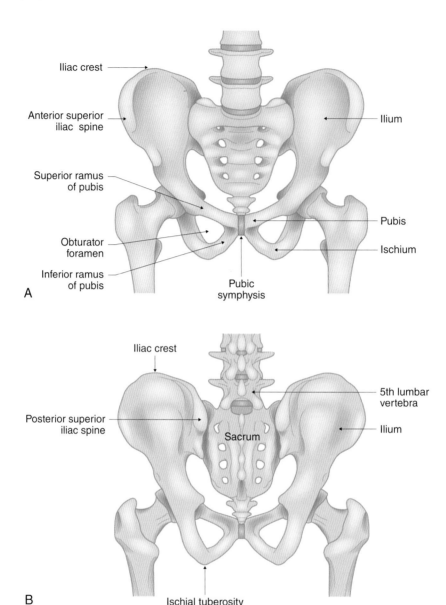

Fig. 5.4 The pelvic girdle anatomical landmarks: (A) anterior view and (B) posterior view.

where it joins with the tendons of the gracilis and sartorius in the PA. The semimembranosus arises from the ischial tuberosity and attaches to the posterior part of the medial tibial condyle.

As its name implies, the biceps femoris has two heads, a short head and a long head. The long head arises from the ischial tuberosity, whereas the short head arises from the linea aspera on the middle third of femur. They both attach to the fibular head. These muscles allow the hip to extend.

ANATOMICAL LANDMARKS
Pelvic Girdle

The iliac crest is the upper margin of the iliac wing (Fig. 5.4).

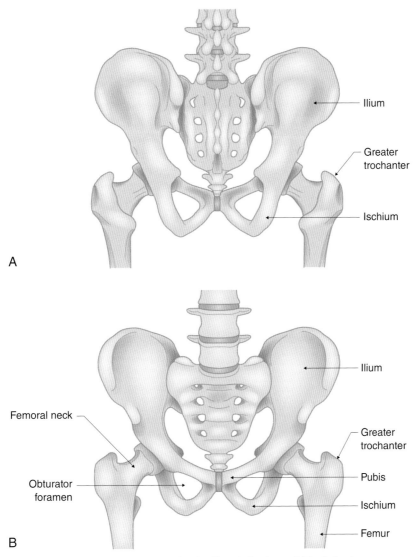

A

B

Fig. 5.5 The hip anatomical landmarks: (A) posterior view and (B) anterior view.

The ASIS is the anterior portion of the iliac crest. The pubic symphysis is the joint between the bodies of the two pubic bones. The PSIS is the posterior portion of the iliac crest, located at the level from the first to second sacral foramina. The sacrum articulates bilaterally with the hip bones. The ischial tuberosity provides support when sitting.

Hip

The neck of the femur connects the head with the shaft. The obturator foramen lies inferior and medial to the acetabulum. It is bordered by the superior pubic ramus and the ischiopubic ramus. It is almost completely covered by the homonymous membrane (Fig. 5.5).

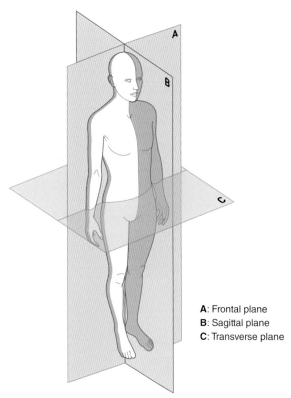

A: Frontal plane
B: Sagittal plane
C: Transverse plane

Fig. 5.6 The hip planes of symmetry of the body: (A) frontal plane, (B) sagittal plane, and (C) transverse plane.

JOINT MOVEMENTS

The Physiological Movements of the Hip

Biomechanics of the hip is very complex due to the multiple joints involved in its range of motion (ROM).

The hip joint has three degrees of freedom, which means it can move the lower limb in the three planes of symmetry of the body: sagittal plane, frontal plane, and transverse plane (Fig. 5.6).

The neutral position of the hip is with the patient supine, the lower limb extended in slightly external rotation; this is the starting position to assess.

- Flexion: lower limb forward and upward in the sagittal plane of the body.
- Extension: lower limb off the bed backward in the sagittal plane of the body.
- Abduction: lower limb raises laterally away from the midline in the frontal plane of the body.
- Adduction: lower limb moves toward the midline in the frontal plane of the body.

There are two methods to assess external and internal rotation.
- External rotation in the transverse plane of the body:
    the hip and the knee are flexed, foot on the bed. Then, the knee moves outward.
- External rotation in the frontal plane of the body:
    the hip and knee are flexed at 90 degrees. Then, the leg moves inward.
- Internal rotation in the transverse plane of the body:
    the hip and the knee are flexed, foot on the bed. Then, the knee moves inward.
- Internal rotation in the frontal plane of the body:
    the hip and knee are flexed at 90 degrees. Then, the leg moves outward.

The normal ROM of the hip from the neutral position.
- To full flexion is 0 to about 90 or 130 degrees, with extended or flexed knee, respectively
- To full extension is 0 to about 10 or 15 degrees, with extended or flexed knee, respectively
- To abduction, 0 to about 45 degrees
- To adduction, 0 to about 30 degrees

From the neutral position where the hip and knee are both flexed at 90 degrees
- To full external rotation, 0 to about 60 degrees
- To full internal rotation, 0 to about 50 degrees

Diagnosis in Western Medicine

HIP PAIN

Hip pain is a common symptom of several conditions, including femoroacetabular impingement (FAI), repetitive strain injuries, sports injuries, and arthritis. It usually manifests itself in the groin. According to our experience, hip pain is often regarded as the consequence of an anatomical alteration, such as FAI or arthritis, rather than being related to a functional disorder, such as altered joint loading.

The most common symptoms are the following:
1. Hip pain felt in the groin and, sometimes, in the gluteal region.
2. Pain radiating along the anterior compartment of the thigh up to the medial aspect of the knee.

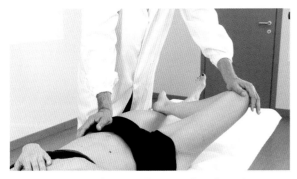

Fig. 5.7 Flexion, abduction, external rotation test.

3. ROM reduced by pain.
4. Stiffness.
5. Positive flexion, abduction, external rotation (FABER) test.

Flexion, Abduction, External Rotation Test

It is used to assess hip mobility.

The patient is supine (Fig. 5.7; Video 5.1). The practitioner stands on the patient's left side.

The hip is flexed, abducted, and externally rotated, with the lateral ankle resting on the contralateral thigh proximal to the knee. While stabilizing the left side of the pelvis on the ASIS, external rotation is performed, and posterior force slightly applied to the bent knee until the end ROM is achieved. The test is considered positive if the patient reports pain over the left groin area.

Rotation Test

The patient is supine with the hip and knee flexed at 90 degrees. The practitioner stands on the patient's right side.

The practitioner holds the patient's ankle with the right hand and brings the hip into external and internal rotation. The practitioner appreciates the range and quality of motion of external rotation and compares them with internal rotation.

If external rotation is better than internal rotation, then there is external rotation dysfunction, and vice versa. In case of external rotation dysfunction, internal

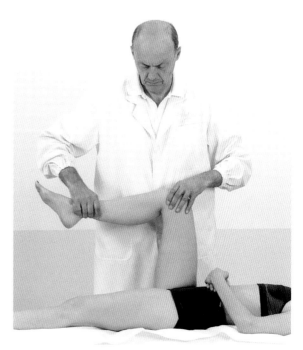

Fig. 5.8 Rotation test—starting position.

rotation can be not only restricted but also painful, and vice versa (Figs. 5.8—5.10; Video 5.2).

TROCHANTERIC BURSITIS

Trochanteric bursitis is the inflammation of the superficial trochanteric bursa lying between the tensor fasciae latae and the greater trochanter.

Trochanteric bursitis is the general term referring to the greater trochanteric pain syndrome (GTPS), which also includes gluteus medius and gluteus minimus tendinopathy, and the snapping hip syndrome (SHS).

Inflammation of the bursa is a slow process, which gets worse over time. Among the most frequent causes are overuse from work or sports, direct trauma, or postural imbalance.

The most common symptoms are the following:
1. Lateral hip pain
2. Pain radiating to the thigh

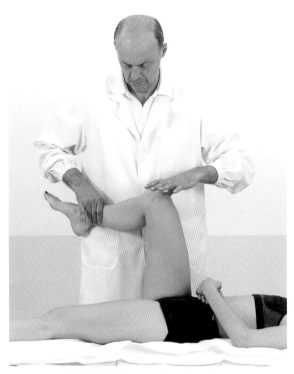

Fig. 5.9 Rotation test—internal rotation.

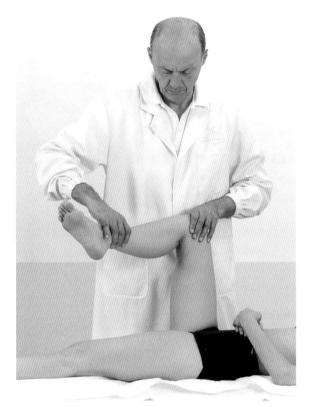

Fig. 5.10 Rotation test—external rotation.

3. Tenderness elicited by palpation over the greater trochanter
4. Pain when climbing the stairs
5. Pain with side-lying on the affected side
6. Pain-related sleep disturbance
7. Symptoms of a pseudosciatica
8. Positive trochanteric bursitis test

Test for Trochanteric Bursitis

It is used to assess trochanteric bursitis.

The patient lies on the left side with the left hip flexed and the right hip extended (Fig. 5.11; Video 5.3). The practitioner stands behind the patient, the left hand on the pelvis with fingers on the greater trochanter and the right hand on the ankle.

The patient is asked to abduct the leg while the practitioner applies a counterforce. The test is considered

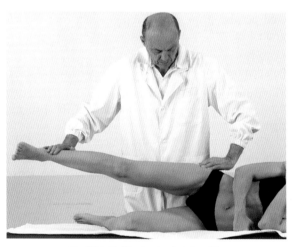

Fig. 5.11 Test for trochanteric bursitis.

positive if the patient reports pain either spontaneously or elicited by palpation over the greater trochanter.

JOINT PAIN, ARTHRITIS, AND STIFFNESS

Patients with hip arthritis and postsurgical outcomes usually complain of pain, weakness, and restricted ROM.

Hip arthritis is a commonly treated condition. Among its most common causes are fractures of the femoral neck, rheumatoid arthritis, septic arthritis, and primary osteoarthritis. Hip arthritis can get progressively worse to the point where a joint replacement is needed.

Diagnosis is based on the patient's medical history, clinical findings, and radiographic examinations.

The most common symptoms are the following:
- Anterior or medial hip pain during weight-bearing activities.
- Morning stiffness.
- ROM reduced by pain, internal and external rotation in particular.
- Radiography shows joint space narrowing, osteophytes, subchondral sclerosis, and bone cysts.

Avascular necrosis (AN) of the femoral head is a pathological condition that results from the loss of blood supply and leads to the collapse of the necrotic segment.

AN can be caused by trauma or nontraumatic events. In the latter case, causes are not easily identified, and therefore it can be defined as a "multifactorial condition." Examples of causes include excessive alcohol consumption, hypercholesterolemia, and therapy with corticosteroids.

The most common symptoms are the following:
1. Pain in the groin that can radiate to the knee or gluteal region.
2. ROM reduced by pain, internal and external rotation in particular.

RED FLAGS IN WESTERN MEDICINE

The presence of heat (calor), redness (rubor), swelling (tumor), pain (dolor), and loss of function (function laesa) determines the need for diagnostic investigations.

Hip trauma is not a common occurrence. Among the signs and symptoms of fracture or dislocation are swelling and deformity of the limb. A fracture affects the continuity of a bone, whereas a dislocation involves a joint.

Patients with rheumatoid arthritis of the hip usually complain of pain throughout the ROM; the hip is usually affected in the later stages of the disease. Both fatigue and general discomfort can also be observed.

Abnormalities uncovered on history taking or physical examination may require medical evaluation, laboratory tests, and imaging investigations, such as X-rays, ultrasound, CT, and MRI.

Red FLags	Pain	Inspection	Other Signs	Neurological Signs	Recommendations
Inflammation	Pain	Redness, swelling, and heat		Functional deficit	Physician evaluation Imaging investigations
Fracture	Spontaneous pain	Deformity and swelling	Movement beyond normal range of motion	Functional deficit	Physician evaluation Imaging investigations
Dislocation	Pain with movement	Deformity and joint swelling	Hematoma	Functional deficit	Physician evaluation Imaging investigations
Rheumatoid arthritis	Pain with or without movement	Redness and swelling	Fatigue and general discomfort	Functional deficit	Physician evaluation Imaging investigations Laboratory tests

Diagnosis in Chinese Medicine

In Chinese medicine, musculoskeletal pain results from the obstruction of Qì and Blood circulation or inadequate Qì and Blood for the nourishment of the secondary channels, especially the Muscle and Connecting channels.

The Muscle and Connecting channels more often involved in hip disorders are listed below:

- Stomach
- Spleen
- Liver
- Gall bladder

An Extraordinary channel, the Yang Qiao Mai, may also be involved.

The channels affected vary according to pain location:

- Stomach: pain is on the anterior side of the hip in the groin area; the pathology is hip pain
- Spleen: pain is on the medial side of the hip in the groin area; the pathology is hip pain
- Liver: pain is on the medial side of the hip in the groin area; the pathology is hip pain
- Gall Bladder: pain is on the lateral side of the hip; the pathology is trochanteric bursitis
- Yang Qiao Mai: pain is on the lateral side of the hip; the pathology is trochanteric bursitis

What matters most is to identify the affected channel where pain is located.

Sometimes, it is not so easy to determine it, and consequently the following data concerning the Muscle channels involved in hip movements should be acquired for a better identification.

- Flexion: ST and SP
- Extension: BL and GB
- Adduction: KI and LR
- Abduction: GB and BL
- Internal Rotation: LR and SP
- External Rotation: BL and GB

The information so acquired on the channel that is likely to be involved, that is, pain location and related movement restriction, can also be integrated with the results from Western medicine orthopedic tests in order to identify which muscle, tendon, and joint are affected in case of:

- Hip pain
- Trochanteric bursitis

ETIOLOGY

Hip pain is usually caused by:

- *Overuse, repetitive strain injury*. Through sports (running, dance, and gymnastics); performing the same movement over and over again causes local Qì stagnation or Qì and Blood deficiency.
- *Trauma, sport injuries*. If mild, they cause local Qì stagnation; if severe, they cause local Blood stasis.
- *Cold*. Local invasion causes Qì stagnation or Blood stasis.

Previous accidents often predispose the hip to more frequent invasions of external pathogenic factors (EPFs), especially Cold.

PATHOLOGY

The Muscle and Connecting channels and the Extraordinary channel Yang Qiao Mai are often affected by Qì stagnation and Blood stasis:

- Qì stagnation manifests itself with widespread pain radiating distally along the pathway of the Muscle channels and could be associated with muscle contracture and stiffness of the antero-medial and lateral thigh, also perceived upon palpation.
- Blood stasis, usually occurring in the Connecting channels, manifests itself with more intense pain localized in the joint or in the lateral thigh area over the TB.

As already mentioned in the fundamentals of acupuncture for MSK pain in the limbs (see Chapter 1), the term *Connecting channels* includes not only the Connecting channel "proper" but also the Connecting channel "area" that covers the whole pathway of the Main channel.

ANTERIOR HIP PAIN

To identify the Muscle and Connecting channels affected, we check the location and characteristics of musculoskeletal pain, palpate the affected area, test the ROM for each hip movement, and perform orthopedic tests to elicit pain.

The Pathways of the Stomach Secondary Channels

In case of hip pain, the Stomach Muscle and Connecting channels are involved.

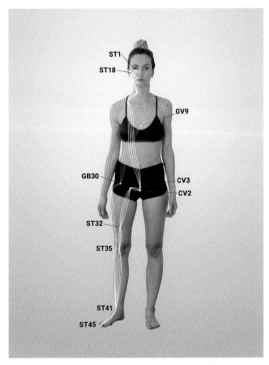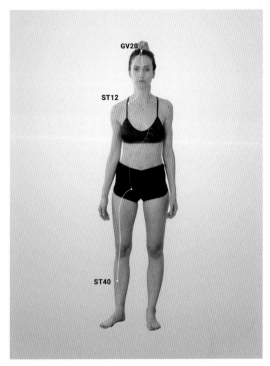

Fig. 5.12 The pathways of the Stomach Muscle and Connecting "proper" channels.

The pathway of the Stomach Muscle and Connecting channels explains pain on the anterior aspect of the hip and groin pain, which could radiate distally to the anterior thigh and knee (Fig. 5.12).

MEDIAL HIP PAIN

To identify the Muscle and Connecting channels affected, we check the location and characteristics of musculoskeletal pain, palpate the affected area, test the ROM for each hip movement, and perform orthopedic tests to elicit pain.

The Pathways of the Spleen Secondary Channels

In case of medial hip pain, the Spleen Muscle and Connecting channels may be involved.

The pathway of the Spleen Muscle and Connecting channels explains pain on the medial aspect of the hip and groin pain, which could radiate distally to the medial aspect of the upper thigh (Fig. 5.13).

The Pathways of the Liver Secondary Channels

In the case of medial hip, the Liver Muscle and Connecting channels may be involved.

The pathways of the Liver Muscle and Connecting channels run more medially than the Spleen channels and explain pain on the medial aspect of the hip and groin pain, which could radiate distally to the upper thigh along the adductor longus (Fig. 5.14).

TROCHANTERIC BURSITIS

To identify the Muscle and Connecting channels affected, we check the location and characteristics of musculoskeletal pain, palpate the affected area, test the ROM for each hip movement, and perform orthopedic tests to elicit pain.

The Pathways of the Gall Bladder Secondary Channels

In the case of trochanteric bursitis, the Gall Bladder Muscle and Connecting channels are involved.

The pathway of the Gall Bladder Muscle channels explains pain on the lateral aspect of the hip, in the greater trochanter, whereas the pathway of the Gall Bladder Connecting channel "proper" does not because it does not ascend to the hip.

Since we now refer to the Gall Bladder Connecting channel "area," we regard the Gall Bladder Connecting channels as channels involved (Fig. 5.15).

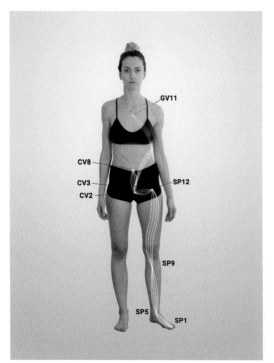
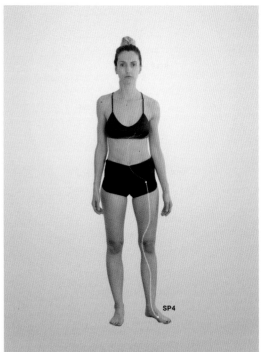

Fig. 5.13 The pathways of the Spleen Muscle and Connecting "proper" channels.

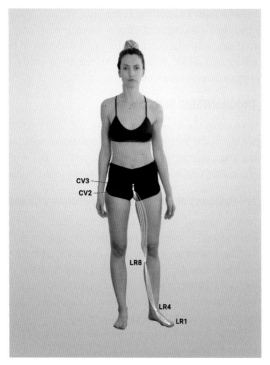
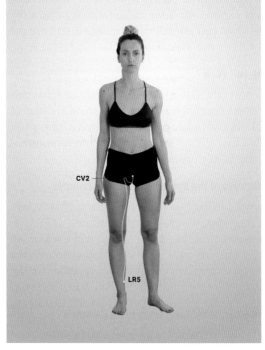

Fig. 5.14 The pathways of the Liver Muscle and Connecting "proper" channels.

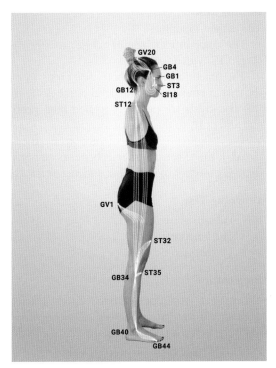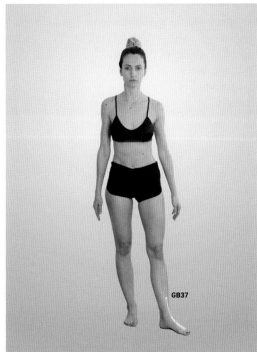

Fig. 5.15 The pathways of the Gall Bladder Muscle and Connecting "proper" channels.

The Pathway of the Yang Qiao Mai

In the case of trochanteric bursitis, the Yang Qiao Mai extraordinary channel may be involved as it starts from the lateral aspect of the heel, at BL62, and ascends along the lateral aspect of the lower extremity by passing over the greater trochanter (Fig. 5.16).

Diagnosis in Osteopathic Medicine

The examination for "somatic dysfunction" is the central concept of the diagnostic process; palpation of the affected area and functionally/anatomically related components of the somatic system is the only way to assess it.

Consequently, the osteopathic diagnostic approach to musculoskeletal hip pain is based on the identification of joint somatic dysfunctions not only of the pelvic girdle and hip but also of the knee and ankle.

Regardless of the condition to be treated, be it hip pain, trochanteric bursitis, arthritis of the hip, or surgical outcomes, all of the recommended tests should be performed to identify the dysfunctions that occur more frequently.

It is therefore evident that the osteopathic diagnosis is developed regardless of the condition to be treated; therefore the osteopathic tests recommended for the pelvic girdle and hip, knee, and ankle will not be repeated when the "injuries" are treated.

TESTS FOR THE MAIN SOMATIC DYSFUNCTIONS

The only way to diagnose somatic dysfunctions of a joint is to assess the passive movements of its articular ends in relation to one another and compare them with the same movements of the joint on the healthy side. Testing of the sacroiliac and hip joints is required.

On the same plane of motion, there is quantitatively and qualitatively equal passive mobility on both sides of a theoretical neutral point that represents the reference point.

When balance is lost and the range and quality of motion are not the same in both directions, then there is somatic dysfunction.

Tests of the Sacroiliac Joint

Tests are performed to assess the most common iliac dysfunctions:

- Anterior rotation of the ilium
- Posterior rotation of the ilium
- Iliac torsion
- Upslip

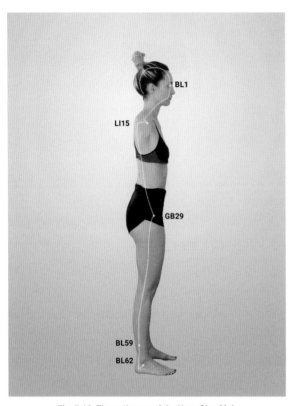

Fig. 5.16 The pathways of the Yang Qiao Mai.

Rolling Test

The patient is supine.

The practitioner stands close to the patient (Fig. 5.17; Video 5.4).

The practitioner holds both iliac crests by placing the thenar eminences at the level of the ASIS. In turn, the iliac crests are passively rotated both posteriorly and anteriorly to the ends of their ROM.

The range and quality of motion are then compared. If the affected side rolls better posteriorly, then there is posterior dysfunction, and vice versa.

Downing Test

It is made up of two tests:

- The lengthening test
- The shortening test

Preparation

The patient is supine with the knees flexed at 90 degrees and feet flat on the bed. The patient is asked to lift the pelvis by contracting the glutes and then the practitioner passively extends the legs on the bed.

The practitioner marks both medial malleoli with two lines for comparison after the test (Figs. 5.18–5.20; Video 5.5).

Downing Lengthening Test

The patient is supine with the legs extended (Fig. 5.21; Video 5.6). The practitioner stands on the patient's right side.

The hip is externally rotated and adducted, the knee slightly bent, and the foot placed on the anterior aspect of the opposite ankle. Then, the leg is returned to the starting position maintaining it in external

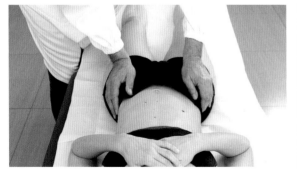
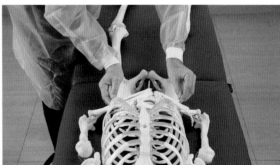

Fig. 5.17 Rolling test.

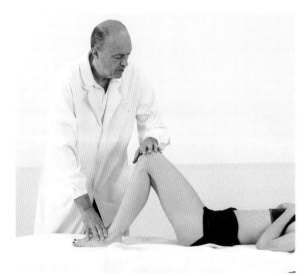

Fig. 5.18 Downing test—starting position.

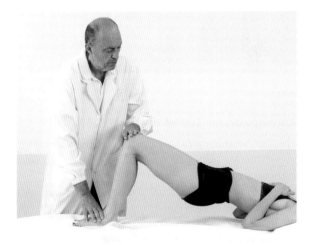

Fig. 5.19 Downing test—intermediate position.

rotation: the two markings are compared, and the tested leg should appear longer than the other. If not, then there is posterior rotation dysfunction.

Anterior rotation dysfunction is often observed on one side and posterior rotation dysfunction on the opposite side, the so-called iliac torsion dysfunction.

Downing Shortening Test

The patient is supine with the legs extended. The practitioner stands on the patient's right side (Fig. 5.22; Video 5.7).

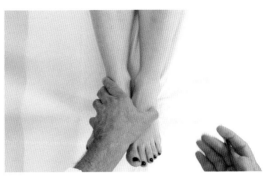

Fig. 5.20 Downing test—final position.

The hip is internally rotated and abducted, the knee flexed and off the bed. Then, the leg is returned to the starting position maintaining it in internal rotation; the two markings are compared, and the tested leg should appear shorter than the other. If not, then there is anterior rotation dysfunction.

As previously mentioned, anterior rotation dysfunction is often observed on one side and posterior rotation dysfunction on the opposite side, the so-called iliac torsion dysfunction.

Upslip: Evaluation of the Anatomical Landmarks

Observation and palpation of "three higher landmarks" on the affected side indicates the presence of an upslip dysfunction.

This traumatic dysfunction can be the result of a sudden vertical force through the outstretched leg and is associated with lifting of the hemipelvis on the affected side.

The patient stands opposite the practitioner (Fig. 5.23A and B):
- Higher iliac crest
- Higher ASIS
- Higher superior ramus of pubis

The patient is supine:
- Higher iliac crest
- Higher ASIS
- Higher superior ramus of pubis

The patient stands in front of the practitioner:
- Higher iliac crest
- Higher PSIS
- Higher ischial tuberosity

The patient is prone:
- Higher iliac crest
- Higher PSIS
- Higher ischial tuberosity

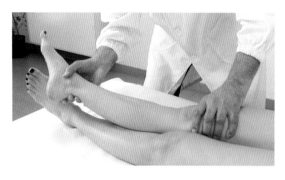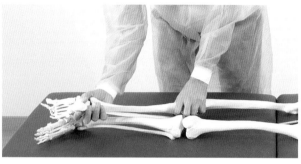

Fig. 5.21 Downing lengthening test.

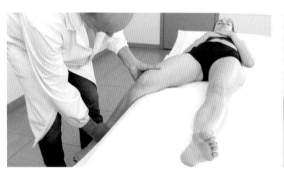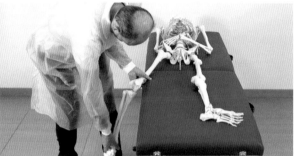

Fig. 5.22 Downing shortening test.

Test of the Pubic Symphysis

Compression Test of the Pubic Symphysis

This test is performed to assess the most common symphysis pubis dysfunction. The patient is supine (Fig. 5.24; Video 5.8).

The practitioner stands close to the patient. The practitioner places the thumbs on the anterior side of each pubic branch close to the pubic symphysis and the other fingers on the ASIS.

While applying concomitant pressure on the ASIS in a backward direction, the thumbs appreciate decoaptation of the pubic symphysis. If decoaptation is not achieved, then there is compression dysfunction. Such a dysfunction may affect iliac mobility and quite often is not associated with pain.

Tests of the Hip Joint

Tests are performed to assess the most common hip dysfunctions:
1. Anterior hip
2. Posterior hip
3. Obturator membrane tension

Anteroposterior Test of the Hip

This test is made up of a sequence of three movements:
- Anterior test: external rotation, abduction, and extension
- Posterior test: internal rotation, adduction, and flexion

The patient is supine with the right knee flexed against the practitioner's thigh. The practitioner stands on the patient's right side, with the knee flexed on the bed.

The practitioner places the web of the right thumb and index finger on the groin and the left hand behind and proximal to the greater trochanter; both hands are positioned on the coxofemoral joint at the level of the femoral neck.

Starting from the neutral position, the practitioner applies a gentle pressure on the coxofemoral joint first in a posterior-outward direction and then in an anterior-inward direction. After each movement, the joint is returned to its neutral position. Finally, the practitioner compares the range and quality of motion achieved in the two directions.

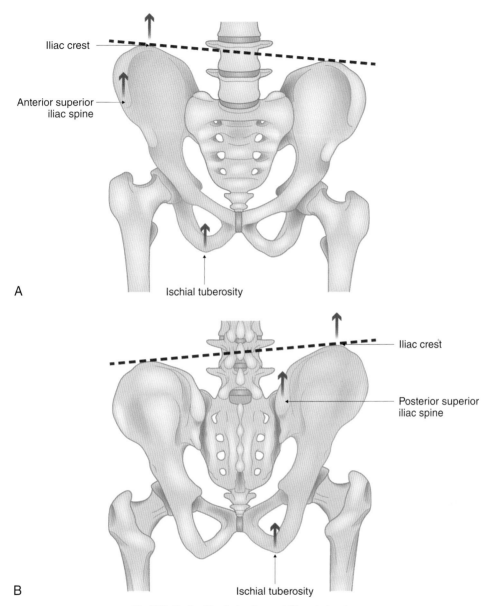

Iliac crest

Anterior superior
iliac spine

Ischial tuberosity

A

Iliac crest

Posterior superior
iliac spine

Ischial tuberosity

B

Fig. 5.23 Upslip: (A) anterior view and (B) posterior view.

If the hip moves more easily in a posterior-outward direction, then there is hip posterior dysfunction, and vice versa (Fig. 5.25; Video 5.9).

Test of the Obturator Membrane

Commonly known as the test of the obturator membrane, it is instead a test of the obturator externus to assess the presence of contractures.

The obturator externus is the most superficial muscle of the pelvic wall and therefore can be palpated. It lies on the obturator membrane, which almost completely closes the obturator foramen. Contractures of the obturator externus result in a decreased joint ROM of the hip and ilium.

The patient is supine with the right knee flexed (Fig. 5.26; Video 5.10).

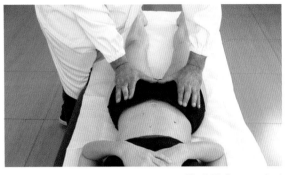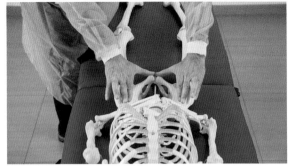

Fig. 5.24 Compression test of the pubic symphysis.

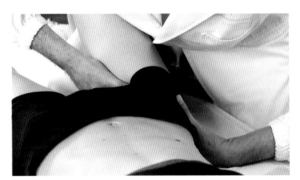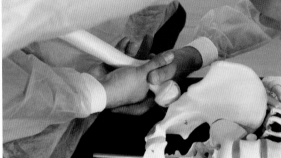

Fig. 5.25 Anteroposterior test of the hip.

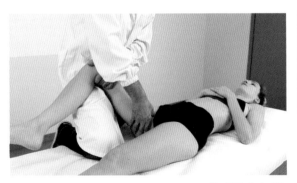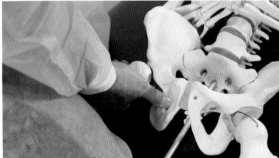

Fig. 5.26 Test of the obturator membrane.

The practitioner stands close to the bed with the right knee flexed on the bed under the patient's knee. The practitioner brings the hip into flexion with slight abduction.

The leg leans relaxed against the practitioner's chest and is held by the left hand. With the thumb of the right hand, the practitioner palpates for the tender point by following the superior border of the adductor longus between the pubic and ischium branches lateral to the pubic symphysis. Tenderness indicates contracture of the obturator externus.

Treatment With the AcuOsteo Method: The Choice of an Integrated Approach

The therapeutic approach of the AcuOsteo method aims to treat those musculoskeletal injuries that do not require consultation with a surgeon or a physician.

Once this fundamental aspect has been defined, treatment envisages the use of acupuncture and osteopathy according to their diagnostic and therapeutic approaches.

We would like to stress that at this point in diagnostic assessment, we do not have to follow the rules of Western medicine, except for some specific cases, such as hip arthritis, posttraumatic and postsurgical pain, and stiffness, which will be covered later.

In addition, we should not be misled by diagnostic imaging investigations and should rely only on the rules of Chinese and osteopathic medicine, which means selecting points according to symptoms and channel pathways and treating all of the somatic dysfunctions encountered.

For didactic purposes, treatment with acupuncture will precede osteopathic treatment, whereas in clinical practice the order is reversed since it may be difficult to perform osteopathic manipulations once the needles have been inserted.

An exception to this methodology is represented by those morbidities where marked stiffness prevents joint mobilization as required by osteopathic manipulations. Specifically, we are referring to the outcomes after immobilization following surgery and fractures.

In these cases, we suggest first using acupuncture, especially the bleeding techniques, and then, at the end of the session and after removing the needles, osteopathy.

In any case, it is always the practitioner's clinical experience that will guide them along the most appropriate pathway to treat each patient's condition.

Osteopathic manipulation in the treatment of "somatic dysfunction" is the central concept of the therapeutic process to treat the affected joints and functionally/anatomically related components of the somatic system.

Consequently, the osteopathic manipulative approach to musculoskeletal hip pain focuses on the treatment of joint somatic dysfunctions not only of the hip but also of the pelvic girdle, knee, and ankle.

Regardless of the condition to be treated, be it trochanteric bursitis, arthritis of the hip, or surgical outcomes, all of the dysfunctions diagnosed should be treated.

It is therefore evident that the osteopathic therapeutic approach does not vary with the condition to be treated and thus the osteopathic manipulations described for the pelvic girdle and hip, as well as those for the knee and ankle, will not be repeated under the paragraphs dedicated to the "injuries."

ACUPUNCTURE TREATMENT

Anterior Hip Pain

The Five Options and Selection of Acupoints

The approach we suggest is widely described in the section dedicated to the fundamentals of acupuncture for MSK pain in the limbs (see Chapter 1).

The most important aspect is the identification of the Ah Shi point(s) to determine which channels are affected. In this specific case, the Stomach Muscle and Connecting channels are involved.

Pricking pain localized on the anterior side of the hip is a sign of Blood stasis to be treated with the bleeding technique, whereas widespread pain radiating along the anterior thigh is a sign of Qì stagnation to be treated with the needling technique.

It is worth reminding that the distal points should be needled one at a time and their effectiveness in terms of pain and ROM tested after each insertion. The same applies to the local points.

Finally, since both options 1 and 2 consist of several steps, it is important to highlight how the selection should be made. Specifically, the practitioner might wonder if all or some of the steps should be followed. The rule we follow is simple: when the result achieved is satisfactory, the remaining steps should be skipped, and the practitioner should move to the following option. Similarly, the use of the points recommended under options 3, 4, and 5 should be carefully evaluated according to the case being treated.

The points and accessory techniques we recommend using are listed below.

Order of Needling

Option One: Distal Points

First Step: Stomach Muscle Channel

ST45. This Jing-Well point activates the Stomach Muscle channel and removes Qì stagnation and Blood stasis with needling and bleeding techniques, respectively.

Second Step: Stomach Connecting Channels

ST40 (Opposite Side). This Luo point activates the Stomach Connecting channels and removes Qì stagnation and Blood stasis in acute and chronic conditions from Excess.

SP4 (Opposite Side). This Luo point activates the Spleen Connecting channels. It is also used in chronic Deficiency conditions with dull pain to tonify Qì and Blood in the internally-externally related Stomach channels. In the latter case, we associate Yuan point ST42 with Luo point SP4, which is the well-known Luo-Yuan point combination. First, as the main point, we needle the Yuan point on the affected side and then, as a secondary point, the Luo point on the internally-externally related channel on the opposite side.

Third Step: Empirical Points

There is no point that is classically recommended.

Fourth Step: Opposite Extremity (Upper/ Lower)

LI15 (Opposite Side). It is located in the shoulder joint that corresponds to the hip joint on the paired channel according to the Six Stages.

Our technique consists of needling the opposite extremity (lower/upper) on the opposite side in acute and chronic conditions.

Alternatively, the most tender point on palpation is selected on the same or opposite side.

Fifth Step: Categories of Traditional Points

ST43 (Affected Side) and LI3 (Opposite Side). A good combination includes the Shu-Stream points on the paired channel according to the Six Stages.

First, we needle the Shu-Stream point on the channel involved on the affected side and then the Shu-Stream point on the coupled channel on the opposite side and opposite extremity (upper/lower).

We use this technique in acute and chronic Excess conditions to treat pain and expel or prevent invasion of EPFs.

ST41. The Jing-River points are used in acute or chronic Excess conditions due to the invasion of an EPF, and they are needled to promote its expulsion from their respective channels. They are also useful to prevent pain exacerbation from seasonal changes or invasion of EPFs.

ST34. The Xi-Cleft points are specifically used in acute conditions for the treatment of Blood stasis in their respective channels. However, they are more effective in the Yin rather than in the Yang channels. That said, our experience teaches that ST34 can be useful in this specific case, and we also use it because it can be considered an adjacent point or a local point if pain radiates to the knee.

ST42. We recommend using this Yuan-Source point in chronic Deficiency conditions with dull pain, in case of weakness, or in the resolution phases of hip pain, to tonify Qì and Blood in the Stomach channels.

In this situation, we can also associate Yuan point ST42 with Luo point SP4, which is the well-known Luo-Yuan point combination of ST42. First, as the main point, we needle the Yuan point on the affected side and then, as a secondary point, the Luo point on the internally-externally related channel on the opposite side.

Sixth Step: Extraordinary Vessels

In our opinion, no Extraordinary Vessel is effective to treat this disorder.

Option Two: Local Points

First Step: Painful Point(s) (Ah Shi)

Ah Shi Point(s). It is difficult to identify a painful point(s) (Ah Shi) because it is usually located deep in the hip. However, being well localized, it corresponds to Blood stasis. In this specific case, we would rather avoid using bleeding or needling techniques and use ST31 instead. Pain radiating from the hip to the anterior thigh and knee corresponds to Qi stagnation and requires needling along pain radiation.

ST31. It can be considered the local point to treat anterior hip pain.

We use 0.30 × 40 mm needles to be inserted deeply in the Ah Shi point(s) and ST31 until the quadriceps muscle sheath is reached.

To ensure the accuracy and precision of local needle placement and manipulation, we prefer the supine position.

Second Step: Anatomically Mirrored Points (Opposite Side)

The points to be needled are located on the opposite side and should correspond as precisely as possible to the anatomical mirror of the Ah Shi point(s) to be treated.

The point(s) may or may not be tender on palpation.

To ensure the accuracy and precision of needle placement and manipulation, we prefer the supine position.

Option Three: Adjacent Points

First Step: Adjacent Points

ST34. It is used to promote the longitudinal flow of local Qì.

As already mentioned above, this point can also be considered a local point if pain radiates to the knee.

ST32. It is an insertion point of the Stomach Muscle channel in the anterior thigh and as such it promotes the longitudinal flow of local Qì. It can also be considered a local point if pain radiates to the knee.

GB29. It is located midway between the ASIS and the greater trochanter, on the anterior aspect of the tensor fasciae latae.

The needle is inserted perpendicularly to the required depth to reach the quadriceps muscle sheath.

LR11. It is a very important point since it releases tension of the adductor longus and therefore reduces joint stiffness. Moreover, it promotes the horizontal flow of local Qì.

SP12. This point is located at the level of the groin area and promotes the horizontal flow of local Qì. Attention should be paid to avoid the risk of needling the femoral artery medially and the femoral nerve laterally.

Option Four: Etiological Points

First Step: According to Patterns

LI4 and LR3 (Bilaterally). They promote the flow of Qì and help remove Blood stasis. Since LR3 is the Shu/Yuan point of the Liver, it also helps nourish muscles and tendons.

ST36 (Bilaterally). It is used to tonify Qì and Blood in chronic Deficiency conditions or the phases of pain resolution that can turn into muscle weakness.

Second Step: General Points

GB34 (Bilaterally). It is the Hui-Gathering point of Sinews and promotes the flow of Qì thus contributing to remove Blood stasis.

BL18 (Bilaterally). It treats all the Excess and Deficiency conditions of the Liver that may favor the onset or duration of musculotendinous symptoms. It harmonizes the flow of Qì and Blood, improves treatment of tendons and muscles, and help restore joint cartilage in case of chondromalacia.

Option Five: Microsystems

First Step: Wrist and Ankle Acupuncture

Lower 4. It roughly corresponds to the pathway of the Stomach channels and controls lower limb mobility (Fig. 5.27).

Second Step: Ear Acupuncture (Fig. 5.28)

Local point: Hip

Zang Fu point: Liver

General points: Subcortex and Shenmen

Acute or Chronic Pain from Excess.

Intense Pain or Range of Motion Reduced by Pain. The principle of treatment is to remove Qì stagnation and

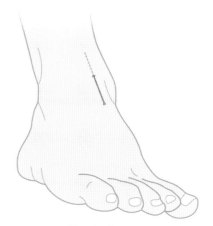

Fig. 5.27 Lower 4.

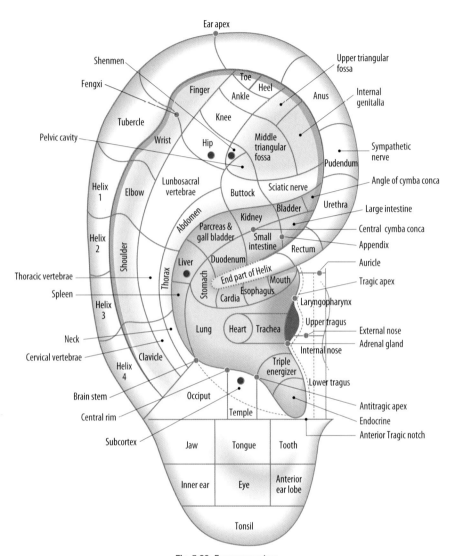

Fig. 5.28 Ear acupuncture.

Blood stasis and expel External or Internal Pathogenic Factors, if any (Box 5.1).

Chronic Pain From Deficiency.

Dull Pain or Muscle Weakness. The principle of treatment is to tonify Qì and Blood, strengthen tissues, and avoid pain exacerbation from physical activities or invasion of EPFs (Box 5.2).

Therapeutic Program, Frequency of Sessions. The frequency of sessions depends on the clinical condition of the patient. If the condition is acute or chronic with intense pain, we recommend sessions twice a week for 2 weeks and then once a week for another 2 weeks. If improvement is observed, sessions are then scheduled once a week until complete pain relief or

BOX 5.1 ACUTE OR CHRONIC PAIN FROM EXCESS ACUPUNCTURE TREATMENT

Option 1 Distal points	• Jing-Well point ST 45 • Luo point ST40 (opposite side) • Point according to the Six Stages LI15 (opposite side) • Shu-Stream point ST43 (affected side) and Shu-Stream point LI3 (opposite side) • Jing-River point ST41 • Xi point ST34
Option 2 Local points	• Ah Shi • ST31 • Anatomically mirrored point(s) (opposite side)
Option 3 Adjacent points	• ST34 • GB29 • LR11 • SP12 • Insertion point ST32
Option 4 Etiological and general points	• LI4 and LR3 (bilaterally) • GB34 (bilaterally) • BL18 (bilaterally)

Option 5
Microsystems
	• W-A acupuncture
	  • Lower 4
	• Ear acupuncture
	  • Hip
	  • Liver
	  • Subcortex and Shenmen

BOX 5.2 CHRONIC PAIN FROM DEFICIENCY ACUPUNCTURE TREATMENT

Option 1 Distal points	• Yuan point ST42 • Luo point SP4 (opposite side) • Point according to the Six Stages LI15 (opposite side) • Jing-River point ST41
Option 2 Local points	• Ah Shi • ST31
Option 3 Adjacent points	• ST34 • GB29 • LR11 • SP12 • Insertion point ST32
Option 4 Etiological and general points	• ST36 • GB34 • LR3

Option 5
Microsystems
	• W-A acupuncture
	  • Lower 4
	• Ear acupuncture
	  • Hip
	  • Liver
	  • Subcortex and Shenmen

at least reduction by 80% to 90%. If not, the whole clinical picture should be reconsidered and the patient referred to another specialist.

If the condition is chronic with dull pain, we recommend sessions once a week for 4 weeks. Afterwards, and if the patient continues to improve, sessions are then scheduled once a week until complete pain relief or at least reduction by 80% to 90%.

Clinical notes

• Improvement following treatment may turn intense pain to dull pain and then to a feeling of weakness. Should this be the case, the principle of treatment has to be changed as follows. It is no longer necessary to remove Qì stagnation and Blood stasis and expel EPFs, if any; instead, Qì and Blood should be tonified to strengthen tissues and avoid pain exacerbation from physical activities or invasion of EPFs.

• Treatment of anterior hip pain can ensure excellent results in terms of disappearance of pain and return to daily activities, even sports.

Medial Hip Pain

The Five Options and Selection of Acupoints

The approach we suggest is widely described in the section dedicated to the fundamentals of acupuncture for MSK pain in the limbs (see Chapter 1).

The most important aspect is the identification of the Ah Shi point(s) to determine which channels are affected. In this specific case, the Spleen and Liver Muscle and Connecting channels are involved.

It is worth reminding that the Liver Muscle and Connecting channels run more medially than the Spleen channels and therefore overlie the region of the hip adductors better than other channels.

Quite often there is no clear evidence as to which channels are involved, either the Spleen or the Liver Muscle and Connecting channels, or both. Therefore, in line with our principle of treatment, we first use the Spleen channels and then test their effectiveness soon after needle insertion. If the result is not satisfactory, we remove the needles or let them in, and move to the Liver channels.

Once the most effective channel is identified, selection of distal points continues along it.

Pricking pain localized on the medial aspect of the hip and in the groin area is a sign of Blood stasis, whereas pain radiating along the thigh is a sign of Qì stagnation. In both cases, we prefer using the needling technique as we will see later.

It is worth reminding that the distal points should be needled one at a time and their effectiveness in terms of pain and ROM tested after each insertion. The same applies to the local points.

Finally, since both options 1 and 2 consist of several steps, it is important to highlight how selection should be made. Specifically, the practitioner might wonder if all or some of the steps should be followed. The rule we follow is simple: when the result achieved is satisfactory, the remaining steps should be skipped, and the practitioner should move to the following option. Similarly, the use of the points recommended under options 3, 4, and 5 should be carefully evaluated according to the case being treated.

The points and accessory techniques we recommend using are listed below.

The Order of Needling

Option One: Distal Points

First Step: Spleen and Liver Muscle Channels

SP1 and LR1. These Jing-Well points activate the Spleen and Liver Muscle channels, and they remove Qì stagnation and Blood stasis with needling and bleeding techniques, respectively.

Second Step: Spleen and Liver Connecting Channels

SP4 and LR5 (Opposite Side). These Luo points activate the Spleen and Liver Connecting channels, and they remove Qì stagnation and Blood stasis in acute or chronic conditions from Excess.

ST40 and GB37 (Opposite Side). These Luo points activate the Stomach and Gall Bladder Connecting channels. They are also used in chronic Deficiency conditions with dull pain to tonify Qì and Blood in their respective internally-externally related channels. In this case, we associate Yuan point SP3 with Luo point ST40 and Yuan point LR3 with Luo point GB37, that is to say the well-known Luo-Yuan point combination. First, as the main point, we needle the Yuan point on the affected side and then, as a secondary point, the Luo point on the internally-externally related channel on the opposite side.

Third Step: Empirical Points

There is no point that is classically recommended.

Fourth Step: Opposite Extremity (Upper/Lower)

LU1 and PC2 (Opposite Side). LU1 is the only point to be located close to the shoulder joint which corresponds to the hip joint on the paired channel according to the Six Stages. In clinical practice, the concept of anatomically mirrored point can lead us to select a tender point located on the Lung Main channel and corresponding exactly to the shoulder joint.

PC2 is located far from the shoulder joint that corresponds to the hip joint on the paired channel according to the Six Stages. In addition, the pathway of the Pericardium Main channel does not reach the shoulder joint, which explains why we would rather avoid using PC2 to treat this condition.

Our technique consists of needling the opposite extremity (lower/upper) on the opposite side in acute and chronic conditions.

Alternatively, the most tender point on palpation is selected on the same or opposite side.

Fifth Step: Categories of Traditional Points

SP3 (Affected Side) and LU9 (Opposite Side); LR3 (Affected Side) and PC7 (Opposite Side). A good combination includes the Shu-Stream points on the paired channel according to the Six Stages.

First, we needle the Shu-Stream point on the channel involved on the affected side and then the Shu-Stream point on the coupled channel on the opposite side and opposite extremity (upper/lower).

We use this technique in acute and chronic Excess conditions to treat pain and expel or prevent invasion of EPFs.

It is worth reminding that in the Yin channels the Shu-Stream point corresponds to the Yuan-Source point. Therefore SP3 and LR3 could also be used in chronic Deficiency conditions, as we will see later.

SP5 and LR4. The Jing-River points are used in acute or chronic Excess conditions due to the invasion of an EPF, and they are needled to promote its expulsion from their respective channels. They are also useful to prevent pain exacerbation from seasonal changes or invasion of EPFs. However, they are more effective in the Yang rather than in the Yin channels.

SP8 and LR6. The Xi-Cleft points are specifically used in acute conditions to treat Blood stasis in their respective channels. We only use SP8 to treat gynecological disorders, not even LR6 has proved to be effective in the treatment of musculoskeletal diseases.

SP3 and LR3. We recommend using these Yuan-Source points in chronic Deficiency conditions with dull pain, in case of weakness, or in the resolution phases of medial hip pain to tonify Qì and Blood in their respective channels.

In this situation, we can also associate Yuan point SP3 with Luo point ST40 and Yuan point LR3 with Luo point GB37, which is the well-known Luo-Yuan point combination. First, as the main point, we needle the Yuan point on the affected side and then, as a secondary point, the Luo point on the Internally-Externally related channel on the opposite side.

SP6. It is the meeting point of the three Yin channels, and as such it promotes the longitudinal flow of Qì and eliminates Blood stasis on those channels.

Sixth Step: Extraordinary Vessels

In our opinion, no Extraordinary Vessel is effective to treat this disorder.

Option Two: Local Points

First Step: Painful Point(s) (Ah Shi)

Ah Shi Point(s). It is difficult to identify a painful point(s) (Ah Shi) because it is usually located deep in the hip. However, being well localized, it corresponds to Blood stasis. Instead, when pain radiates from the hip to the medial thigh, it indicates Qì stagnation. In both cases, we would rather avoid using bleeding or needling techniques and use SP12, LR11, and LR12 instead.

SP12. It can be considered the local point to treat medial hip pain on the Spleen channels.

This point is located at the level of the groin area and is used to promote the longitudinal flow of local Qì. Attention should be paid to avoid the risk of needling the femoral artery medially and the femoral nerve laterally.

We also use it because it is an insertion point of the Spleen Muscle channel in the hip.

LR11 and LR12. They can be considered local points to treat medial hip pain on the Liver channels. They are used to promote the longitudinal flow of local Qì.

LR11 is located lateral to the adductor longus and is used to release its contracture. In anatomical terms, LR12 corresponds to the iliopsoas and is used to release its contracture.

We use 0.30 × 40 mm needles to be inserted deeply in both points until the muscle sheath is reached. Electroacupuncture stimulation can be taken into consideration and used between these two points.

To ensure the accuracy and precision of local needle placement and manipulation, we prefer the supine position.

Second Step: Anatomically Mirrored Points (Opposite Side)

The points to be needled are located on the opposite side and should correspond as precisely as possible to the anatomical mirror of the Ah Shi point(s) to be treated. The point(s) may or may not be tender on palpation.

To ensure the accuracy and precision of needle placement and manipulation, we prefer the supine position.

Option Three: Adjacent Points

First Step: Adjacent Points

ST31. It is used to promote the horizontal flow of local Qì.

GB29. It is used to promote the horizontal flow of local Qì.

SP10. Located in the belly of the vastus medialis of the quadriceps, it is used to promote the longitudinal flow of local Qì and remove Blood stasis.

LR8. It is the insertion point of the Liver Muscle channel in the knee and as such it promotes the longitudinal flow of local Qì.

Option Four: Etiological Points

First Step: According to Patterns

LI4 and LR3 (Bilaterally). They promote the flow of Qì and help remove Blood stasis. Since LR3 is the Shu/Yuan point of the Liver, it also helps nourish muscles and tendons.

ST36 (Bilaterally). It is used to tonify Qì and Blood in chronic Deficiency conditions or the phases of pain resolution that can turn into muscle weakness.

Second Step: General Points

GB34 (Bilaterally). It is the Hui-Gathering point of Sinews and promotes the flow of Qì thus contributing to remove Blood stasis.

BL18 (Bilaterally). It treats all Excess and Deficiency conditions of the Liver that may favor the onset or duration of musculotendinous symptoms. It harmonizes the flow of Qì and Blood and enhances treatment of tendons and muscle.

Option Five: Microsystems

First Step: Wrist and Ankle Acupuncture

Lower 2. It roughly corresponds to the pathway of the Spleen and Liver channels (Fig. 5.29).

Lower 4. It controls lower limb mobility (Fig. 5.30).

Second Step: Ear Acupuncture (Fig. 5.31)

Local point: Hip

Zang Fu point: Liver

General points: Subcortex and Shenmen

Acute or Chronic Pain From Excess.

Intense Pain or Range of Motion. Reduced by Pain. The principle of treatment is to remove Qì stagnation and Blood stasis and expel EPFs, if any (Box 5.3).

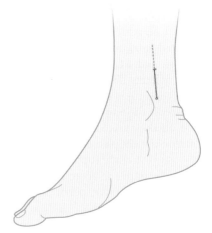

Fig. 5.29 Lower 2.

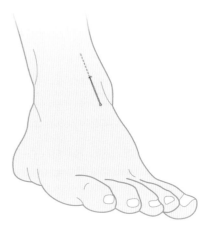

Fig. 5.30 Lower 4.

Chronic Pain From Deficiency.

Dull *Pain or Muscle Weakness.* The principle of treatment is to tonify Qì and Blood, strengthen tissues, and avoid pain exacerbation from physical activities or invasion of EPFs (Box 5.4).

Therapeutic Program, Frequency of Sessions. The frequency of sessions depends on the clinical condition of the patient. If the condition is acute or chronic with intense pain, we recommend sessions twice a week for 2 weeks and then once a week for another 2

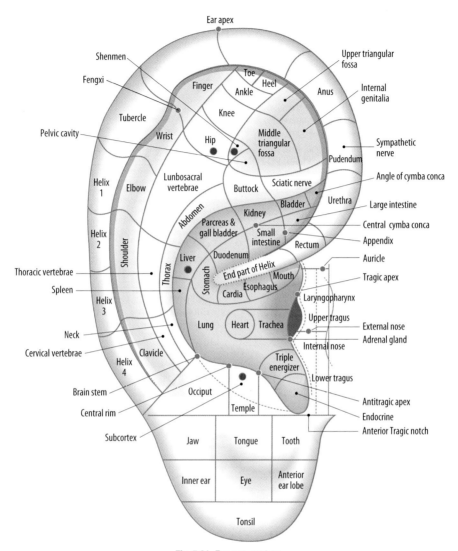

Fig. 5.31 Ear acupuncture.

weeks. If improvement is observed, sessions are then scheduled once a week until complete pain relief or at least reduction by 80% to 90%. If not, the whole clinical picture should be reconsidered and the patient referred to another specialist.

If the condition is chronic with dull pain, we recommend sessions once a week for 4 weeks. Afterwards, and if the patient continues to improve, sessions are then scheduled once a week until complete pain relief or at least reduction by 80% to 90%.

BOX 5.3 ACUTE OR CHRONIC PAIN FROM EXCESS ACUPUNCTURE TREATMENT

Option 1 Distal points	• Jing-Well point SP1, LR1 • Luo point SP4, LR5 (opposite side) • Point according to the Six Stages LU1 (opposite side) • Shu-Stream point SP3, LR3 (affected side) and Shu-Stream point LU9, PC7 (opposite side) • Jing-River point SP5, LR4 • SP6
Option 2 Local points	• Ah Shi • SP12 • LR11 • LR12 • Anatomically mirrored point(s) (opposite side)
Option 3 Adjacent points	• ST31 • SP10 • Insertion point LR8
Option 4 Etiological and general points	• LI4 and LR3 (bilaterally) • GB34 (bilaterally) • BL18 (bilaterally)

Option 5
Microsystems
	• W-A acupuncture
	  • Lower 2
	  • Lower 4
	• Ear acupuncture
	  • Hip
	  • Liver
	  • Subcortex and Shenmen

BOX 5.4 CHRONIC PAIN FROM DEFICIENCY ACUPUNCTURE TREATMENT

Option 1 Distal points	• Yuan point SP3, LR3 • Luo point ST40, GB37 (opposite side) • Point according to the Six Stages LU1 (opposite side) • Jing-River point SP5, LR4 • SP6
Option 2 Local points	• Ah Shi • SP12 • LR11 • LR12
Option 3 Adjacent points	• ST31 • SP10 • Insertion point LR8
Option 4 Etiological and general points	• ST36 (bilaterally) • GB34 (bilaterally) • LR3 (bilaterally) • BL18 (bilaterally)

Option 5
Microsystems
	• W-A acupuncture
	  • Lower 2
	  • Lower 4
	• Ear acupuncture
	  • Hip
	  • Liver
	  • Subcortex and Shenmen

Clinical notes

- Improvement following treatment may turn intense pain to dull pain and then to a feeling of weakness. Should this be the case, the principle of treatment has to be changed as follows. It is no longer necessary to remove Qì stagnation and Blood stasis and expel EPFs, if any; instead, Qì and Blood should be tonified to strengthen tissues and avoid pain exacerbation from physical activities or invasion of EPFs.
- Treatment of medial hip pain can ensure excellent results in terms of disappearance of pain and return to daily activities, even sports.

Trochanteric Bursitis

As already mentioned in the section dedicated to Western medicine, trochanteric bursitis is inflammation of the superficial trochanteric bursa lying between the tensor fasciae latae and the greater trochanter.

The Five Options and Selection of Acupoints

The approach we suggest is widely described in the section dedicated to the fundamentals of acupuncture for MSK pain in the limbs (see Chapter 1).

The most important aspect is the identification of the Ah Shi point(s) to determine which channels are affected. In this specific case, the Gall Bladder Muscle and Connecting channels are involved and, according to our experience, the Yang Qiao Mai Extraordinary channel may also be involved.

Pricking pain localized on the lateral side of the hip is a sign of Blood stasis to be treated with the bleeding technique, whereas widespread pain radiating along the lateral thigh is a sign of Qì stagnation to be treated with the needling technique.

It is worth reminding that the distal points should be needled one at a time and their effectiveness in terms of pain and ROM tested after each insertion. The same applies to the local points.

Finally, since both options 1 and 2 consist of several steps, it is important to highlight how selection should be made. Specifically, the practitioner might wonder if all or some of the steps should be followed. The rule we follow is simple: when the result achieved is satisfactory, the remaining steps should be skipped, and the practitioner should move to the following option. Similarly, the use of the points recommended under options 3, 4, and 5 should be carefully evaluated according to the case being treated.

The points and accessory techniques we recommend using are listed below.

The Order of Needling

Option One: Distal Points

First Step: Gall Bladder Muscle Channel

GB44. This Jing-Well point is used to activate the Gall Bladder Muscle channel and remove Qì stagnation and Blood stasis with needling and bleeding techniques, respectively.

Second Step: Gall Bladder Connecting channels

GB37 (Opposite Side). This Luo point activates the Gall Bladder Connecting channels and removes Qì stagnation and Blood stasis in acute and chronic conditions from Excess.

LR5 (Opposite Side). This Luo point activates the Liver Connecting channels. It is also used in chronic Deficiency conditions with dull pain to tonify Qì and Blood in the internally-externally related Gall Bladder channels. In the latter case, we associate Yuan point GB40 with Luo point LR5, which is the well-known Luo-Yuan combination. First, as the main point, we needle the Yuan point on the affected side and then, as a secondary point, the Luo point on the internally-externally related channel on the opposite side.

Our technique consists of needling LR5 from oblique to transverse in proximal direction along the pathway of the Liver Main Channel.

Third Step: Empirical Points

There is no point that is classically recommended.

Fourth Step: Opposite Extremity (Upper/Lower)

TB14 (Opposite Side). It is located in the shoulder joint that corresponds to the hip joint on the paired channel according to the Six Stages.

It is worth remembering that the painful point on the great trochanter is not exactly in the hip joint; it is in fact slightly distally located and this means we could palpate the arm in a downward direction along the Triple Energizer Main channel to find another or more tender point(s).

Our technique consists of needling the opposite extremity (lower/upper) on the opposite side in acute and chronic conditions.

Alternatively, the most tender point on palpation is selected on the same or opposite side.

Fifth Step: Categories of Traditional Points

GB41 (Affected Side) and TB3 (Opposite Side). A good combination includes the Shu-Stream points on the paired channel according to the Six Stages.

First, we needle the Shu-Stream point on the channel involved on the affected side and then the Shu-Stream point on the coupled channel on the opposite side and opposite extremity (upper/lower).

We use this technique in acute and chronic Excess conditions to treat pain and expel or prevent the invasion of EPFs.

GB38. The Jing-River points are used in acute or chronic Excess conditions due to the invasion of an EPF, and they are needled to promote its expulsion from their respective channels. They are also useful to prevent pain exacerbation from seasonal changes or invasion of EPFs.

GB36. The Xi-Cleft points are specifically used in acute conditions to remove Blood stasis from their respective channels. However, they are more effective in the Yin rather than in the Yang channels; that is why we would rather avoid using GB36 to treat this condition.

GB40. We recommend using this Yuan-Source point in chronic Deficiency conditions with dull pain, in case of weakness, or in the resolution phases of trochanteric bursitis to tonify Qì and Blood in the Gall Bladder channels.

In this situation, we can also associate Yuan point GB40 with Luo point LR5, which is the well-known Luo-Yuan point combination. First, as the main point, we needle the Yuan point on the affected side and then, as a secondary point, the Luo point on the internally-externally related channel on the opposite side.

Sixth Step: Extraordinary Vessels

BL62 (Affected Side) and SI3 (Opposite Side). BL62 is the opening point of the Yang Qiao Mai, while SI3 is the coupled point and opening point of the Governing Vessel (Du Mai). The Yang Qiao Mai is used in Excess conditions with muscle spasms, tightness, and pain affecting the lateral aspect of the thigh.

When the Yang Qiao Mai is used, we also needle BL59, which is its Xi-Cleft point. First, as the main point, the opening point of the Yang Qiao Mai is needled on the same side and then, as a secondary point, the coupled point on the opposite side.

Option Two: Local Points

First Step: Painful Point(s) (Ah Shi)

Ah Shi Point(s). We identify the most painful point(s) (Ah Shi) that is usually located at the level of the lateral hip on the greater trochanter: palpation reveals either the Ah Shi point(s) corresponding to Blood stasis and therefore to be bled or an area of widespread pain corresponding to Qì stagnation and requiring needling. In this area, pain radiates distally along the lateral thigh.

When the bleeding technique is chosen, the cupping therapy should be used to bleed the most painful point (Ah Shi) on the greater trochanter. Afterwards, another four points should be bled, so as to create a circle about 1 cun away from the first point or, alternatively, another two or three points located distally about 1 cun away from the first point (Fig. 5.32; Video 5.11).

Alternatively, a choice can be made between two needling techniques:

The needle is inserted perpendicularly to the required depth to reach the bursa and then four needles are inserted obliquely, so as to create a circle about 1 cun away from the first needle;

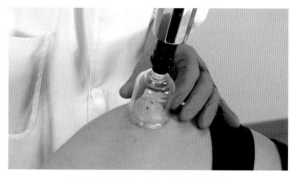

Fig. 5.32 Bleeding of the Ah Shi point(s).

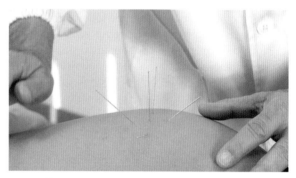

Fig. 5.33 Needing of the Ah Shi point(s)_concentric.

the tips of the needles are directed towards the perpendicular needle (Fig. 5.33; Video 5.12).

Two or three needles are inserted perpendicularly to the required depth to reach the bursa and the tensor fasciae latae; the distance between the needles is 1 cun; needle insertion starts from the area above the trochanter and follows distal pain radiation in a longitudinal direction (Fig. 5.34; Video 5.13).

We use one or more 0.30 x 40 mm needles; the diameter and length of the needle to be used depend on the patient physique.

Electroacupuncture stimulation can be taken into consideration and used between two points. In acute or exacerbation of chronic conditions due to invasion of EPFs, Cold in particular, moxa on the needle can be added to help expel them. Attention should be paid to avoid burning of the underlying skin due to the horizontal insertion of the needles, keeping in mind that

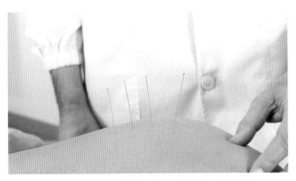

Fig. 5.34 Needing of the Ah Shi point(s)_longitudinal.

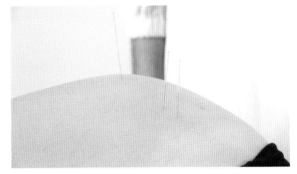

Fig. 5.35 Needing of the Ah Shi point and Jiankua.

too much heat can increase the ongoing inflammatory process.

To ensure the accuracy and precision of local needle placement and manipulation, we prefer the side-lying position on the unaffected side with the affected hip slightly flexed.

Second Step: Anatomically Mirrored Points (Opposite Side)

The points to be needled are located on the opposite side and should correspond as precisely as possible to the anatomical mirror of the Ah Shi point(s) to be treated. The point(s) may or may not be tender on palpation.

To ensure the accuracy and precision of needle placement and manipulation, we prefer the side-lying position on the affected side with the affected hip slightly flexed.

Option Three: Adjacent Points

First Step: Adjacent Points

GB29. It is located midway between the ASIS and the greater trochanter, on the anterior aspect of the tensor fasciae latae. The needle is inserted perpendicularly to the required depth to reach the quadriceps sheath.

Jiankua. This Extraordinary point was suggested by W. Reaves,[1] who named it "posterior" GB29. It is located midway between the lateral tibial crest and the greater trochanter, on the posterior aspect of the tensor fasciae latae, and is often tender on palpation.

One or two needles are inserted perpendicularly, at a distance of 1 cun, until the gluteus medius sheath is reached (Fig. 5.35; Video 5.14).

We use a 0.30 × 40 mm or a 0.32 × 70 mm needle: the diameter and length of the needle to be used depend on the patient physique.

Electroacupuncture stimulation can be taken into consideration and used between two points.

GB31. It is a very important point, especially when pain radiates to the lateral thigh, since it is located on the ITB and as such it promotes the longitudinal flow of local Qì.

BL54 and ST31. They help promote the horizontal flow of local Qì.

GB30. It is the insertion point of Gall Bladder muscle channel in the hip, and as such it promotes the longitudinal flow of local Qì.

Option Four: Etiological Points

First Step: According to Patterns

LI4 and LR3 (Bilaterally). They promote the flow of Qì and help remove Blood stasis. Since LR3 is the Shu/Yuan point of the Liver, it also helps nourish muscles and tendons.

ST36 (Bilaterally). It is used to tonify Qì and Blood in chronic Deficiency conditions or the phases of pain resolution that can turn into muscle weakness.

Second Step: General Points

GB34 (Bilaterally). It is the Hui-Gathering point of Sinews and promotes the flow of Qì thus contributing to remove Blood stasis.

BL18 (Bilaterally). It treats all Excess and Deficiency conditions of the Liver that may favor the onset or duration of musculotendinous symptoms. It harmonizes the flow of Qì and Blood and enhances the treatment of tendons and muscle.

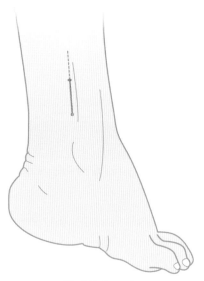

Fig. 5.36 Lower 5.

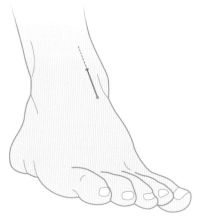

Fig. 5.37 Lower 4.

Option Five: Microsystems

First Step: Wrist and Ankle Acupuncture
Lower 5. It roughly corresponds to the pathway of the Gall Bladder channels (Fig. 5.36).

Lower 4. It controls lower limb mobility (Fig. 5.37).

Second Step: Ear Acupuncture (Fig. 5.38)
Local point: Hip
Zang Fu point: Liver
General points: Subcortex and Shenmen

Acute or Chronic Pain From Excess.
Intense Pain or Range of Motion Reduced by Pain. The principle of treatment is to remove Qì stagnation and Blood stasis and expel EPFs, if any (Box 5.5).
Chronic Pain From Deficiency.
Dull Pain or Muscle Weakness. The principle of treatment is to tonify Qì and Blood, strengthen tissues, and avoid pain exacerbation from physical activities or invasion of EPFs (Box 5.6).

Therapeutic Program, Frequency of Sessions
The frequency of sessions depends on the clinical condition of the patient. If the condition is acute or chronic with intense pain, we recommend sessions twice a week for 2 weeks and then once a week for another 2 weeks. If improvement is observed, sessions are then scheduled once a week until complete pain relief or at least reduction by 80% to 90%.

Response to treatment may take longer than expected, and therefore treatment should be continued and some more weekly sessions scheduled.

Finally, if expected outcomes are not achieved, the whole clinical picture should be reconsidered and the patient referred to another specialist.

If the condition is chronic with dull pain, we recommend sessions once a week for 4 weeks. Afterwards, and if the patient continues to improve, sessions are then scheduled once a week until complete pain relief or at least reduction by 80% to 90%.

Clinical notes

- Improvement following treatment may turn intense pain to dull pain and then to a feeling of weakness. Should this be the case, the principle of treatment has to be changed as follows. It is no longer necessary to remove Qì stagnation and Blood stasis; instead, Qì and Blood should be tonified to strengthen tissues and avoid pain exacerbation from physical activities.
- Sometimes, temporary worsening of symptoms is observed, especially when cupping is used.
- Sometimes, results do not meet patient expectations of care; an explanation for the poorer outcome could be the fact that trochanteric bursitis may be due to dysfunctions not only of the pelvic girdle, hip, and lower limb, but also of the lumbar spine. Should this be the case, then further investigation would be mandatory.

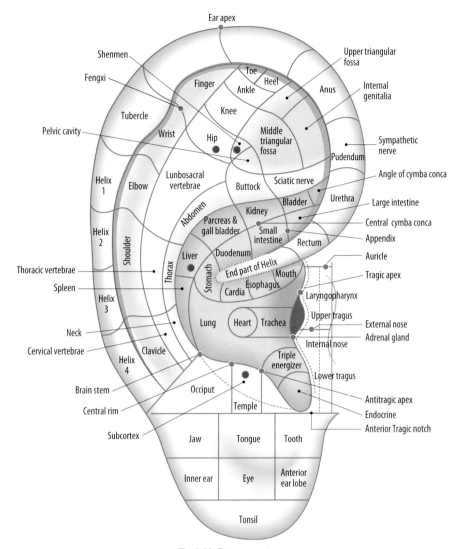

Fig. 5.38 Ear acupuncture.

OSTEOPATHIC MANIPULATIVE TREATMENT

This section deals with osteopathic manipulations to treat dysfunctions of the pelvic girdle and hip joint.

As already mentioned in the section dedicated to the fundamentals of osteopathy for MSK pain in the limbs (see Chapter 1), the key point of the osteopathic therapeutic process is the treatment not only of the somatic dysfunctions of the pelvic girdle and hip but also of those that are functionally and anatomically related.

Consequently, the osteopathic manipulative approach to musculoskeletal hip pain is based on the identification of joint somatic dysfunctions not only of the pelvic girdle and hip but also of the knee and ankle.

BOX 5.5 ACUTE OR CHRONIC PAIN FROM EXCESS ACUPUNCTURE TREATMENT

Option 1 Distal points	• Jing-Well point GB44 • Luo point GB37 (opposite side) • Point according to the Six Stages TE14 (opposite side) • Shu-Stream point GB41 (affected side) and Shu-Stream point, TE3 (opposite side) • Jing-River point GB38
Option 2 Local points	• Ah Shi • Anatomically mirrored point(s) (opposite side)
Option 3 Adjacent points	• GB29 • Jiankua • GB31 • BL54 • ST31 • Insertion point GB30
Option 4 Etiological and general points	• LI4 and LR3 (bilaterally) • GB34 (bilaterally) • BL18 (bilaterally)

Option 5
Microsystems
	• W-A acupuncture
	  • Lower 5
	  • Lower 4
	• Ear acupuncture
	  • Hip
	  • Liver
	  • Subcortex and Shenmen

BOX 5.6 CHRONIC PAIN FROM DEFICIENCY ACUPUNCTURE TREATMENT

Option 1 Distal points	• Yuan point GB40 • Luo point LR5 (opposite side) • Point according to the Six Stages TE14 (opposite side) • Jing-River point GB38
Option 2 Local points	• Ah Shi
Option 3 Adjacent points	• GB29 • Jiankua • GB31 • BL54 • ST31 • Insertion point GB30
Option 4 Etiological and general points	• ST36 • GB34 • LR3

Option 5
Microsystems
	• W-A acupuncture
	  • Lower 5
	  • Lower 4
	• Ear acupuncture
	  • Hip
	  • Liver
	  • Subcortex and Shenmen

Regardless of the condition to be treated, be it hip pain, trochanteric bursitis, arthritis of the hip, or surgical outcomes, all of the dysfunctions identified should be treated.

Somatic Dysfunctions of the Sacroiliac Joint

Anterior Rotation of the Ilium: Treatment

Anterior rotation dysfunction: anterior rotation is better than posterior rotation, that is, after the Downing shortening test, the tested leg does not appear shorter than the other (Fig. 5.39).

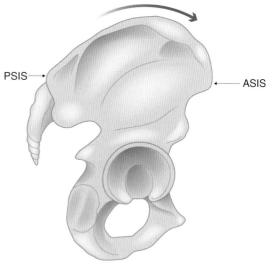

Fig. 5.39 Anterior rotation of the ilium.

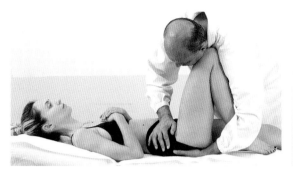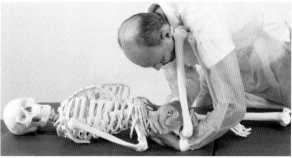

Fig. 5.40 Anterior rotation of the ilium MET treatment.

In this case, a muscle energy technique (MET) is used instead of performing a thrust.

The patient is supine. The practitioner stands on the patient's left side.

With the left hand, the practitioner hooks the ischium and searches for the sacroiliac restrictive barrier while flexing the hip and, at the same time, controlling the ASIS spine with the right hand. The patient is then asked to extend the hip by pushing against the practitioner's shoulder while the practitioner applies a counterforce to create an isometric contraction.

The position is held for three seconds and followed by a 3-second period of postisometric relaxation. Then, the practitioner flexes the hip again to engage a new restrictive barrier.

This process needs to be repeated thrice (Fig. 5.40; Video 5.15).

Posterior Rotation of the Ilium: Treatment

Posterior rotation dysfunction: posterior rotation is better than anterior rotation, that is, after the Downing lengthening test, the tested leg does not appear longer than the other (Fig. 5.41).

In this case, a MET is used instead of performing a thrust.

The patient is prone. The practitioner stands on the patient's left side. The practitioner holds the knee at 90 degrees with the right hand and the PSIS with the left hand.

The hip is extended until the practitioner engages the sacroiliac restrictive barrier. The patient is then asked to flex the hip by pushing against the practitioner's hand while the practitioner applies a counterforce to create an isometric contraction.

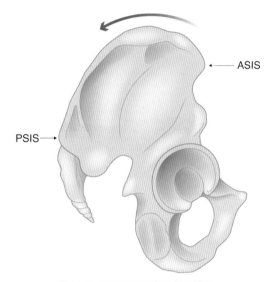

Fig. 5.41 Posterior rotation of the ilium.

The position is held for 3 seconds and followed by a 3-second period of postisometric relaxation. Then, the practitioner extends the hip again to engage a new restrictive barrier.

This process needs to be repeated thrice (Fig. 5.42; Video 5.16).

Iliac Torsion: Treatment

It is a dysfunction frequently observed as characterized by the concomitant presence of the two previous dysfunctions, that is, anterior rotation dysfunction of one ilium and posterior rotation dysfunction of the other ilium.

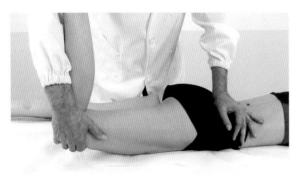
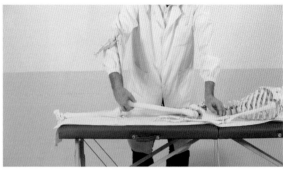

Fig. 5.42 Posterior rotation of the ilium MET treatment.

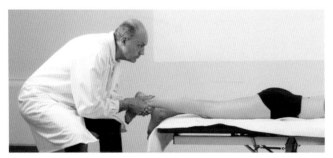
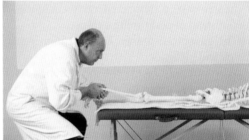

Fig. 5.43 Upslip treatment.

Also in this case we would rather use a MET following the sequences described in the two previous paragraphs.

Upslip: Treatment

A lifting of the hemipelvis is observed on the right side.

The patient is prone with the feet off the bed. The practitioner stands next to the patient's feet to hold the right ankle with both hands.

By flexing on the knees, the practitioner aligns with the longitudinal axis of the lower limb affected. While adding gradual traction on the ankle, tension on the hip is increased and the hip joint slightly extended.

When the correct point of tension is reached, the thrust is performed at the end of the expiration (Fig. 5.43; Video 5.17).

Somatic Dysfunction of the Pubic Symphysis

Compression of the Pubic Symphysis: Treatment

The pubic symphysis is compressed.

Treatment consists of three steps:
1. Isometric contraction of the hip adductor muscles.

    The patient is supine with knees flexed, feet flat on the bed and the practitioner's fist between the knees.

    The practitioner stands close to the patient.

    The patient is asked to move the knees inward squeezing the fist, thus creating an isometric contraction of the hip adductor muscles.
2. Isometric contraction of the hip abductor muscles.

    The practitioner applies resistance to either side of the knees.

    The patient is asked to push out against the resistance, creating an isometric contraction of the hip abductor muscles.
3. Isometric contraction of the hip adductor muscles.

The practitioner applies resistance to the inside of both knees.

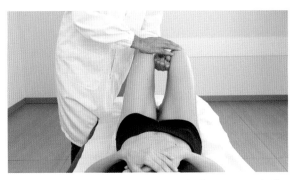

Fig. 5.44 Compression of the pubic symphysis treatment_starting position.

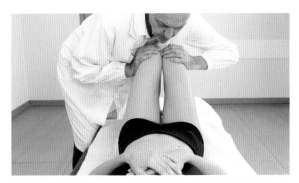

Fig. 5.45 Compression of the pubic symphysis treatment_intermediate position.

The patient is asked to squeeze in against the resistance, thus creating an isometric contraction of the hip adductor muscles (Figs. 5.44—5.46; Video 5.18).

Somatic Dysfunctions of the Hip Joint

Anterior Hip: Treatment

Anterior dysfunction: the hip slides more easily in an anterior-inward direction rather than in a posterior-outward direction.

The patient is supine with the right hip and knee flexed. The practitioner stands on the patient's left side and places the web of the right thumb and index finger at the level of the groin, and the left hand on the lateral aspect of the knee.

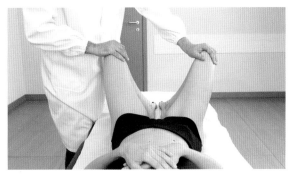

Fig. 5.46 Compression of the pubic symphysis treatment_final position.

Starting from the neutral position, the practitioner applies a gentle pressure with the right hand on the coxofemoral joint in a posterior-outward direction to engage the restrictive barrier.

A coupled thrust is then performed by pushing the hip posteriorly and outward with the right hand while adducting the knee with the left hand (Fig. 5.47; Video 5.19).

Posterior Hip: Treatment

Posterior dysfunction: the hip slides more easily in a posterior-outward direction rather than in an anterior-inward direction.

The patient is supine. The practitioner stands on the patient's right side.

The hip is abducted and slightly extended, and the knee flexed against the practitioner's side. The practitioner's web of the left thumb and index finger is behind and proximal to the greater trochanter, the

right hand on the inner thigh, and the forearm along the medial aspect of the knee.

Starting from the neutral position, the practitioner applies a gentle pressure with the left hand on the coxofemoral joint in an anterior-inward direction to engage the restrictive barrier.

A coupled thrust is then performed by pushing the hip anteriorly and inward with the left hand while abducting the knee with the right hand (Fig. 5.48; Video 5.20).

Tension of the Obturator Membrane: Treatment

A contracture of the obturator externus is observed.

The patient is supine with the right knee flexed. The practitioner stands close to the bed with the right knee flexed on the bed under the patient's knee. The practitioner brings the hip into flexion with slight abduction.

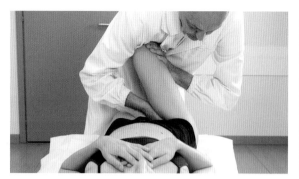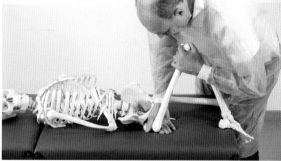

Fig. 5.47 Anterior hip treatment.

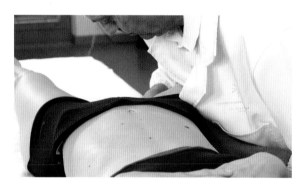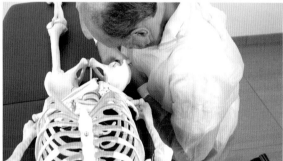

Fig. 5.48 Posterior hip treatment.

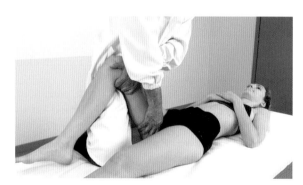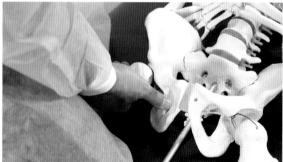

Fig. 5.49 Tension of the obturator membrane treatment.

The leg leans relaxed against the practitioner's chest and is held by the left hand. With the thumb of the right hand, the practitioner palpates for the tender point by following the superior border of the adductor longus between the pubic and ischium branches lateral to the pubic symphysis.

The practitioner progressively slightly increases adduction and flexion until tenderness disappears and then holds this position for 90 seconds.

At the same time, a mild amount of pressure is progressively applied with the thumb, while the muscle first and then the membrane slowly relax (Fig. 5.49; Video 5.21).

Therapeutic Program, Frequency of Sessions

The AcuOsteo Method of treatment combines acupuncture and osteopathic manipulations, and, in principle, both therapeutic techniques are used during each session and at the same time.

If the condition is acute or chronic with intense pain, we recommend sessions twice a week for 2 weeks and then once a week for another 2 weeks. If improvement is observed, sessions are then scheduled once a week until complete pain relief or at least reduction by 80% to 90%.

In practice, however, since the osteopathic approach differs from acupuncture in that it follows a mechanical principle and aims to restore proper joint mobility, we opt for a parsimonious use of osteopathic manipulations over acupuncture; there may be no need to repeat them in every session.

Osteopathic maneuvers are therefore performed in case of persistent somatic dysfunction. That is why the patient should always be reevaluated at the beginning of each session to assess joint conditions and compare them with preexisting dysfunction.

REFERENCE

1. Reaves W, Bong C. *The Acupuncture Handbook of Sports Injuries & Pain*. 3rd ed. Hidden Needle Press; 2013.

BIBLIOGRAPHY

Baldry PE. *Acupuncture, Trigger Points and Musculoskeletal Pain*. 3rd ed. Elsevier; 2005.

Buckup K. *Test Ortopedici*. Verduci Editore; 1997.

Cipriano JJ. *Test Ortopedici e Neurologici*. Verduci Editore; 1998.

De Seze S, Ryckewaert A. *Malattie dell'osso e delle articolazioni*. Aulo Gaggi Editore; 1979.

Audouard M. *Osteopatia, l'Arto Inferiore*. Editore Marrapese; 1989.

Giusti R. *Glossary of Osteophatic Terminology*. 3rd ed. American Association of Colleges of Osteophatic Medicine; 2017.

Greenman PE. *Principles of Manual Medicine*. 2nd ed. Williams & Wilkins; 1996.

Guolo F. *Atlante di Tecniche di Energia Muscolare*. Piccin; 2014.

Hoppenfeld S. *L'Esame Obiettivo dell'Apparato Locomotore*. Aulo Gaggi Editore; 1985.

Legge D. *Close to the Bone*. Sydney College Press; 2010.

Maciocia G. *The Practice of Chinese Medicine*. 3rd ed. Elsevier; 2022.

Misulis KE, Head TC. *Neurologia di Netter*. Elsevier, Masson; 2008.

Nicholas AS, Nicholas EA. *Atlas of Osteophatic Thechniques*. Lippincott Williams & Wilkins; 2012.

Qiao W. *Wrist and Ankle and Balance Acupuncture, Italian Chine School of Acupuncture-A.M.A.B. (Association of Medical Acupuncturist of Bologna)*. Seminar; 2007.

Romoli M. *Auricular Acupuncture Diagnosis*. Churchill Livingstone Elsevier; 2009.

Tan RT. In: Besinger JW, ed. *Dr. Tan's Strategy of Twelve Magical Points*. 2003.

Tixa S. *Atlas d'Anatomie Palpatoire, tome 2, Membre Inferior*. 3e éd. Elsevier Masson; 2005.

Tixa S, Ebenegger B. *Atlas de Techniques articulaires ostéopathiques, tome 3, Les Membres*. 2e éd. Elsevier Masson; 2016.

Chapter 6

The Knee

Medial, Lateral, and Anterior Pain

Knee pain can occur medially, laterally, or anteriorly, and more rarely posteriorly. Among the most common causes of medial pain are medial meniscus tear and medial collateral ligament (MCL) sprain, often due to trauma, as well as pes anserinus syndrome (PES) resulting from postural imbalance. Lateral pain is a common sign of insertional tendonitis of biceps femoris and iliotibial band syndrome (ITBS), often stemming from sports-related repetitive microtraumas.

Pain located anteriorly can result from patellofemoral pain syndrome (PFPS; patellofemoral joint dysfunction and chondromalacia patella) and patellar tendonitis, which are often due to mechanical overloading following sports-related repetitive microtraumas and postural imbalance.

Anatomy and Biomechanics According to Western Medicine

JOINTS AND MUSCLES

The knee joint mainly allows for flexion and extension in the sagittal plane and also allows for a small degree of internal and external rotation. It is formed by four bones and an extensive network of ligaments and muscles.

Four bones make up the knee joint:
- Femur
- Tibia
- Patella
- Fibula

The femur connects the hip to the knee and is the largest and strongest bone in the body. The distal aspect of the femur includes the medial and lateral condyles and forms the proximal articulating surface for the knee. The two condyles are connected anteriorly by the trochlear groove where the patella is located.

The tibia has two condyles, also known as the tibial plateau. They are separated by the intercondylar eminence. The two condyles articulate with the femoral condyles through the two menisci.

The patella is a flat, inverted, triangular bone, situated at the front of the knee joint. It lies in the trochlear groove. It is attached to the quadriceps tendon above and the patellar tendon below. The quadriceps femoris causes the patella to slide up and down the trochlear groove.

The space between the patella and femur varies according to the pressure applied on the knee, which is the degree of flexion: the more the knee is flexed, the more the patellar pressure on the femur increases and the space decreases. An increase in pression and subsequent decrease in space may cause chondromalacia.

The fibula runs alongside the tibia and provides a surface for the lateral collateral ligament (LCL) and the biceps femoris tendon to attach to.

These bones articulate through the tibiofemoral and patellofemoral joints as follows:
- The medial and lateral condyles of the femur articulate with the tibia to form the tibiofemoral joint, which is the weight-bearing joint of the knee.
- The anterior part of the distal femur articulates with the patella to form the patellofemoral joint.
- The medial part of the head of the fibula articulates with the lateral condyle of the tibia to form the tibiofibular joint (Figs. 6.1 and 6.2).

Between the femoral and tibial condyles, the medial and lateral menisci, two structures of fibrocartilage, are C-shaped and O-shaped, respectively. Each meniscus consists of an anterior horn, a body, and a posterior horn. Each anterior horn is attached in front of the intercondylar eminence, and each posterior horn is attached behind the intercondylar eminence. Fibrocartilage is tough cartilage made of thick fibers, and it cushions the space between the femur and tibia.

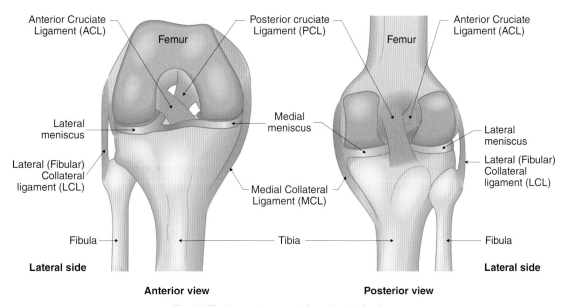

Fig. 6.1 The knee anatomy: anterior and posterior view.

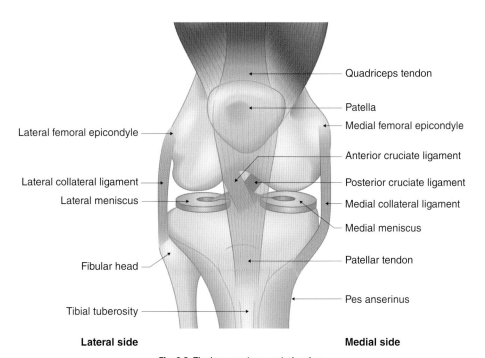

Fig. 6.2 The knee anatomy: anterior view.

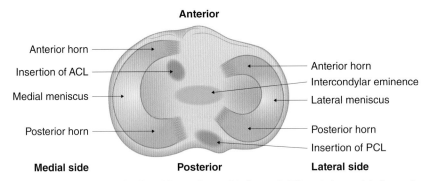

Fig. 6.3 The menisci: superior view. *ACL,* anterior cruciate ligament; *PCL,* posterior cruciate ligament.

The surface of each meniscus is concave superiorly (Fig. 6.3) and flat inferiorly to provide a congruous surface for the femoral condyles and the tibial plateau, respectively.

The menisci deepen the articular surface of the tibia, act as shock absorbers, correct the lack of congruence between the articular surfaces of the femur and tibia, evenly distribute the load from the femur to the tibia when walking, and increase joint stability.

The medial meniscus is also attached to the MCL and the joint capsule; the lateral meniscus has no attachment to the LCL. The fact that only the anterior and posterior horns are attached to the tibia allows for some mobility of the menisci, and on account of their cartilaginous structure, they also have some degree of deformation. Consequently, under joint load, the menisci "move backward" with knee flexion, and "move forward" with extension, pushed by the femoral condyles.

For the same reason, in external rotation the medial meniscus "moves backward" and the lateral meniscus "moves forward," and vice versa in internal rotation (Fig. 6.4).

Because of its peculiar C-shape anatomy providing attachment to ligaments and tendons, the medial meniscus is inherently less mobile and therefore less compliant than the lateral meniscus, which explains why it is more commonly injured.

The major ligaments in the knee joint are the collateral and cruciate ligaments. Collateral ligaments are two strap-like ligaments that prevent hyperextension, adduction, abduction, and rotations.

- The MCL adheres to the joint capsule. It runs from the medial epicondyle of the femur to the medial condyle and the superior part of the medial tibia. It is formed by a femoral band and a tibial band, which provide attachment to the posterior medial body of the medial meniscus. It is oblique, downward and forward oriented. Its primary function is to resist valgus force, but it also resists lateral rotation of the tibia on the femur. Due to its physiology, the MCL is subjected to increased tension during external rotation, that is, when it provides stabilization to the knee. This explains why the MCL sprain is the most commonly observed among external rotation injuries that, in turn, are the most frequently encountered.
- The LCL is entirely separated from the articular capsule. It runs from the lateral epicondyle of the femur to the lateral surface of the fibular head. Its primary function is to resist varus force.

Cruciate ligaments connect the femur and the tibia, and in doing so, they form a cross, hence the term "cruciate" from the Latin "cross."

- The anterior cruciate ligament (ACL) is the major stabilizing ligament of the knee. It originates from the anteromedial surface of the intercondylar eminence, just behind the attachment of the anterior horn of the medial meniscus. Then, it ascends superolaterally and posteriorly, up to the posteromedial aspect of the lateral femoral condyle. It is oblique, upward, backward, and outward oriented. It prevents the femur from sliding

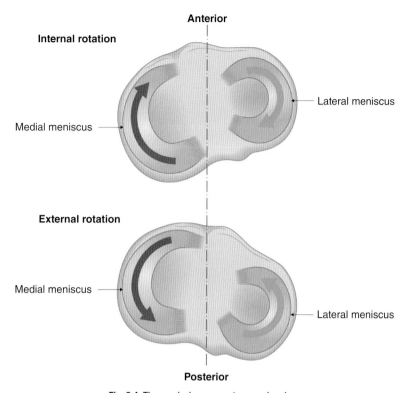

Internal rotation

Anterior

Medial meniscus

Lateral meniscus

External rotation

Medial meniscus

Lateral meniscus

Posterior

Fig. 6.4 The menisci movements: superior view.

backward on the tibia (or the tibia sliding forward on the femur). It also resists rotary forces medially and laterally, as well as valgus and varus forces.

• The posterior cruciate ligament (PCL) originates from the posterior surface of the tibia, just behind the attachment of the two posterior horns of the menisci. Then, it ascends superiorly and anteriorly and attaches to the lateral aspect of the medial femoral condyle. It is oblique, upward, forward, and inward oriented. It prevents the femur from moving too far forward on the tibia (or the tibia sliding backward on the femur). It also resists rotary forces, as well as valgus and varus forces. The PCL is the knee's basic stabilizer and provides a central axis about which the knee rotates.

Finally, we should mention the patellar tendon, which is a continuation of the quadriceps femoris tendon distal to the patella. It attaches to the tibial tuberosity (Figs. 6.5 and 6.6).

The knee muscles that are more relevant to our study include the following:

The tensor fasciae latae is a muscle that originates from the tibial crest and the anterior superior iliac spine (ASIS). Then, it attaches distally to the iliotibial band (ITB) and lies adjacent to the lateral tibial condyle. This muscle allows the knee to extend.

The quadriceps femoris consists of four muscles: the vastus lateralis, medialis, and intermedius, which originate from the linea aspera of the femur, and the rectus femoris, which originates from the ASIS and the superior acetabulum. These four muscles unite and attach to the patella through the quadriceps tendon. In turn, the patellar tendon originates from the patella and attaches to the tuberosity of the tibia. This is the main muscle that allows the knee to extend.

The sartorius originates from the ASIS and attaches below to the medial tibial condyle, where it joins with the tendons of the gracilis and semitendinosus in the pes anserinus. This muscle allows the knee to flex and internally rotate.

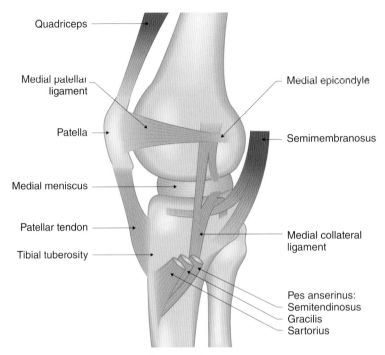

Quadriceps

Medial patellar
ligament

Patella

Medial meniscus

Patellar tendon

Tibial tuberosity

Medial epicondyle

Semimembranosus

Medial collateral
ligament

Pes anserinus:
Semitendinosus
Gracilis
Sartorius

Fig. 6.5 The knee anatomy: medial view.

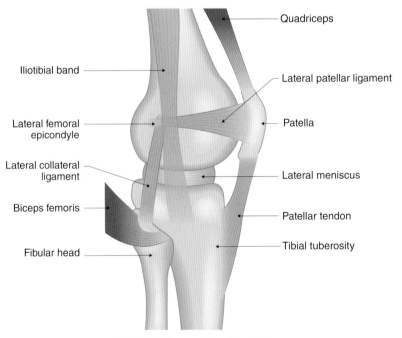

Iliotibial band

Lateral femoral
epicondyle

Lateral collateral
ligament

Biceps femoris

Fibular head

Quadriceps

Lateral patellar ligament

Patella

Lateral meniscus

Patellar tendon

Tibial tuberosity

Fig. 6.6 The knee anatomy: lateral view.

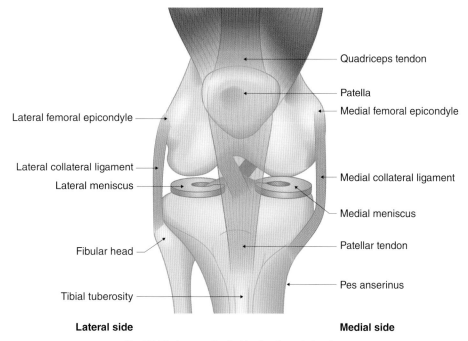

Fig. 6.7 The knee anatomical landmarks: anterior view.

The hamstrings are a group of three muscles: the semitendinosus, semimembranosus, and biceps femoris.

- The semitendinosus originates from the ischial tuberosity and attaches below to the medial tibial condyle, where it joins with the tendons of the gracilis and sartorius in the pes anserinus.
- The semimembranosus originates from the ischial tuberosity and attaches to the posterior surface of the medial tibial condyle.
- As its name implies, the biceps femoris has two heads, a short head and a long head. The long head originates from the ischial tuberosity, whereas the short head originates from the linea aspera on the middle third of femur. They both attach to the fibular head.

These muscles allow the knee to flex. The semitendinosus and semimembranosus allow the knee to internally rotate and the biceps femoris to externally rotate.

The gracilis originates from the inferior ramus of pubis and attaches to the medial tibial condyle, where it joins with the tendons of the semitendinosus and sartorius in the pes anserinus. This muscle allows the knee to flex and internally rotate.

ANATOMICAL LANDMARKS

The most useful anatomical landmarks are listed as follows (Figs. 6.7–6.9):

- Patella: it has an anterior and a posterior surface, three borders, and an apex. The superior, medial, and lateral borders give attachment to the quadriceps femoris; the apex gives attachment to the patellar tendon.
- Tibial tuberosity: it is a bony prominence located on the anterior surface of the proximal tibial shaft.
- Medial and lateral condyles: they are located at the distal end of the femur. An epicondyle projects from each condyle and serves as an attachment site for the collateral ligaments.
- Fibular head: located in the proximal part of the fibula, it is a large, pointed bone.

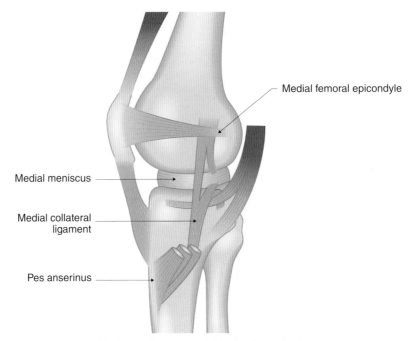

Fig. 6.8 The knee anatomical landmarks: medial view.

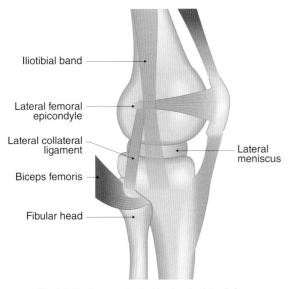

Fig. 6.9 The knee anatomical landmarks: lateral view.

- The peripheral border of each meniscus, between the femoral and tibial condyles: it is thick, convex, and attached to the inside of the joint capsule.

JOINT MOVEMENTS

The Physiological Movements of the Knee Joint

Biomechanics of the knee allows for a large degree of flexion and extension and also for a small degree of internal and external rotation. Adduction and abduction are passive and small movements.

The neutral position to assess the physiological movements of the knee is with the patient lying supine, the lower limb extended.

- Flexion
  Hip and knee flexed at 90 degrees: the leg moves toward the thigh.
- Extension
  Hip and knee extended: the popliteal fossa touches the bed.
- External Rotation
  Hip and knee flexed at 90 degrees: the tibia rotates outward.
- Internal Rotation
  Hip and knee flexed at 90 degrees: the tibia rotates inward.

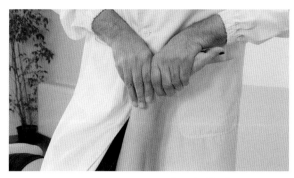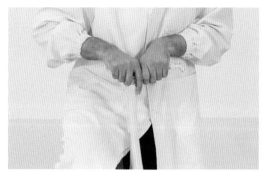

Fig. 6.10 The Apley's compression test: starting position.

Lateral movements are tested with the knee slightly flexed.
- Abduction (valgus): the leg moves outward and the knee joint is angled outward.
- Adduction (varus): the leg moves inward and the knee joint is angled inward.

The normal range of motion of the knee from the neutral position to full extension is 180 degrees.

The normal range of motion of the knee from the neutral position, where the knee is slightly flexed:
- To abduction is 0 to about 10 to 15 degrees
- To adduction is 0 to about 10 to 15 degrees

The normal range of motion of the knee from the neutral position, where the hip and knee are flexed at 90 degrees:
- To full flexion is about 140 degrees
- To full external rotation is 0 to about 30 to 40 degrees
- To full internal rotation is 0 to about 10 degrees

Diagnosis in Western Medicine

MEDIAL PAIN

Medial knee pain is commonly seen in our clinical practice. We define it as a feeling of physical suffering on the inner side of the knee.

Medial Meniscus Tear

There are two types of medial meniscus tear. Menisci can tear due to traumatic injury, mainly resulting from playing contact sports or degenerative (nontraumatic) wear.

The most common symptoms are the following:
- Tenderness on palpation over the medial joint line

- Pain during external rotation of the foot and lower leg
- Weakened or hypotrophied quadriceps muscle
- Positive Apley's compression test

The Apley's Compression Test

It is used to assess medial and lateral meniscus tear. The patient is prone with the right knee flexed at 90 degrees. The practitioner stands on the patient's right side with the hands on the plantar aspect of the foot and heel. Then, the practitioner roots the patient's thigh to the bed with the right knee.

The aim of the test is to trap the menisci between the tibia and the femur while internally and externally rotating the tibia and, at the same time, compressing the knee to elicit pain.

Pain over the medial and lateral compartments is considered positive for medial and lateral meniscus, respectively (Figs. 6.10–6.12; Video 6.1).

Medial Collateral Ligament Sprain

There are several causes of MCL sprains, and there is a spectrum of severity ranging from a stretch or partial tear, up to a complete rupture of the ligament. It is one of the most common knee injuries, mainly resulting from a direct trauma to the knee or excessive outward twist.

MCL sprains are graded according to their level of severity: grades I, II, and III.

Grade I and II symptoms:
- Mild medial pain
- Little swelling
- Tenderness on palpation

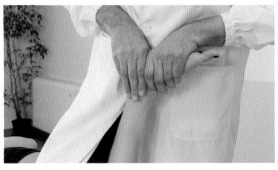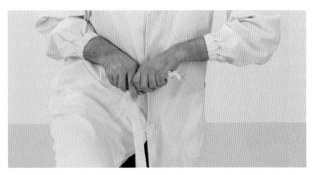

Fig. 6.11 The Apley's compression test: internal rotation.

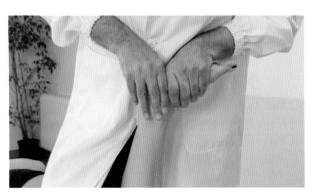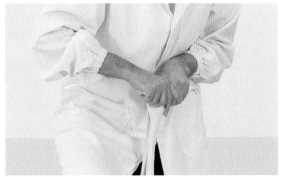

Fig. 6.12 The Apley's compression test: external rotation.

- Possible mild instability
- Possible positive Apley's distraction test

Grade III:

- Severe medial pain
- Marked swelling
- Tenderness on palpation
- Knee gives way into valgus
- Gross instability
- Positive Apley's distraction test

The Apley's Distraction Test

It is used to assess MCL and LCL sprains. The patient is prone with the right knee flexed at 90 degrees. The practitioner stands on the patient's right side. The practitioner roots the patient's thigh to the bed with the right knee and holds the ankle with the hands. Then, the practitioner applies moderate traction along the axis of the tibia and moves the ankle into external rotation. The aim of the test is to reach a point of tension on the medial and lateral collateral ligaments to elicit pain.

The test is considered positive for a sign of MCL sprain if external rotation elicits pain in the medial compartment. It is instead a sign of LCL sprain if internal rotation elicits pain in the lateral compartment (Figs. 6.13–6.15; Video 6.2).

Pes Anserinus Syndrome

This condition is an inflammation of the pes anserinus bursa, which is located where the three tendons (sartorius, gracilis, and semitendinosus muscles) attach to the lower leg. Their attachment looks like a "goose foot," which explains the name pes anserinus.

Symptoms appear on the medial side of the tibial shaft near the proximal end.

The most common symptoms are the following:

- Pain slowly developing on the inside of the knee
- Inner knee pain increasing with exercise or climbing stairs
- Swelling or tenderness on the pes anserinus bursa
- Possible limited range of motion

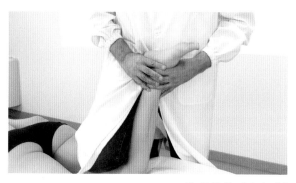 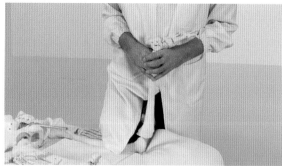

Fig. 6.13 The Apley's distraction test: starting position.

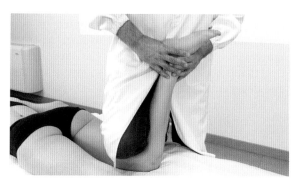 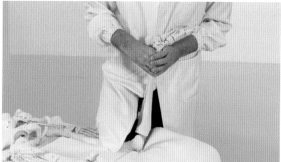

Fig. 6.14 The Apley's distraction test: external rotation.

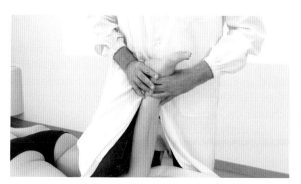 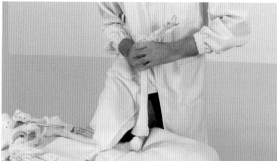

Fig. 6.15 The Apley's distraction test: internal rotation.

- Weakness
- Postural imbalance

Pes Anserinus Syndrome Test

There is no specific test, and it can only be assessed by palpation. The patient is supine. Palpation with the index finger starts from the medial midportion of the tibia close to the medial border and ascends the leg up to the three tendons attached to the tibia below the tibial condyle. The tender area is of variable size. The test is considered positive if the patient reports pain over the tendon attachment to the tibia.

ANTERIOR PAIN

Anterior knee pain presents over the anterior aspect of the knee and may result from several conditions. This handbook will only deal with the most common conditions observed in our clinical practice.

Patellofemoral Pain Syndrome

PFPS is a broad term used to refer to pain arising from the patellofemoral joint itself or adjacent soft tissues. It is a chronic pain that increases when running, walking up and down stairs, sitting, or squatting.

The patient usually refers to it as anterior knee pain, which gets worse with activities loading the patellofemoral joint. The differential diagnosis of PFPS includes chondromalacia patellae, patellofemoral joint dysfunction, and patellar tendinopathy. Patellofemoral pain may be a sign of chondromalacia patella, but not everyone with PFPS will have chondromalacia patella.

The most common symptoms of chondromalacia patellae are the following:
- Anterior knee pain, increasing with common daily activities loading the joint
- Pain when walking up and down the stairs
- Tenderness on palpation under the lateral or medial side of the patella
- Moderate swelling
- Crepitation
- Positive patellar grind test

Patellar Grind Test

It is used to assess chondromalacia patellae. The patient is supine with the right knee and hip extended. The practitioner stands on the patient's right side. The practitioner places the web of the left thumb and index finger on the superior border of the patella, while the right hand holds the leg. The patient is then asked to contract the quadriceps femoris gently and gradually, while the practitioner applies a counterforce on the superior aspect of the patella to prevent it from moving upward. The test is considered positive if the patient reports pain under the patella (Fig. 6.16; Video 6.3).

Patellar Tendonitis

Patellar tendonitis is one of the causes of anterior knee pain, commonly found in young athletes. It

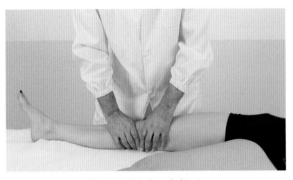

Fig. 6.16 Patellar grind test.

can develop when the tendon is injured or overused, and pain increases with loading, repetitive movements, or sports. It can be classified as reactive, that is, a noninflammatory response, traumatic, and degenerative.

The most common symptoms are the following:
- Pain in the tendon below the patella
- Load-related pain increasing with the demand on the knee extensors
- Positive patellar tendonitis test

Patellar Tendonitis Test

There is no specific test, and it can only be assessed by palpation. The patient is supine. The practitioner stands on the patient's right side.

First, the practitioner examines the affected tendon along its pathway or where it attaches to the anterior tibial apophysis to see if it is thicker and more swollen than the other. The thicker it is, the more severe and chronic the condition is.

Then, the tendon is palpated by pinching it with the thumb and index finger, starting from the lateral and medial sides of the proximal portion and moving downward to its tibial attachment.

The test is considered positive if the patient reports pain over the tendon itself or its attachment to the tibia. Pain can be one sided or bilateral.

LATERAL PAIN

Lateral knee pain presents over the lateral aspect of the knee and can be the result of several conditions. This handbook will only deal with the most common diseases observed in our clinical practice.

Insertional Tendonitis of Biceps Femoris

Insertional tendonitis of biceps femoris is a common and disabling condition that is more frequently observed in young patients. Tendonitis of biceps femoris refers to tendon inflammation that may lead to degeneration and calcifications of the tendon itself. It is a disease of multifactorial etiology, often caused by or associated with overuse or work- or sports-related repetitive movements.

The most common symptoms are the following:
- Pain on the posterolateral side of the knee
- Pain during active and passive knee flexion at 90 degrees
- Difficulty in performing sports-related activities
- Positive resisted knee flexion test

Resisted Knee Flexion Test

It is used to assess insertional tendonitis of biceps femoris. The patient is prone with the right knee flexed at 90 degrees.

The practitioner stands on the patient's left side with the left index finger on the insertion of the biceps femoris into the fibula, while the right hand holds the ankle and brings it into external rotation.

The practitioner tries to bring the knee into extension while the patient applies resistance that should progressively decrease (eccentric contraction). The aim of the test is to apply tension on the biceps tendon to elicit pain.

The test is considered positive if the patient reports pain when the insertion of the biceps femoris into the fibula is palpated, either at rest or during resistance to extension (Fig. 6.17; Video 6.4).

Iliotibial Band Syndrome

ITBS is a common overuse injury that usually causes pain and tenderness on palpation of the lateral femoral epicondyle. It is considered to be multifactorial in its etiology and is typically seen in runners and cyclists. Sliding of the ITB on the lateral femoral epicondyle can create excess friction resulting in inflammation.

The most common symptoms are the following:
- Sharp pain located on the outside of the knee that increases as the heel strikes the floor
- The pain gets worse with exercise

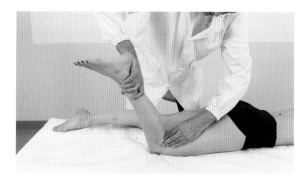

Fig. 6.17 Resisted knee flexion test.

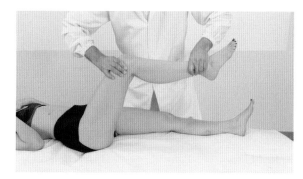

Fig. 6.18 The Noble test.

- Feeling a click, pop, or snap on the femoral epicondyle due to the band rubbing or "flicking" over the bony surface when the joint bends.
- Exercise-related tenderness over the lateral femoral epicondyle
- Positive Noble test

The Noble Test

It is used to assess ITBS. The patient is supine with the right knee flexed at 90 degrees. The practitioner stands on the patient's left side with the right index and middle fingers applying firm pressure on the ITB at the level of the lateral epicondyle of the femur. Then, the patient is asked to actively extend the knee. The test is considered positive if palpable snapping or localized pain at 30 degrees of flexion is reported (Fig. 6.18; Video 6.5).

JOINT PAIN, ARTHRITIS, AND STIFFNESS

Patients with knee arthritis and postsurgical outcomes usually complain of pain, weakness, and restricted range of motion. Swelling of posterior knee should not be underestimated and could be caused by a Baker cyst.

Also known as a popliteal cyst, it is a fluid-filled sac that can form in the back of the knee. Knee injuries can often lead to a developing Baker cyst. Some Baker cysts are asymptomatic, while others can sometimes cause pain, swelling, and stiffness. In the most severe cases, the cyst can even burst.

A partial or a complete tear of the cruciate ligaments, the ACL in particular, is commonly reported. It results from excessive strain with simultaneous external rotation of the knee.

The most common symptoms are the following:
- Severe pain
- Hematoma
- Swelling
- Knee instability

Among the most common causes of knee arthritis are fracture or rheumatoid arthritis; primary

osteoarthritis, septic arthritis, crystal arthropathy are also to be mentioned. Diagnosis is based on the patient's medical history, along with clinical and radiographic examinations. The most common complications that may occur after surgery or as a result of fracture include:
- Knee stiffness with possible loss of motion (flexion, extension)
- Late-onset osteoarthritis
- Failed fusion
- Persistent pain

RED FLAGS IN WESTERN MEDICINE

The presence of heat (calor), redness (rubor), swelling (tumor), pain (dolor), and loss of function (function laesa) determines the need for diagnostic investigations. Knee trauma is a common occurrence.

Patients with rheumatoid arthritis of the knee usually complain of pain throughout the range of motion,

Red Flags	Pain	Inspection	Other Signs	Neurological Signs	Recommendations
Inflammation	Pain	Redness, swelling, and heat	–	Functional deficit	Physician evaluation Imaging investigations
Fracture	Spontaneous pain	Deformity and swelling	Movement beyond normal range of motion	Functional deficit	Physician evaluation Imaging investigations
Grade 3 MCL sprain	Severe medial pain	Joint swelling	Marked medial edema	Functional deficit Knee tilts outward (valgus)	Physician evaluation Imaging investigations
Complete tear of the cruciate ligament	Severe pain	Joint swelling	Hematoma	Knee instability	Physician evaluation Imaging investigations
Rheumatoid arthritis	Pain with or without movement	Redness and swelling	Fatigue and general discomfort	Functional deficit	Physician evaluation Imaging investigations Laboratory tests

but usually the knee is not affected. Both fatigue and general discomfort can also be observed.

The use of imaging techniques is mandatory in case of a grade 3 MCL sprain or a complete tear of the cruciate ligament.

Special attention should be paid if concomitant symptoms are observed, such as numbness, tingling, paresthesia (abnormal sensation), muscle weakness, decreased tendon reflexes, and pain, mainly at night.

Abnormalities uncovered on history taking or physical examination may require medical evaluation, laboratory tests, and imaging investigations, such as x-rays, US, CT, and MRI.

Diagnosis in Chinese Medicine

In Chinese Medicine, musculoskeletal pain results from the obstruction of Qì and Blood circulation or inadequate Qì and Blood for the nourishment of the secondary channels, especially the Muscle and Connecting channels.

The Muscle and Connecting channels more often involved in knee disorders are listed below:
- Spleen
- Liver
- Stomach
- Gall Bladder
- Bladder

Two Extraordinary channels may also be involved.
- Yin Qiao Mai
- Yang Qiao Mai

The channels affected vary according to pain location:
- Spleen: pain is on the medial aspect of the knee, with pathologies being medial meniscus tear (anterior horn and body), MCL sprain and PES.
- Liver: pain is on the medial aspect of the knee, with pathologies being medial meniscus tear (body and posterior horn) and MCL sprain.
- Yin Qiao Mai: pain is on the medial aspect of the knee, with pathologies being medial meniscus tear and MCL sprain.
- Stomach: pain is on the anterior aspect of the knee, with pathologies being PFPS (patellofemoral joint dysfunction and chondromalacia patellae) and patellar tendonitis.
- Gall Bladder: pain is on the lateral aspect of the knee, with pathologies being insertional tendonitis of biceps femoris and ITBS.

- Bladder: pain is on the posterolateral aspect of the knee, the pathology is insertional tendonitis of biceps femoris.
- Yang Qiao Mai: pain is on the lateral aspect of the knee, with pathologies being insertional tendonitis of biceps femoris and ITBS.

What matters most is to identify the affected channel where pain is located. Sometimes, it is not so easy to determine it, and consequently, the following data concerning the Muscle channels involved in elbow movements should be acquired for a better identification.
- Extension: ST
- Flexion: BL, GB, SP, and LR
- External rotation: GB
- Internal rotation: SP and LR
- Abduction: GB
- Adduction: SP, LR and KI

The information so acquired on the channel which is likely to be involved, that is, pain location and related movement restriction, can also be integrated with the results from Western medicine orthopedic tests to identify which muscle, tendon, and joint are affected in case of:
- Medial meniscus tear
- MCL sprain
- PES
- PFPS (patellofemoral joint dysfunction and chondromalacia patellae) and patellar tendonitis
- Insertional tendonitis of biceps femoris
- ITBS

ETIOLOGY

Knee pain is usually caused by:
- *Overuse, repetitive strain injury*. Through work (paver) or sports (soccer, basketball or running); performing the same movement over and over again causes local Qì stagnation or Qì and Blood deficiency.
- *Trauma, sport injuries*. If mild, they cause local Qì stagnation; if severe, they cause local Blood stasis.
- *Cold and Dampness*. Local invasion causes Qì stagnation or Blood stasis.

Previous accidents often predispose the knee to more frequent invasions of external pathogenic factors (EPFs), especially Cold.

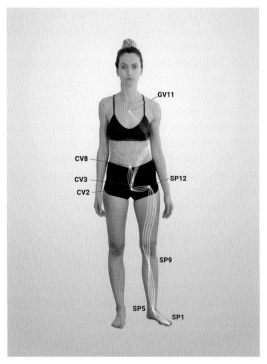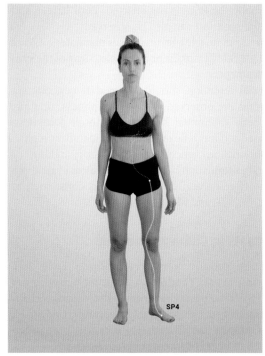

Fig. 6.19 The pathways of the Spleen Muscle and Connecting "proper" channels.

PATHOLOGY

The Muscle and Connecting channels, and the Extraordinary channels Yin and Yang Qiao Mai are often affected by Qì stagnation and Blood stasis:

- Qì stagnation manifests itself with widespread pain radiating proximally or distally along the pathway of the Muscle channels and could be associated with muscle contracture and stiffness of the quadriceps and hamstrings (in particular of the biceps femoris), also perceived upon palpation.
- Blood stasis, usually occurring in the Connecting channels, manifests itself with more intense pain localized in the joint or, more frequently, in the site of muscle insertion and ligament with consequent limited range of motion or joint stiffness.

As already mentioned in the fundamentals of acupuncture for MSK pain in the limbs (see Chapter 1), the term Connecting channels includes not only the Connecting channel "proper" but also the Connecting channel "area" that covers the whole pathway of the Main channel.

MEDIAL MENISCUS TEAR, MEDIAL COLLATERAL LIGAMENT SPRAIN, AND PES ANSERINUS SYNDROME

To identify the channels affected, whether Muscle, Connecting channels, or the Extraordinary channel, we check the location and characteristics of musculoskeletal pain, palpate the affected area, test the range of motion for each knee movement, and perform orthopedic tests to elicit pain.

The Pathways of the Spleen Secondary Channels

In case of medial meniscus tear, MCL sprain, and PES, the Spleen Muscle and Connecting channels are involved (Fig. 6.19).

The pathway of the Spleen Muscle and Connecting channels explains pain on the medial aspect of the knee, which could radiate distally to the medial aspect of the leg.

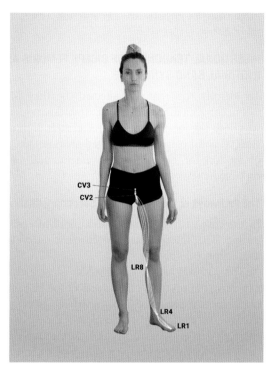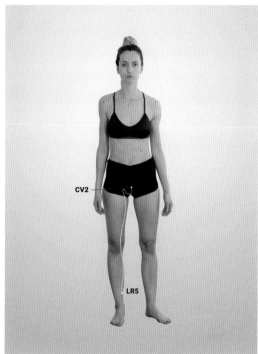

Fig. 6.20 The pathways of the Liver Muscle and Connecting "proper" channels.

According to our experience, the Spleen channels are more likely to be involved in case of anterior horn medial meniscus tear and PES, whereas they overlap with the Liver channels when the body of the medial meniscus is involved or, more rarely, a collateral ligament sprain occurs.

The Pathways of the Liver Secondary Channels

In case of medial meniscus tear and MCL sprain, the Liver Muscle and Connecting channels are involved (Fig. 6.20).

The pathway of the Liver Muscle and Connecting channels explains pain on the medial aspect of the knee, which could radiate distally to the medial aspect of the leg.

According to our experience, the Liver channels are more likely to be involved in case of MCL sprain and posterior horn medial meniscus tear, whereas they overlap with the Spleen channels when the body of the medial meniscus is involved.

The Pathway of the Yin Qiao Mai

In case of medial meniscus tear, MCL sprain, and pes anserinus, the Yin Qiao Mai extraordinary channel may be involved (Fig. 6.21).

The pathway of the Yin Qiao Mai extraordinary channel may explain pain or tension on the medial aspect of the knee, which can radiate distally or proximally to the medial aspect of the leg or thigh, respectively.

PATELLOFEMORAL PAIN SYNDROME (PATELLOFEMORAL JOINT DYSFUNCTION AND CHONDROMALACIA PATELLAE) AND PATELLAR TENDONITIS

To identify the Muscle and Connecting channels affected, we check the location and characteristics of musculoskeletal pain, palpate the affected area, test the range of motion for each knee movement, and perform orthopedic tests to elicit pain.

The Pathways of the Stomach Secondary Channels

In case of PFPS and patellar tendonitis, the Stomach Muscle and Connecting channels are involved (Fig. 6.22).

The pathway of the Stomach Muscle and Connecting channels explains pain on the anterior aspect of the knee, which could slightly radiate

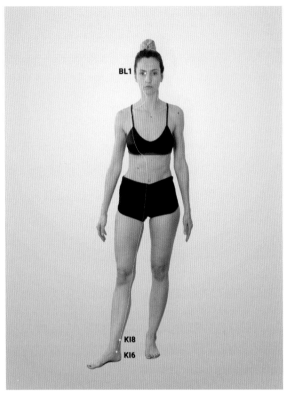

Fig. 6.21 The pathways of the Yin Qiao Mai.

proximally or distally to the anterior aspect of the thigh or leg, respectively.

INSERTIONAL TENDONITIS OF BICEPS FEMORIS AND ILIOTIBIAL BAND SYNDROME

To identify the channels affected, be they Muscle, Connecting channels, or the Extraordinary channel, we check the location and characteristics of musculoskeletal pain, palpate the affected area, test the range of motion for each knee movement, and perform orthopedic tests to elicit pain.

The Pathways of the Gall Bladder Secondary Channels

In the case of insertional tendonitis of biceps femoris and ITBS, the Gall Bladder Muscle and Connecting channels are involved.

The pathway of the Gall Bladder Muscle channels explains pain on the lateral aspect of the knee, which could radiate proximally to the lateral aspect of the thigh or distally to the lateral aspect of the leg, whereas the pathway of the Gall Bladder Connecting channel "proper" does not because it does not ascend to the knee (Fig. 6.23).

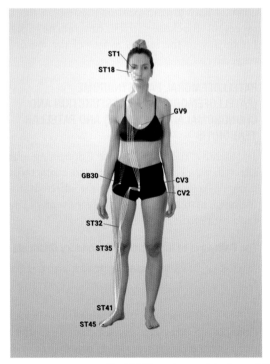

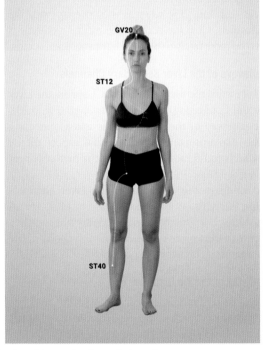

Fig. 6.22 The pathways of the Stomach Muscle and Connecting "proper" channels.

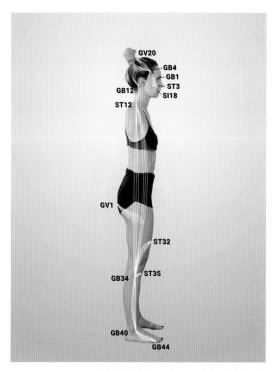 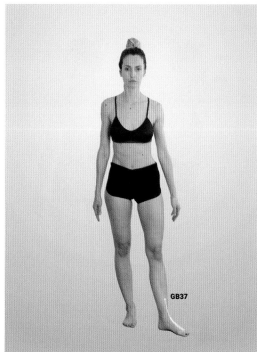

Fig. 6.23 The pathways of the Gall Bladder Muscle and Connecting "proper" channels.

Since we are now referring to the Gall Bladder Connecting channel "area," we regard the Gall Bladder Connecting channels as channels involved.

The Pathways of the Bladder Secondary Channels

In case of insertional tendonitis of biceps femoris, the Bladder Muscle and Connecting channels may be involved.

According to our experience, the Bladder channels are involved in case of insertional tendonitis of biceps femoris when pain is on the posterolateral aspect of the knee.

The pathway of the Bladder Muscle and Connecting channels explains pain on the posterolateral aspect of the knee, which could slightly radiate proximally, or more rarely distally, to the posterolateral aspect of the thigh or leg, respectively (Fig. 6.24).

The Pathway of the Yang Qiao Mai

In case of insertional tendonitis of biceps femoris and ITBS, the Yang Qiao Mai extraordinary channel may be involved.

The pathway of the Yang Qiao Mai extraordinary channel may explain pain or tension on the lateral aspect of the knee, which can radiate distally or proximally to the lateral aspect of the leg or thigh, respectively (Fig. 6.25).

Diagnosis in Osteopathic Medicine

The examination for "somatic dysfunction" is the central concept of the diagnostic process; palpation of the affected area and functionally/anatomically related components of the somatic system is the only way to assess it.

Consequently, the osteopathic diagnostic approach to musculoskeletal knee pain is based on the identification of joint somatic dysfunctions not only of the knee but also of the hip, pelvic girdle and ankle.

Regardless of the condition to be treated, be it medial meniscus tear, MCL strain or tear, PES, PFPS, patellar tendonitis, insertional tendonitis of biceps femoris, ITBS, arthritis of the knee, or surgical outcomes, all the recommended tests should be performed to identify the dysfunctions that occur more frequently.

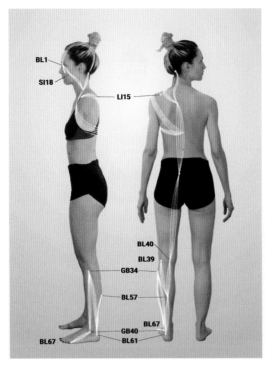 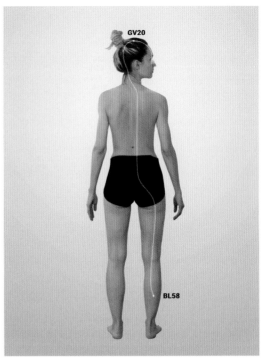

Fig. 6.24 The pathways of the Bladder Muscle and Connecting "proper" channels.

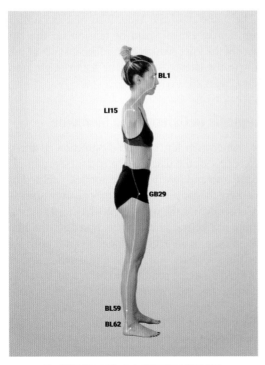

Fig. 6.25 The pathways of the Yang Qiao Mai.

It is therefore evident that the osteopathic diagnosis is developed regardless of the condition to be treated; therefore the osteopathic tests recommended for the knee, hip, pelvic girdle, and ankle will not be repeated when the "injuries" are treated.

TESTS FOR THE MAIN SOMATIC DYSFUNCTIONS

The only way to diagnose somatic dysfunctions of a joint is to assess the passive movements of its articular ends in relation to one another and compare them with the same movements of the joint on the healthy side. Testing of all knee joints is required.

On the same plane of motion, there is passive mobility quantitatively and qualitatively equal on both sides of a theoretical neutral point that represents the reference point.

When the balance is lost and the range and quality of motion are not the same in both directions, then there is somatic dysfunction.

Tests of the Tibiofemoral Joint

Tests are performed to assess the most common tibial dysfunctions:

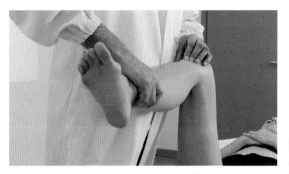 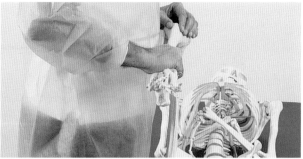

Fig. 6.26 Internal-external rotation test of the tibia_starting position.

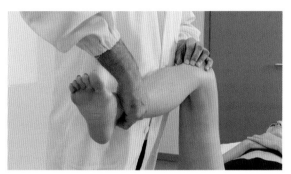 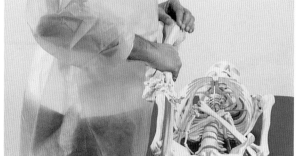

Fig. 6.27 Internal-external rotation test of the tibia—internal rotation.

- External rotation of the tibia
- Internal rotation of the tibia
- Abduction of the tibia
- Adduction of the tibia
- Anterior tibia
- Posterior tibia

Internal-External Rotation Test of the Tibia

The patient is supine close to the bed edge with the right hip and knee flexed at 90 degrees. The practitioner stands on the patient's right side. The practitioner holds the ankle with the right hand and maintains it in neutral rotation, while placing the left thumb and index finger on the anterior tibial apophysis:

The internal-external rotation test is then performed by rotating the leg with the right hand.

The practitioner appreciates the range and quality of motion for tibial internal rotation and then compares them with external rotation, and vice versa.

If the knee rotates more easily in internal rotation, then there is internal rotation dysfunction, and vice versa (Figs. 6.26–6.28; Video 6.6).

Adduction-Abduction Test of the Tibia

The patient is supine close to the bed edge with the right hip and knee slightly flexed and abducted off the bed. The practitioner stands on the patient's right side and holds the patient's ankle between the thighs to apply distal traction and produce knee decoaptation. The thenar eminences and fingers are on the lateral and medial joint spaces and on the popliteal fossa, respectively.

- The adduction test is then performed by pushing the tibia externally with the right hand.
- The abduction test is then performed by pushing the tibia internally with the left hand.

The practitioner appreciates the range and quality of motion for tibial adduction and then compares them with tibial abduction and vice versa.

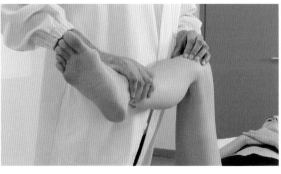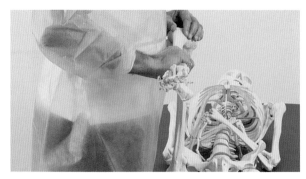

Fig. 6.28 Internal-external rotation test of the tibia—external rotation.

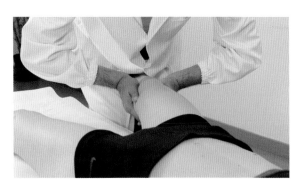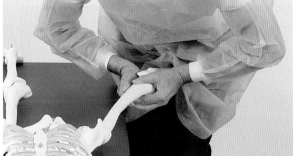

Fig. 6.29 Tibial adduction-abduction test_starting position.

If the tibia moves more easily in adduction than in abduction, then there is adduction dysfunction, and vice versa (Figs. 6.29–6.31; Video 6.7).

Anterior Test of the Tibia

The patient is supine close to the bed edge with the right knee flexed at 90 degrees and foot flat on the bed.

The practitioner sits on the foot and holds the knee by placing the thenar eminences on the tibia, the thumbs on the femoral condyles, and the other fingers on the popliteal fossa:

The anterior test is then performed by pulling the tibia forward with the fingers.

The practitioner appreciates the range and quality of anterior motion and then compares them with posterior motion.

If the tibia moves more easily anteriorly than posteriorly, then there is tibial anterior dysfunction (Fig. 6.32; Video 6.8).

Posterior Test of the Tibia

The patient is supine close to the bed edge with the right knee flexed at 90 degrees and foot flat on the bed. The practitioner sits on the foot and holds the knee by placing the thenar eminences on the tibia, the thumbs on the femoral condyles, and the other fingers on the popliteal fossa:

The posterior test is then performed by pushing the tibia backward with the thenar eminences.

The practitioner appreciates the range and quality of posterior motion and then compares them with anterior motion.

If the tibia moves more easily posteriorly than anteriorly, then there is tibial posterior dysfunction (Fig. 6.33; Video 6.9).

Test of the Proximal Tibiofibular Joint

A test is performed to assess the most common fibular dysfunctions:

- Anterior fibula
- Posterior fibula

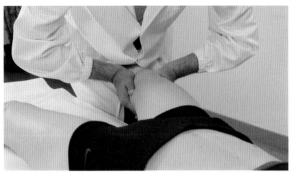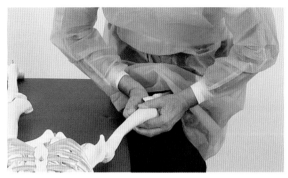

Fig. 6.30 Tibial adduction-abduction test_adduction.

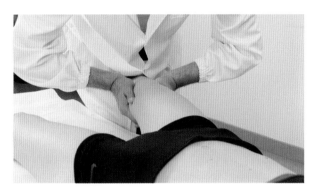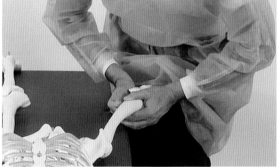

Fig. 6.31 Tibial adduction-abduction test_abduction.

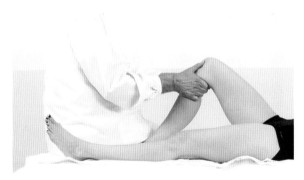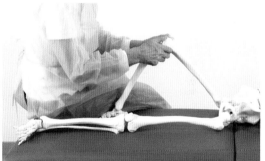

Fig. 6.32 Anterior test of the tibia.

Anteroposterior Test of the Fibula

The patient is supine close to the bed edge with the right knee flexed at 90 degrees and foot flat on the bed.

The practitioner sits on the foot to stabilize the leg and holds the tibia with the right hand, while the left thumb, index finger, and middle finger hold the fibular head:

- The anterior test is performed by pulling the fibula forward with the fingers.

- The posterior test is performed by pushing the fibula backward with the thumb.

The practitioner appreciates the range and quality of anterior motion and then compares them with posterior motion.

If the fibula moves more easily anteriorly than posteriorly, then there is fibular anterior dysfunction, and vice versa (Figs. 6.34–6.36; Video 6.10).

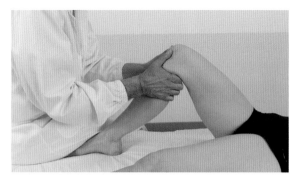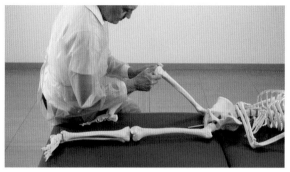

Fig. 6.33 Posterior test of the tibia.

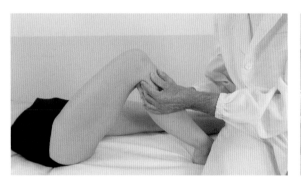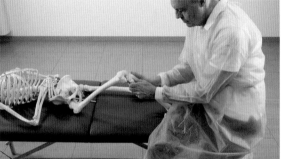

Fig. 6.34 Anteroposterior test of the fibula_starting point.

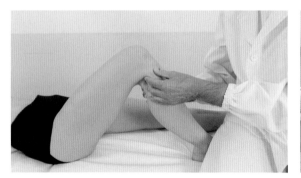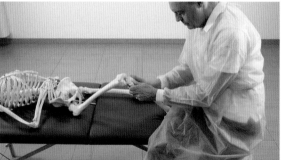

Fig. 6.35 Anteroposterior test of the fibula_anterior test.

Test of the Medial Meniscus

A test is performed to assess the most common medial meniscus dysfunction:

- Anterior medial meniscus

The Retreating Test of the Medial Meniscus

The patient is supine with the right knee and hip flexed at 90 degrees. The practitioner stands on the patient's right side. The left thumb is on the anterior

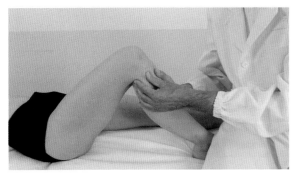
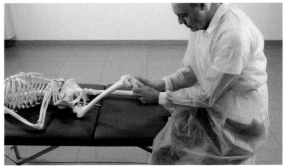

Fig. 6.36 Anteroposterior test of the fibula_posterior test.

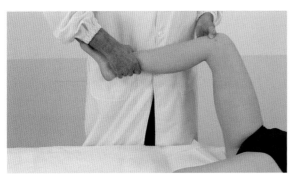
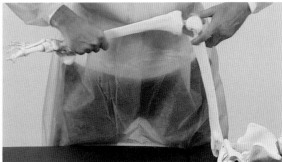

Fig. 6.37 The retreating medial meniscus test_starting position.

horn of the medial meniscus and the right hand holds the ankle. The right hand moves the leg from the neutral position into internal rotation, while the left hand keeps the knee still and the left thumb applies pressure.

During extension and passive external rotation of the leg, the anterior horn of the medial meniscus should move backward. The test is considered positive if the patient reports pain with movement, meaning that the medial meniscus is not free to move backward and stays fixed in the anterior position.

A positive test is a sign of anterior dysfunction of the medial meniscus (Figs. 6.37 and 6.38; Video 6.11).

Test of the Patella

A test is performed to assess the most common patellar dysfunction.

- Superolateral patella

Superolateral-Inferomedial Test of the Patella

The patient is supine close to the bed edge with the right leg extended. The practitioner stands on the patient's right side. The practitioner places the web of the left and right thumb and index finger on the superior and inferior border of the patella, respectively.

- The superolateral test is performed by pushing the patella superiorly and laterally with the right hand.
- The inferomedial test is performed by pushing the patella inferiorly and medially with the left hand.

The practitioner appreciates the range and quality of motion of the two movements.

If the patella moves more easily superiorly and laterally, then there is superolateral dysfunction. On the contrary, if it moves more easily inferiorly and medially, then there is inferomedial dysfunction (Fig. 6.39; Video 6.12).

Treatment With the AcuOsteo Method: The Choice of an Integrated Approach

The therapeutic approach of the AcuOsteo method aims to treat those musculoskeletal injuries that do not require consultation with a surgeon or a physician.

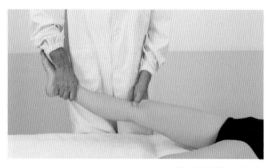
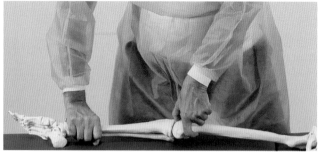

Fig. 6.38 The retreating medial meniscus test_final position.

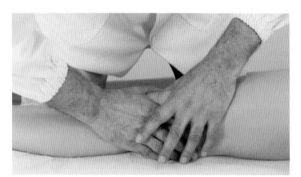
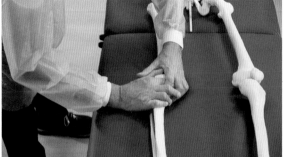

Fig. 6.39 Superolateral-inferomedial test of the patella.

Once this fundamental aspect has been defined, treatment envisages the use of acupuncture and osteopathy according to their diagnostic and therapeutic approaches.

We would like to stress that at this point in diagnostic assessment, we do not have to follow the rules of Western medicine, except for some specific cases, such as arthritis of the knee, posttraumatic and postsurgical pain, and stiffness, which will be covered later.

In addition, we should not be misled by diagnostic imaging investigations and should rely only on the rules of Chinese and osteopathic medicine, which means selecting points according to symptoms and channel pathways and treating all of the somatic dysfunctions encountered.

For didactic purposes, treatment with acupuncture will precede osteopathic treatment, whereas in clinical practice the order is reversed since it may be difficult to perform osteopathic manipulations once the needles have been inserted.

An exception to this methodology is represented by those morbidities where marked stiffness prevents joint mobilization as required by osteopathic manipulations. Specifically, we are referring to the outcomes after immobilization following surgery, fractures, and knee dislocation.

In these cases, we suggest first using acupuncture, especially the bleeding techniques, and then, at the end of the session and after removing the needles, osteopathy.

In any case, it is always the practitioner's clinical experience that will guide them along the most appropriate pathway to treat each patient's condition.

Osteopathic manipulation in the treatment of "somatic dysfunction" is the central concept of the therapeutic process to treat the affected joints and functionally/anatomically related components of the somatic system.

Consequently, the osteopathic manipulative approach to musculoskeletal knee pain focuses on the treatment of joint somatic dysfunctions not only of the knee but also of the hip, pelvic girdle and ankle.

Regardless of the condition to be treated, be it medial meniscus tear, MCL sprain, PES, PFPS, patellar tendonitis, insertional tendonitis of biceps femoris, ITBS, arthritis of the knee, or postsurgical outcomes, all the dysfunctions diagnosed should be treated.

It is therefore evident that the osteopathic therapeutic approach does not vary with the condition to be treated; thus the osteopathic manipulations described for the knee, as well as those for the hip, pelvic girdle and ankle, will not be repeated under the paragraphs dedicated to the "injuries."

ACUPUNCTURE TREATMENT

Medial Meniscus Tear, Medial Collateral Ligament Sprain, and Pes Anserinus Syndrome

Although medial meniscus tear and MCL sprain are two different types of injuries, an injury to the MCL is likely to occur in conjunction with injury to the medial meniscus and vice versa, due to the MCL being attached to the body of the medial meniscus.

This is why these two injuries will be covered together in this chapter, keeping in mind that both Spleen and Liver channels have also proved to be often involved.

Specifically, the Spleen channels are involved in case of anterior horn medial meniscus tear, PES, and more rarely MCL sprain and the Liver channels in case of MCL sprain and posterior horn medial meniscus tear.

The Spleen and Liver channels overlap when tears of the medial meniscus body and collateral ligament sprains occur, though these latter more rarely.

According to our experience, posterior horn medial meniscus tear is reported less frequently; although the Kidney channels could be indicated in this specific case, these channels have not proved to be so effective as the Liver channels in clinical practice.

The Five Options and Selection of Acupoints

The approach we suggest is widely described in the section dedicated to the fundamentals of acupuncture for MSK pain in the limbs (see Chapter 1).

The most important aspect is the identification of the Ah Shi point(s) to determine which channels are affected. In this specific case, the Spleen and

Liver Muscle and Connecting channels are involved and, according to our experience, the Yin Qiao Mai Extraordinary channel may also be involved.

It is worth reminding that the Spleen Muscle and Connecting channels run more anteriorly than the Liver ones.

In line with our principle of treatment, in case of medial meniscus tears involving the body, we first use the Spleen channels and then test their effectiveness soon after needle insertion. If the result is not satisfactory, we remove the needles or let them in, and move to the Liver channels.

On the contrary, in case of MCL sprain, we first use the Liver channels and then test their effectiveness soon after needle insertion. If the result is not satisfactory, we remove the needles or let them in, and move to the Spleen channels.

Once the most effective channel is identified, selection of distal points continues.

Pricking pain localized on the medial aspect at the level of the joint space is a sign of Blood stasis to be treated with the bleeding technique, whereas widespread pain radiating along the thigh and leg is a sign of Qì stagnation to be treated with the needling technique.

Joint swelling is a sign of Dampness to be treated with the bleeding and cupping therapy.

It is worth reminding that the distal points should be needled one at a time, and their effectiveness in terms of pain and range of motion tested after each insertion. The same applies to the local points.

Finally, since both options 1 and 2 consist of several steps, it is important to highlight how selection should be made. Specifically, the practitioner might wonder if all or some of the steps should be followed. The rule we follow is simple: when the result achieved is satisfactory, the remaining steps should be skipped, and the practitioner should move to the following option. Similarly, the use of the points recommended under options 3, 4, and 5 should be carefully evaluated according to the case being treated.

The points and accessory techniques we recommend are listed below.

Order of Needling

Option One: Distal Points
First Step: Spleen and Liver Muscle Channels
SP1 and LR1. These Jing-Well points activate the Spleen and Liver Muscle channels, and they remove

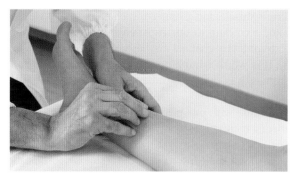

Fig. 6.40 Needling of the LR5 starting position.

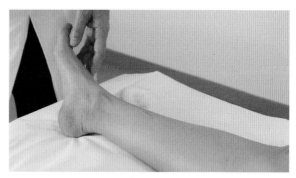

Fig. 6.41 Needling of the LR5 final position.

Qì stagnation and Blood stasis with needling and bleeding techniques, respectively.

Second Step: Spleen and Liver Connecting Channels

SP4 and LR5 (Opposite Side). These Luo points activate the Spleen and Liver Connecting channels, and they remove Qì stagnation and Blood stasis in acute or chronic conditions from Excess (Figs. 6.40 and 6.41; Video 6.13).

ST40 and GB37 (Opposite Side). These Luo points activate the Stomach and Gall Bladder Connecting channels. They are also used in chronic Deficiency conditions with dull pain to tonify Qì and Blood in their respective internally-externally related channels. In this case, we associate Yuan point SP3 with Luo point ST40 and Yuan point LR3 with Luo point GB37, which is the well-known Luo-Yuan point combination. First, as the main point, we needle the Yuan point on the affected side and then, as a secondary point, the Luo point on the internally-externally related channel on the opposite side.

Third Step: Empirical Points

There is no point that is classically recommended.

Fourth Step: Opposite Extremity (Upper/Lower)

LU5 and PC3 (Opposite Side). They are located in the elbow joint, which corresponds to the knee joint on the paired channels according to the Six Stages. Our technique consists of needling the opposite extremity (lower/upper) on the opposite side in acute and chronic conditions. Alternatively, the most tender point on palpation is selected on the same or opposite side.

Fifth Step: Categories of Traditional Points

SP3 (Affected Side) and LU9 (Opposite Side); LR3 (Affected Side) and PC7 (Opposite Side). A good combination includes the Shu-Stream points on the paired channel according to the Six Stages.

First, we needle the Shu-Stream point on the channel involved on the affected side and then the Shu-Stream point on the coupled channel on the opposite side and opposite extremity (upper/lower). We use this technique in acute and chronic Excess conditions to treat pain and expel or prevent invasion of EPFs.

It is worth remembering that in the Yin channels the Shu-Stream point corresponds to the Yuan-Source point. Therefore SP3 and LR3 could also be used in chronic Deficiency conditions, as we will see later.

SP5 and LR4. The Jing-River points are used in acute or chronic Excess conditions due to the invasion of an EPF, and they are needled to promote its expulsion from their respective channels. They are also useful to prevent pain exacerbation from seasonal changes or invasion of EPFs. However, they are more effective in the Yang rather than in the Yin channels.

SP8 and LR6. The Xi-Cleft points are specifically used in acute conditions to treat Blood stasis in their respective channels. We only use SP8 to treat gynecological disorders; not even LR6 has proved to be effective in the treatment of musculoskeletal diseases.

SP3 and LR3. We recommend using these Yuan-Source points in chronic Deficiency conditions with dull pain, in case of weakness, or in the resolution phases of medial meniscus tear, MCL sprain, and PES to tonify Qì and Blood in their respective channels.

In this situation, we can also associate Yuan point SP3 with Luo point ST40 and Yuan point LR3 with Luo point GB37, which is the well-known Luo-Yuan point combination. First, as the main point, we needle the Yuan point on the affected side and then, as a secondary point, the Luo point on the internally-externally related channel on the opposite side.

SP6. It is the meeting point of the three Yin channels, and as such it promotes the longitudinal flow of Qi and eliminates Blood stasis on those channels.

Sixth Step: Extraordinary Vessels

KI6 (Affected Side) and LU7 (Opposite Side). KI6 is the opening point of the Yin Qiao Mai, while LU7 is the coupled and opening point of the Directing Vessel (Ren Mai). The Yin Qiao Mai extraordinary channel could be involved in the medial knee pain from Excess conditions with spasms, tightness, and muscle pain affecting the medial aspect of the knee, which could radiate to the medial side of thigh and leg.

When the Yin Qiao Mai is used, we also needle KI8, which is its Xi-Cleft point. First, as the main point, the opening point of the Yin Qiao Mai is needled on the same side and then, as a secondary point, the coupled point on the opposite side.

Option Two: Local Points

First Step: Painful Point(s) (Ah Shi)

Ah Shi Point(s). We identify the most painful point(s) (Ah Shi), which is located at the level of the medial aspect of the knee (usually in the joint space or along the collateral ligament); palpation reveals the Ah Shi point(s) corresponding to Blood stasis or Qi stagnation, which is the point to be bled or needled, respectively.

When the bleeding technique is chosen and if the anatomical structure of the knee allows us to, the cupping therapy should be used to bleed the most painful point(s) (Ah Shi), paying attention not to damage the tendinous tissue with the lancet or the soft tissues with a too strong cupping (Figs. 6.42 and 6.43; Video 6.14).

As far as acupuncture is concerned, when we treat the body of the medial meniscus or the MCL, we prefer inserting the needle under the collateral ligament into the superficial region of the body of the meniscus along the medial joint space. Two needles are inserted from oblique to transverse, one from before

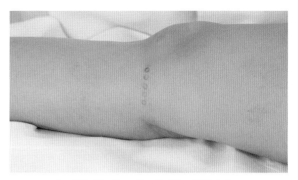

Fig. 6.42 Bleeding of the Ah Shi point(s)starting.

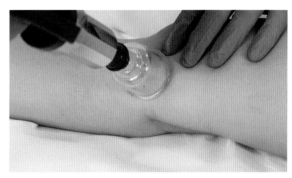

Fig. 6.43 Bleeding of the Ah Shi point(s)final.

the ligament and in posterior direction, and the other from behind the ligament, approximately where LR8 is located, in anterior direction. Needle insertion should be smooth providing next to no resistance.

More attempts are likely to be required before achieving correct positioning, since the tip of the needle may easily hit against the ligamentous surfaces (Fig. 6.44; Video 6.15).

We use 0.30 × 40 mm needles and prefer positioning a pillow under the knee joint to release ligament tension.

Electroacupuncture stimulation can be taken into consideration and used between the two points on the sides of the medial ligament.

Medial Xiyan and Lateral Xiyan (ST35). These two points are called "Calf's nose—Eyes of the knee" because they are located in the two depressions, medial and lateral to the patellar ligament depicted as a "nose."

From the anatomical point of view, they correspond to the anterior horns of the medial and lateral meniscus, and therefore they may be painful when palpated or during the tests for meniscal disorders.

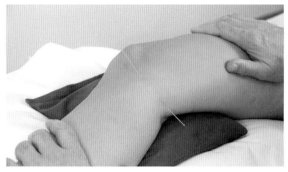

Fig. 6.44 Needling of the Ah Shi point(s) and LR8.

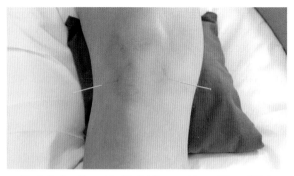

Fig. 6.45 Needling of the Medial Xiyan and lateral Xiyan (ST35).

To treat the anterior horn of the medial meniscus, we use the medial point Xiyan. The point is needled perpendicularly, to a depth of 1 to 2 cun toward BL40, to reach the meniscal surface. When the medial Xiyan is used, we always associate it with the lateral Xiyan corresponding to the anterior horn of the lateral meniscus (Fig. 6.45; Video 6.16).

We use 0.30 × 40 mm needles and prefer positioning a pillow under the knees to widen the joint space, thus making needling of the medial and lateral Xiyan easier.

Electroacupuncture stimulation can be taken into consideration and used between the medial and lateral Xiyan.

Both in acute and chronic conditions, moxa on the needle can be useful to resolve internal Dampness and to treat invasion of EPFs, Cold, and Dampness in particular. However, attention should be paid since too much heat can increase the ongoing inflammatory.

Heding. It is a point positioned in the middle of the superior border of the patella and could be useful in case of meniscus tear with joint swelling. We often needle another two points located at the same level as the Heding point on the sides of the quadriceps tendon.

Moderate cupping therapy could be used to bleed these three points in case of swelling to resolve Dampness.

LR8. It is the local point in case of posterior horn medial meniscus tear: the needle is inserted perpendicularly to the required depth to reach the meniscal surface. We also use it because it is an insertion point of the Liver Muscle channel in the knee, as we will see later.

SP9. It is the local point in case of PES. It can be also considered a local point to treat medial meniscus and collateral ligament disorders, although in reality it is only adjacent to them. We also use it because it is an insertion point of the Spleen Muscle channel in the knee, as we will see later.

To ensure the accuracy and precision of local needle placement and manipulation, we prefer the supine position.

Second Step: Anatomically Mirrored Points (Opposite Side)

The points to be needled are located on the opposite side and should correspond as precisely as possible to the anatomical mirror of the Ah Shi point(s) to be treated. The point(s) may or may not be tender on palpation.

To ensure the accuracy and precision of needle placement and manipulation, we prefer the supine position.

Option Three: Adjacent Points
First Step: Adjacent Points

LR7. It is a very important point since it releases tendon tension and therefore reduces joint stiffness.

KI10. It is used to promote the horizontal flow of local Qì.

ST36. It is used to promote the horizontal flow of local Qì.

SP10. Located in the belly of the vastus medialis of the quadriceps, it is used to promote the longitudinal flow of local Qì and remove Blood stasis. Releasing this muscle tension can improve postural balance of the knee, thus reducing inflammation and pain.

SP9. It is a very important point since it is the insertion point of the Spleen Muscle channel in the knee and as such it promotes the longitudinal flow of local Qì. It also helps promote the horizontal flow of local Qì when the Liver channels are affected.

In addition, this point is located at the level of the pes anserinus, which consists of the conjoined tendons of the sartorius, gracilis, and semitendinosus muscles. Releasing this muscle tension can improve postural balance of the knee, thus reducing inflammation and pain.

LR8. It is an important point since it is the insertion point of the Liver Muscle channel in the knee and as such it promotes the longitudinal flow of local Qì. In addition, it also helps promote the horizontal flow of local Qì when the Spleen channels are affected.

Option Four: Etiological Points

First Step: According to Patterns
LI4 and LR3 (bilaterally). They promote the flow of Qì and help remove Blood stasis. Since LR3 is the Shu/Yuan point of the Liver, it also helps nourish muscles and tendons.

ST36 (Bilaterally). It is used to tonify Qì and Blood in chronic Deficiency conditions or the phases of pain resolution that can turn into muscle weakness. In addition, it could be useful to apply moxa on the needle.

SP9. It is a very important point in case of joint swelling since it resolves Dampness.

Second Step: General Points
GB34 (Bilaterally). It is the Hui-Gathering point of Sinews and is specifically used for medial meniscus tear, MCL sprain, and PES. In addition, it promotes the flow of Qì thus contributing to remove Blood stasis.

BL18 (Bilaterally). It treats all Excess and Deficiency conditions of the Liver that may favor the onset or duration of musculotendinous symptoms. It harmonizes the flow of Qì and Blood and enhances treatment of tendons and muscle.

BL20 (Bilaterally). They transform "impure" fluids thus contributing to resolve Dampness in case of joint swelling.

Option Five: Microsystems

First Step: Wrist and Ankle Acupuncture
Lower 2. It roughly corresponds to the pathway of the Spleen and Liver channels (Fig. 6.46).

Lower 4. It controls lower limb mobility (Fig. 6.47).

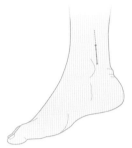

Fig. 6.46 Lower 2.

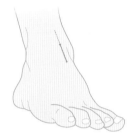

Fig. 6.47 Lower 4.

Second Step: Ear Acupuncture Fig. 6.48
Local point: Knee
Zang Fu point: Liver
General points: Subcortex and Shenmen
Acute or Chronic Pain from Excess
Intense Pain or Range of Motion Reduced by Pain. The principle of treatment is to remove Qì stagnation and Blood stasis and expel EPFs or internal pathogenic factors (IPFs), if any (Box 6.1).
Chronic Pain From Deficiency
Dull Pain or Muscle Weakness. The principle of treatment is to tonify Qì and Blood, strengthen tissues, and avoid pain exacerbation from physical activities or invasion of EPFs (Box 6.2).

Therapeutic Program, Frequency of Sessions

The frequency of sessions depends on the clinical condition of the patient. If the condition is acute or chronic with intense pain, we recommend sessions twice a week for 2 weeks and then once a week for another 2 weeks. If improvement is observed, sessions are then scheduled once a week until complete pain relief or at least reduction by 80% to 90%. If not, the whole clinical picture should be reconsidered and the patient referred to another specialist.

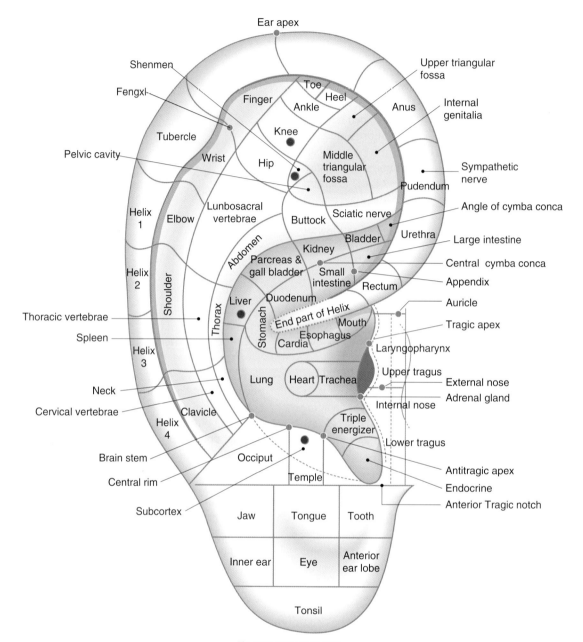

Fig. 6.48 Ear acupuncture.

If the condition is chronic with dull pain, we recommend sessions once a week for 4 weeks. Afterwards, and if the patient continues to improve, sessions are then scheduled once a week until complete pain relief or at least reduction by 80% to 90%.

Patellofemoral Pain Syndrome (Patellofemoral Joint Dysfunction And Chondromalacia Patellae) and Patellar Tendonitis

Although PFPS and patellar tendonitis are two different disorders, they will be covered together in this

BOX. 6.1 ACUTE OR CHRONIC PAIN FROM EXCESS ACUPUNCTURE TREATMENT

Option 1 Distal points	• Jing-Well point SP1 and LR1 • Luo point SP4 and LR5 (opposite side) • Point according to the Six Stages LU5 and PC3 (opposite side) • Shu-Stream point SP3 and LR3 (affected side), and Shu-Stream point LU9 and PC7 (opposite side) • Jing-River point SP5 and LR4 • SP6
Option 2 Local points	• Ah Shi • Medial and lateral Xiyan (ST35) • Heding • Anatomically mirrored point(s) (opposite side)
Option 3 Adjacent points	• LR7 • KI10 • ST36 • SP10 • Insertion points SP9 and LR8
Option 4 Etiological and general points	• LI4 and LIV-3 (bilaterally) • GB34 (bilaterally) • BL18 (bilaterally) • BL20 (bilaterally) • SP9 (bilaterally)

Option 5 Microsystems	• W-A acupuncture
	  • Lower 2
	  • Lower 4
	• Ear acupuncture
	  • Knee
	  • Liver
	  • Subcortex and Shenmen

BOX. 6.2 CHRONIC PAIN FROM DEFICIENCY ACUPUNCTURE TREATMENT

Option 1 Distal points	• Yuan points SP3 and LR3 • Luo point ST40 and GB37 (opposite side) • Point according to the Six Stages LU5 and PC3 (opposite side) • Jing-River point SP5 and LR4 • SP6
Option 2 Local points	• Ah Shi • Medial and lateral Xiyan (ST35) • Heding
Option 3 Adjacent points	• LR7 • KI10 • ST36 • SP10 • Insertion points SP9 and LR8
Option 4 Etiological and general points	• ST36 • GB34 (bilaterally) • LR3 (bilaterally) • BL18 (bilaterally)

Option 5 Microsystems	• W-A acupuncture
	  • Lower 2
	  • Lower 4
	• Ear acupuncture
	  • Knee
	  • Liver
	  • Subcortex and Shenmen

chapter, with the therapeutic protocol being always the same as far as the distal, adjacent, and etiological points are concerned. Needless to say, local points and techniques to be used vary according to the different disorders to treat.

The Five Options and Selection of Acupoints

The approach we suggest is widely described in the section dedicated to the fundamentals of acupuncture for MSK pain in the limbs (see Chapter 1).

The most important aspect is the identification of the Ah Shi point(s) to determine which channels are affected. In this specific case, the Stomach Muscle and Connecting channels are involved.

Pricking pain localized deeply under the patella, on the patellar tendon junction at the anterior tibial

Clinical Notes

- Treatment of knee injuries and disorders often achieves excellent outcomes, although imaging techniques may show anatomical changes in joint structures, such as meniscal tear or ligament sprain. Sometimes, temporary worsening of symptoms is observed, especially when cupping is used.
- Improvement following treatment may turn intense pain to dull pain and then to a feeling of weakness. Should this be the case, the principle of treatment has to be changed as follows. It is no longer necessary to remove Qì stagnation and Blood stasis and expel EPFs, if any; instead, Qì and Blood should be tonified to strengthen tissues and avoid pain exacerbation from physical activities or invasion of EPFs.
- Treatment of medial meniscus tear and collateral ligament sprain can ensure excellent results in terms of disappearance of pain and return to daily activities, even sports.

tuberosity is a sign of Blood Stasis to be treated with the bleeding technique, whereas any anterior pain radiating from patella along the thigh and leg is a sign of Qì stagnation and therefore needling is the most appropriate technique.

Joint swelling is a sign of Dampness to be treated with the bleeding and cupping therapy.

It is worth reminding that the distal points should be needled one at a time and their effectiveness in terms of pain and range of motion tested after each insertion. The same applies to the local points.

Finally, since both options 1 and 2 consist of several steps, it is important to highlight how selection should be made. Specifically, the practitioner might wonder if all or some of the steps should be followed. The rule we follow is simple: when the result achieved is satisfactory, the remaining steps should be skipped, and the practitioner should move to the following option. Similarly, the use of the points recommended under options 3, 4, and 5 should be carefully evaluated according to the case being treated.

The points and accessory techniques we recommend using are listed below.

The Order of Needling

Option One: Distal Points

First Step: Stomach Muscle Channel

ST45. This Jing-Well point activates the Stomach Muscle channel and removes Qì stagnation and Blood stasis with needling and bleeding techniques, respectively.

Second Step: Stomach Connecting Channels

ST40 (Opposite Side). This Luo point activates the Stomach Connecting channels and removes Qì stagnation and Blood stasis in acute and chronic conditions from Excess.

SP4 (Opposite Side). This Luo point activates the Spleen Connecting channels and is also used in chronic Deficiency conditions with dull pain to tonify Qì and Blood in the internally-externally related Stomach channels. In the latter case, we associate Yuan point ST42 with Luo point SP4, which is the well-known Luo-Yuan point combination. First, as the main point, we needle the Yuan point on the affected side and then as a secondary point the Luo point on the internally-externally related channel on the opposite side.

Third Step: Empirical Points

There is no point which is classically recommended.

Fourth Step: Opposite Extremity (Upper/Lower)

LI11 (Opposite Side). It is located in the elbow joint, which corresponds to the knee joint on the paired channel according to the Six Stages. Our technique consists of needling the opposite extremity (lower/upper) on the opposite side in acute and chronic conditions. Alternatively, the most tender point on palpation is selected on the same or opposite side.

Fifth Step: Categories of Traditional Points

ST43 (Affected Side) and LI3 (Opposite Side). A good combination includes the Shu-Stream points on the paired channel according to the Six Stages.

First, we needle the Shu-Stream point on the channel involved on the affected side and then the Shu-Stream point on the coupled channel on the opposite side and opposite extremity (upper/lower).

We use this technique in acute and chronic Excess conditions to treat pain and expel or prevent invasion of EPFs.

ST41. The Jing-River points are used in acute or chronic Excess conditions due to the invasion of an

EPF, and they are needled to promote its expulsion from their respective channels. They are also useful to prevent pain exacerbation from seasonal changes or invasion of EPFs.

ST34. The Xi-Cleft points are specifically used in acute conditions for the treatment of Blood stasis in their respective channels. However, they are more effective in the Yin rather than in the Yang channels. That said, our experience teaches that ST34 can be useful in this specific case and we also use it because it is an adjacent point of the knee, as we will see later.

ST42. We recommend using this Yuan-Source point in chronic Deficiency conditions with dull pain, in case of weakness, or in the resolution phases of PFPS and patellar tendonitis, to tonify Qì and Blood in the Stomach channels.

In this situation, we can also use Yuan point ST42 with Luo point SP4, which is the well-known Luo-Yuan point combination of ST42. First, as the main point, we needle the Yuan point on the affected side and then as a secondary point the Luo point on the internally-externally related channel on the opposite side.

Sixth Step: Extraordinary Vessels

In our opinion, no Extraordinary Vessel is effective to treat this disorder.

Option Two: Local Points

First Step: Painful Point(s) (Ah Shi)

Ah Shi Point(s). We identify the most painful point(s) (Ah Shi), which is located at the level of the anterior aspect of the knee, usually deep under the patella. Pain radiates from the patella to the thigh or along the patellar tendon. Palpation reveals the Ah Shi point(s) corresponding to Blood stasis or Qì stagnation, which is the point(s) to be bled or needled, respectively.

However, to make the treatment as effective as possible, a distinction is to be made among the various clinical conditions.

Medial Xiyan and Lateral Xiyan (ST35). In case of patellofemoral joint dysfunction and chondromalacia patellae, our first choice is to use "the eyes of the knee," the medial and lateral Xiyan, especially when pain is reported to be under the patella.

How the needle is inserted is very important: the patient is supine with the knee extended. The needle

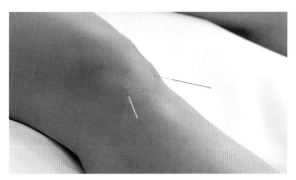

Fig. 6.49 Needling of the Medial and lateral Xiyan (ST35).

is inserted trying to enter the patellofemoral joint, which means under the patella but above the femoral trochlea. Direction of the needle is oblique, from medial Xiyan toward ST34, and from lateral Xiyan toward SP10. Needle insertion should be smooth providing next to no resistance.

Sometimes, more attempts may be required before achieving correct positioning, since the tip of the needle may easily hit against the bone surfaces. Should it be the case, the degree of knee flexion can be modified (Fig. 6.49; Video 6.17).

Use a 0.30 × 40 mm needle to achieve an insertion depth from 1. to 1.5 cun.

Electroacupuncture stimulation can be taken into consideration and used between the medial and lateral Xiyan.

In acute or exacerbation of chronic conditions due to invasion of EPFs, Cold in particular, moxa on the needle can be added to help expel them. Attention should be paid to avoid burning of the underlying skin due to the horizontal insertion of the needles, keeping in mind that too much heat can increase the ongoing inflammatory process.

Lateral Xiyan point (ST35) is a very important point: in addition to being a local point, it is also the insertion point of the Stomach Muscle channel in the knee and as such it promotes the longitudinal flow of local Qì.

To treat patellar tendonitis, again we use the two medial and lateral Xiyan points ("the eyes of the knee"), or two points located slightly distally, but needle insertion is different from the one previously described. The patient is supine, with the knee extended; the needle

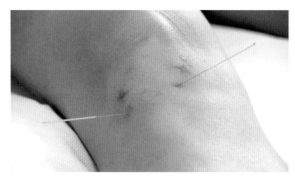

Fig. 6.50 Needling of the Medial Xiyan and lateral Xiyan (ST35).

is inserted perpendicularly, from the two sides of the tendon but passing below it. Needle insertion should be smooth providing next to no resistance.

Sometimes, more attempts may be required before achieving correct positioning, since the tip of the needle may easily hit against the tendon surface. Consequently, once the needle is inserted, caution is mandatory to avoid eliciting pain and increasing inflammation. Modification of the degree of knee flexion, using a pillow, may be of help (Fig. 6.50; Video 6.18).

We use a 0.30 × 40 mm needle to reach an insertion depth ranging from 1 to 1.5 cun. Electroacupuncture stimulation can be taken into consideration and used between these two points. In acute and chronic conditions, moxa on the needle can be useful to promote the flow of Qì and Blood and to resolve Dampness.

A moxa stick or moxa on the needle can also be useful to promote the flow of Qì and Blood in chronic Deficiency conditions and resolution phases of PFPS and patellar tendonitis.

Attention should be paid to avoid burning of the underlying skin due to the horizontal insertion of the needles, keeping in mind that too much heat can increase the ongoing inflammatory process.

It should be kept in mind that once the needles are inserted, their effectiveness in terms of pain and range of motion can no longer be tested.

In case of pain localized on the osteotendinous junction at the anterior tibial tuberosity palpation reveals the Ah Shi point(s) corresponding to Blood stasis or Qì stagnation, which is the point to be bled or needled, respectively.

When the bleeding technique is chosen and if the anatomical structure of the tibial tuberosity allows us to, the cupping therapy should be used to bleed the most painful point(s) (Ah Shi), paying attention not to damage the tendinous tissue with the lancet or the soft tissues with a too strong cupping.

Heding. It is a point positioned in the middle of the superior border of the patella and could be painful on palpation. It is useful in case of PFPS. We often needle another two points located at the same level as the Heding point on the sides of the quadriceps tendon.

Moderate cupping therapy could be used to bleed these three points in case of swelling to resolve Dampness.

To ensure the accuracy and precision of local needle placement and manipulation, we prefer the supine position.

Second Step: Anatomically Mirrored Points (Opposite Side)

The points to be needled are located on the opposite side and should correspond as precisely as possible to the anatomical mirror of the Ah Shi point(s) to be treated.

The point(s) may or may not be tender on palpation.

To ensure the accuracy and precision of needle placement and manipulation, we prefer the supine position.

Option Three: Adjacent Points

First Step: Adjacent Points

ST36. It is used to promote the longitudinal flow of local Qì.

ST34. As mentioned above, this is not only a Xi-Cleft point but also an adjacent point in case of anterior knee pain.

SP10. This point removes Blood Stasis and nourishes Blood. In addition, it is located in the belly of the vastus medialis of the quadriceps.

Releasing tension in this muscle significantly contributes to the correct patellar alignment over the femoral trochlea, thus reducing inflammation and pain.

LR7. It is a very important point since it releases tendon tension and therefore, reduces joint stiffness. Moreover, it promotes the horizontal flow of local Qì.

SP9. This point is located at the level of the pes anserinus, which consists of the conjoined tendons of the sartorius, gracilis, and semitendinosus muscles. Releasing this muscle tension can improve the postural balance of the knee, thus reducing inflammation and pain.

Option Four: Etiological Points

First Step: According to Patterns

LI4 and LR3 (Bilaterally). They promote the flow of Qì and help remove Blood stasis. Since LR3 is the Shu/Yuan point of the Liver, it also helps nourish muscles and tendons.

ST36 (Bilaterally). It could be used with moxa on the needle to tonify Qì and Blood in chronic Deficiency conditions or the phases of pain resolution that can turn into muscle weakness. In addition, it is useful to treat this point with moxa on the needle on affected side, when pain is caused by invasion of Cold, to expel it, or Dampness, to resolve it.

SP9. It is a very important point in case of joint swelling since it resolves Dampness.

Second Step: General Points

GB34 (Bilaterally). It is the Hui-Gathering point of Sinews and is specifically used for patellar tendonitis. In addition, it promotes the flow of Qì thus contributing to remove Blood stasis.

BL18 (Bilaterally). It treats all the Excess and Deficiency conditions of the Liver that may favor the onset or duration of musculotendinous symptoms. It harmonizes the flow of Qì and Blood, improves treatment of tendons and muscles, and help restore joint cartilage in case of chondromalacia.

BL20 (Bilaterally). It transforms "impure" fluids thus contributing to resolve Dampness in case of swelling.

Option Five: Microsystems

First Step: Wrist and Ankle Acupuncture

Lower 3. It controls the medial border of patella (Fig. 6.51).

Lower 4. It roughly corresponds to the pathway of the Stomach channels and controls lower limb mobility (Fig. 6.52).

Second Step: Ear Acupuncture (Fig. 6.53)
Local point: Knee
Zang Fu point: Liver
General points: Subcortex and Shenmen

Acute or Chronic Pain from Excess
Intense Pain or Range of Motion Reduced by Pain. The principle of treatment is to remove Qì stagnation

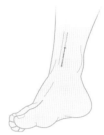

Fig. 6.51 Lower 3.

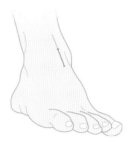

Fig. 6.52 Lower 4.

and Blood stasis and expel EPFs or IPFs, if any (Box 6.3).

Chronic Pain From Deficiency
Dull Pain or Muscle Weakness. The principle of treatment is to tonify Qì and Blood, strengthen tissues, and avoid pain exacerbation from physical activities or invasion of EPFs (Box 6.4).

Therapeutic Program, Frequency of Sessions

The frequency of sessions depends on the clinical condition of the patient. If the condition is acute or chronic with intense pain, we recommend sessions twice a week for 2 weeks and then once a week for another 2 weeks. If improvement is observed, sessions are then scheduled once a week until complete pain relief or at least reduction by 80% to 90%. If not, the whole clinical picture should be reconsidered and the patient referred to another specialist.

If the condition is chronic with dull pain, we recommend sessions once a week for 4 weeks. Afterwards, and if the patient continues to improve, sessions are then scheduled once a week until complete pain relief or at least reduction by 80% to 90%.

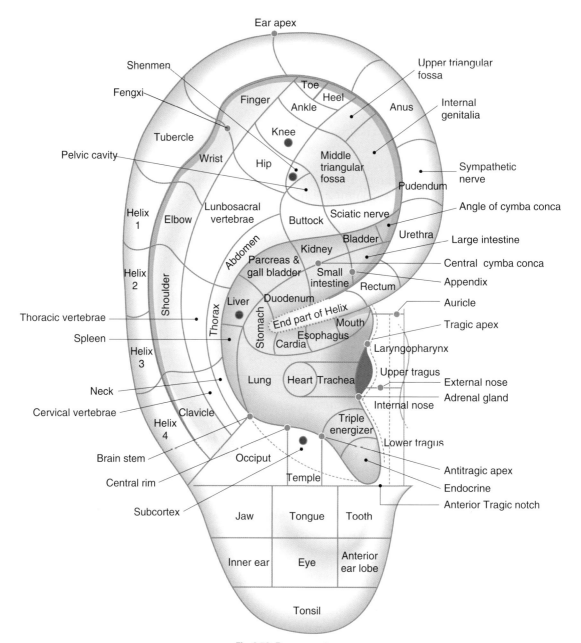

Fig. 6.53 Ear acupuncture.

Insertional Tendonitis of Biceps Femoris and Iliotibial Band Syndrome

Although insertional tendonitis of biceps femoris on the fibular head and ITBS are two different disorders, they will be covered together in this chapter, since the Gall Bladder channels are affected and treated successfully in both cases. The Bladder channels, instead, are involved only in case of insertional tendonitis of biceps femoris, when pain is on the posterolateral aspect of the knee, which occurs more rarely.

BOX. 6.3 ACUTE OR CHRONIC PAIN FROM EXCESS ACUPUNCTURE TREATMENT

Option 1 Distal points	• Jing-Well point ST45 • Luo point ST40 (opposite side) • Point according to the Six Stages LI11 (opposite side) • Shu-Stream point ST43 (affected side) and Shu-Stream point LI3 (opposite side) • Jing-River point ST41 • Xi-Cleft point ST34
Option 2 Local points	• Ah Shi • Medial and lateral Xiyan (ST35) • Heding • Anatomically mirrored point(s) (opposite side)
Option 3 Adjacent points	• ST36 • ST34 • SP10 • SP9 • LR7 • Insertion point Lateral Xiyan (ST35)
Option 4 Etiological and general points	• LI4 and LR3 (bilaterally) • GB34 (bilaterally) • BL18 (bilaterally)

Option 5
Microsystems
	• W-A acupuncture
	  • Lower 3
	  • Lower 4
	• Ear acupuncture
	  • Knee
	  • Liver
	  • Subcortex and Shenmen

BOX. 6.4 CHRONIC PAIN FROM DEFICIENCY ACUPUNCTURE TREATMENT

Option 1 Distal points	• Yuan point ST42 • Luo point SP4 (opposite side) • Point according to the Six Stages LI11 (opposite side) • Jing-River point ST41
Option 2 Local points	• Ah Shi • Medial and lateral Xiyan (ST35) • Heding
Option 3 Adjacent points	• ST36 • ST34 • SP10 • SP9 • LR7 • Insertion point lateral Xiyan (ST35)
Option 4 Etiological and general points	• ST36 • GB34 • LR3 • BL18

Option 5
Microsystems
	• W-A acupuncture
	  • Lower 3
	  • Lower 4
	• Ear acupuncture
	  • Knee
	  • Liver
	  • Subcortex and Shenmen

The Five Options and Selection of Acupoints

The approach we suggest is widely described in the section dedicated to the fundamentals of acupuncture for MSK pain in the limbs (see Chapter 1).

The most important aspect is the identification of the Ah Shi point(s) to determine which channels are affected. In this specific case, the Gall Bladder and Bladder Muscle and Connecting channels are involved.

Therefore, when a combination of two points (GB and BL) is presented, the first point to be needled or bled is the GB point, which treats lateral pain, followed by the BL point to treat posterior pain.

Once the most effective channel is identified, selection of distal points continues.

Sharp pain localized in the distal lateral aspect of the thigh in case of ITBS or at the level of the insertion of the biceps on the fibular head in case of its tendonitis is a sign of Blood stasis to be treated with the bleeding technique, whereas widespread pain radiating along the lateral aspect of the thigh and leg is a sign of Qì stagnation to be treated with the needling technique.

Clinical Notes

- Treatment of knee injuries and disorders often achieves excellent outcomes, although imaging techniques may show anatomical changes in joint structures, such as damage to femoral and patellar cartilage.
- Sometimes, temporary worsening of symptoms is observed, especially when cupping is used.
- Improvement following treatment may turn intense pain to dull pain and then to a feeling of weakness. Should this be the case, the principle of treatment has to be changed as follows. It is no longer necessary to remove Qì stagnation and Blood stasis and expel EPFs, if any; instead, Qì and Blood should be tonified to strengthen tissues and avoid pain exacerbation from physical activities or invasion of EPFs.
- Treatment of PFPS and patellar tendonitis can ensure excellent results in terms of disappearance of pain and return to daily activities, even sports.

It is worth reminding that the distal points should be needled one at a time and their effectiveness in terms of pain and range of motion tested after each insertion. The same applies to the local points.

Finally, since both options 1 and 2 consist of several steps, it is important to highlight how selection should be made. Specifically, the practitioner might wonder if all or some of the steps should be followed. The rule we follow is simple: when the result achieved is satisfactory, the remaining steps should be skipped, and the practitioner should move to the following option. Similarly, the use of the points recommended under options 3, 4, and 5 should be carefully evaluated according to the case being treated.

The points and accessory techniques we recommend are listed below.

The Order of Needling

First Step: Gall Bladder and Bladder Muscle Channels

GB44 and BL67. These Jing-Well points activate the Gall Bladder and Bladder Muscle channels, and

they remove Qì stagnation and Blood stasis with needling and bleeding techniques, respectively.

Second Step: Gall Bladder and Bladder Connecting Channels

GB37 and BL58 (Opposite Side). These Luo points activate the Gall Bladder and Bladder Connecting channels, and they remove Qì stagnation and Blood stasis in acute and chronic conditions from Excess.

LR5 and KI4 (Opposite Side). These Luo points activate the Liver and Kidney Connecting channels. They are also used in chronic Deficiency conditions with dull pain to tonify Qì and Blood in their respective internally-externally related channels. In this case, we associate Yuan point GB40 with Luo point LR5 and Yuan point BL64 with Luo point KI4, which is the well-known Luo-Yuan point combination. First, as the main point, we needle the Yuan point on the affected side and then as a secondary point, the Luo point on the internally-externally related channel on the opposite side.

Third Step: Empirical Points

There is no point which is classically recommended.

Fourth Step: Opposite Extremity (Upper/Lower)

TE10 and SI8 (Opposite Side). They are located in the elbow joint, which corresponds to the knee joint on the paired channel according to the Six Stages.

It is worth remembering that the painful point on the ITB is not exactly in the knee joint; it is in fact slightly proximally located and this means we could palpate the arm in an upward direction along the Triple Energizer Main channel to find another or more tender point(s).

In clinical practice, in case of ITBS syndrome, the anatomical mirror concept can lead us to select a point, which may be tender or not, on the area corresponding to the lateral arm, which could correspond to the lateral thigh, although it is not located on the Triple Energizer Main channel.

In line with our principle of treatment, we first needle TE10 or some other more proximal point(s) and then test their effectiveness soon after insertion. If the result is not satisfactory, we remove the needles and move to option 2.

Our technique consists of needling the opposite extremity (lower/upper) on the opposite side if pain is intense in acute and chronic conditions.

Alternatively, the most tender point on palpation is selected on the same or opposite side.

Fifth Step: Categories of Traditional Points

GB41 (Affected Side) and TE3 (Opposite Side); BL65 (Affected Side) and SI3 (Opposite Side). A good combination includes the Shu-Stream points on the paired channel according to the Six Stages selected according to the affected area.

First, we needle the Shu-Stream point on the channel involved on the affected side and then the Shu-Stream point on the coupled channel on the opposite side and opposite extremity (upper/lower).

We use this technique in acute and chronic Excess conditions to treat pain and expel or prevent invasion of EPFs.

GB38 and BL60. The Jing-River points are used in acute or chronic Excess conditions due to the invasion of an EPF, and they are needled to promote its expulsion from their respective channels. They are also useful to prevent pain exacerbation from seasonal changes or invasion of EPFs.

GB36 and BL63. The Xi-Cleft points are specifically used in acute conditions to treat Blood stasis in their respective channels. However, they are more effective in the Yin rather than in the Yang channels; that is why we would rather avoid using them to treat this condition.

GB40 and BL64. We recommend using these Yuan-Source points in chronic Deficiency conditions with dull pain, in case of weakness, or in the resolution phases of insertional tendonitis of biceps femoris and ITBS to tonify Qì and Blood in their respective channels.

In this situation, we can also use Yuan point GB40 with Luo point LR5 and Yuan point BL64 with Luo point KI4, which is the well-known Luo-Yuan point combination. First, as the main point, we needle the Yuan point on the affected side and then, as a secondary point, the Luo point on the internally-externally related channel on the opposite side.

Sixth Step: Extraordinary Vessels

BL62 (Affected Side) and SI3 (Opposite Side). BL62 is the opening point of the Yang Qiao Mai, while SI3 is the coupled point and opening point of the Governing Vessel (Du Mai).

The Yang Qiao Mai could be useful to treat this Excess condition.

When the Yang Qiao Mai is used, we also needle BL59, which is its Xi-Cleft point.

First, as the main point, the opening point of the Yang Qiao Mai is needled on the same side and then, as a secondary point, the coupled point on the opposite side.

Option Two: Local Points

First Step: Painful Point(s) (Ah Shi)

Ah Shi Point(s). We identify the most painful point(s) (Ah Shi), which is usually located from 2 to 4 cm proximally to the knee joint space, on the lateral aspect of the femoral condyle, in case of ITBS, or at the level of the insertion of the biceps femoris on the fibular head, laterally or posteriorly, in case of insertional tendonitis.

Palpation reveals either the Ah Shi point(s) corresponding to Blood stasis and therefore to be bled or an area of widespread pain radiating corresponding to Qì stagnation and requiring needling. In this area, pain radiates proximally to the thigh or distally to the leg.

When the bleeding technique is chosen and if the anatomical structure of the fibular head allows us to, the cupping therapy should be used to bleed the most painful point(s) (Ah Shi) paying attention not to damage the tendinous tissue with the lancet or the soft tissues with a too strong cupping.

Both in acute and chronic conditions, a moxa stick can be useful to promote the flow of Qì and Blood. However, attention should be paid since too much heat can increase the ongoing inflammatory.

GB33 and "Anterior" GB33. They are the most important points in case of ITBS. The "anterior" GB33, name suggested by W. Reaves,[1] is located at the same level of GB33, just in front of the ITB. Both needles should be inserted passing under the ITB, moving from its posterior and anterior margins with an oblique to transverse angle. GB33 is inserted from posterior with an anterior direction, while "anterior" GB33 is inserted from anterior with a posterior direction.

To make the insertion easier, the patient is in side-lying position, lying on the healthy side, with a pillow between the knees. The knee should be so flexed as to make it easier to insert the needles under the ITB. Sometimes it is not easy to locate the anterior access to insert the needle under the tibial band. Should this be

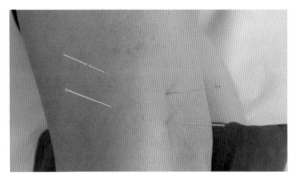

Fig. 6.54 Needling of the GB33 and anterior GB33.

the case, we suggest inserting it perpendicularly until the underlying fascia is reached.

Another two needles positioned at 1 or 2 cun proximally to the previous ones and inserted in the same way may be useful (Fig. 6.54; Video 6.19).

We use 0.30 × 40 mm needles. Electroacupuncture stimulation can be taken into consideration and used between these two points.

GB34. It can be considered the local point to treat insertional tendonitis of biceps femoris, although it is only adjacent to the osteotendinous junction. We also use it because it is an insertion point of the Gall Bladder Muscle channel in the knee, as we will see later.

BL39. It can be considered the local point to treat insertional tendonitis of biceps femoris when pain is on the posterolateral aspect of the knee although it is only adjacent to the osteotendinous junction. We also use it because it is an insertion point of the Bladder Muscle channel in the knee, as we will see later.

To ensure the accuracy and precision of needle placement and manipulation of local needles, we prefer the supine position with the knee flexed, the thigh lying on a pillow.

Second Step: Anatomically Mirrored Point(s) (Opposite Side)

The points to be needled are located on the opposite side and should correspond as precisely as possible to the anatomical mirror of the Ah Shi point(s) to be treated. The point(s) may or may not be tender on palpation.

To ensure the accuracy and precision of needle placement and manipulation, we prefer the supine position with the knee flexed, the thigh lying on a pillow.

Option Three: Adjacent Points

First Step: Adjacent Points

GB31. It is a very important point in case of ITBS, especially if pain radiates proximally along the lateral thigh. It is in fact located on the ITB and as such it promotes the longitudinal flow of local Qì.

The needle is inserted perpendicularly until it reaches the ITB.

GB33. It is an important point in case of insertional tendonitis of biceps femoris since it relaxes the tendons and reduces joint stiffness.

GB34. It is a very important point in both conditions since it is the insertion point of the Gall Bladder Muscle channel in the knee and as such it promotes the longitudinal flow of local Qì.

BL39. It is a very important point in case of insertional tendonitis of biceps femoris since it is the insertion point of the Bladder Muscle channel in the knee and as such it promotes the longitudinal flow of local Qì.

BL40. It is an important adjacent point in case of insertional tendonitis of biceps femoris when pain is on the posterolateral aspect of the knee, since it promotes the horizontal flow of local Qì. Being the insertion point of the Bladder Muscle channel in the knee, it also promotes the longitudinal flow of local Qì.

Option Four: Etiological Points

First Step: According to Patterns

LI4 and LR3 (Bilaterally). They promote the flow of Qì and help remove Blood stasis. Since LR3 is the Shu/Yuan point of the Liver, it also helps nourish muscles and tendons.

ST36 (Bilaterally). It is used to tonify Qì and Blood in chronic Deficiency conditions or the phases of pain resolution that can turn into muscle weakness.

Second Step: General Points

GB34 (Bilaterally). It is the Hui-Gathering point of Sinews and is used for insertional tendonitis of biceps femoris and ITBS. In addition, it promotes the flow of Qì thus contributing to remove Blood stasis.

BL18 (Bilaterally). It treats all Excess and Deficiency conditions of the Liver that may favor the onset or duration of musculotendinous symptoms. It

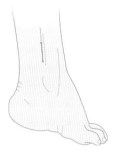

Fig. 6.55 Lower 5.

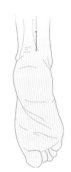

Fig. 6.56 Lower 6.

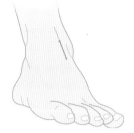

Fig. 6.57 Lower 4.

harmonizes the flow of Qì and Blood and enhances the treatment of tendons and muscle.

Option Five: Microsystems

First Step: Wrist and Ankle Acupuncture
Lower 5. It roughly corresponds to the pathway of the Gall Bladder channels (Fig. 6.55).

Lower 6. It roughly corresponds to the pathway of the Bladder channels (Fig. 6.56).

Lower 4. It controls lower limb mobility (Fig. 6.57).
Second Step: Ear Acupuncture (Fig. 6.58)
Local point: Knee
Zang Fu point: Liver
General points: Subcortex and Shenmen
Acute or Chronic Pain from Excess
Intense Pain or Range of Motion Reduced by Pain. The principle of treatment is to remove Qì stagnation and Blood stasis and expel EPFs, if any (Box 6.5).
Chronic Pain From Deficiency
Dull Pain or Muscle Weakness. The principle of treatment is to tonify Qì and Blood, strengthen tissues, and

avoid pain exacerbation from physical activities or invasion of EPFs (Box 6.6).

Therapeutic Program, Frequency of Sessions
The frequency of sessions depends on the clinical condition of the patient. If the condition is acute or chronic with intense pain, we recommend sessions twice a week for 2 weeks and then once a week for another 2 weeks. If improvement is observed, sessions are then scheduled once a week until complete pain relief or at least reduction by 80% to 90%. Response to treatment of trochanteric bursitis may take longer than expected, and therefore treatment should be continued for another week and two more sessions scheduled. Finally, if expected outcomes are not achieved, the whole clinical picture should be reconsidered and the patient referred to another specialist. If the condition is chronic with dull pain, we recommend sessions once a week for 4 weeks. Afterwards, and if the patient continues to improve, sessions are then scheduled once a week until complete pain relief or at least reduction by 80% to 90%.

OSTEOPATHIC MANIPULATIVE TREATMENT
This paragraph will deal with osteopathic manipulations to treat knee joint dysfunctions.

As already mentioned in the section dedicated to the fundamentals of osteopathy for MSK pain in the limbs (see Chapter 1), the key concept of the osteopathic therapeutic process is the treatment not only of the somatic dysfunctions of the knee but also of those that are functionally and anatomically related.

Consequently, the osteopathic manipulative approach to musculoskeletal knee pain is based on the identification of joint somatic dysfunctions not only of the knee but also of the hip, pelvic girdle and ankle.

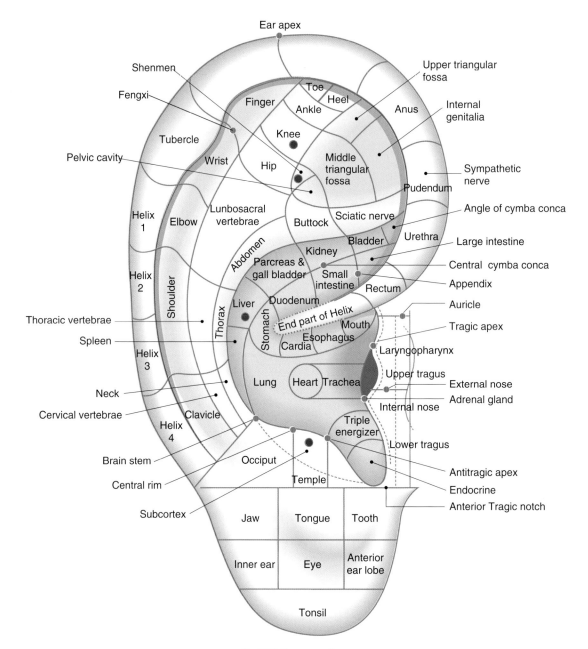

Fig. 6.58 Ear acupuncture.

Regardless of the condition to be treated, be it medial meniscus tear or MCL sprain, PES, PFPS, patellar tendonitis, insertional tendonitis of biceps femoris, ITBS, arthritis of the knee or surgical outcomes, all the dysfunctions identified should be treated.

Somatic Dysfunctions of the Tibiofemoral Joint

External Rotation of the Tibia: Treatment

External rotation dysfunction: knee external rotation is better than internal rotation.

BOX 6.5 ACUTE OR CHRONIC PAIN FROM EXCESS ACUPUNCTURE TREATMENT

Option 1 Distal point	• Jing-Well point GB44 and BL67 • Luo point GB37 and BL58 (opposite side) • Point according to the Six Stages TE10 and SI8 (opposite side) • Shu-Stream point GB41 and BL65 (affected side), and Shu-Stream point TE3 and SI3 (opposite side) • Jing-River point GB38 and BL60
Option 2 Local points	• Ah Shi • GB33 and "anterior" GB33 • GB34 • BL39 • Anatomically mirrored point(s) (opposite side)
Option 3 Adjacent points	• GB31 • GB33 • Insertion point GB34, BL39, and BL40
Option 4 Etiological and general points	• LI4 and LR3 (bilaterally) • GB34 (bilaterally) • BL18 (bilaterally)

Option 5
Microsystems
	• W-A acupuncture
	  • Lower 4
	  • Lower 5
	• Ear acupuncture
	  • Knee
	  • Liver
	  • Subcortex and Shenmen

BOX. 6.6 CHRONIC PAIN FROM DEFICIENCY ACUPUNCTURE TREATMENT

Option 1 Distal points	• Yuan point(s) GB40 and BL64 • Luo point LR5 and KI4 (opposite side) • Point according to the Six Stages TE10 and SI8 (opposite side) • Jing-River point GB38 and BL60
Option 2 Local points	• Ah Shi • GB33 and "anterior" GB33 • GB34 • BL39
Option 3 Adjacent points	• GB31 • GB33 • Insertion point GB34, BL39, and BL40
Option 4 Etiological and general points	• ST36 (bilaterally) • GB34 (bilaterally) • LR3 (bilaterally) • BL18 (bilaterally)

Option 5
Microsystems
	• W-A acupuncture
	  • Lower 4
	  • Lower 5
	• Ear acupuncture
	  • Knee
	  • Liver
	  • Subcortex and Shenmen

We can choose between two techniques depending on full hip and knee flexion, that is, if it can or cannot be achieved.

First Technique

The patient is supine close to the bed edge with the right knee and hip flexed at 90 degrees. The practitioner stands on the patient's right side, holds the patient's ankle with the right hand, and places the left hand on the knee:

The practitioner moves the tibia into external rotation and applies a compression force on the tibia with the chest, while flexing and internally rotating the knee with the right hand.

After joint decoaptation and rebalancing, the thrust is performed by forcing the knee and hip into internal rotation and flexion with the right hand, which pushes the ankle toward the gluteal muscles from above downward (Figs. 6.59 and 6.60; Video 6.20).

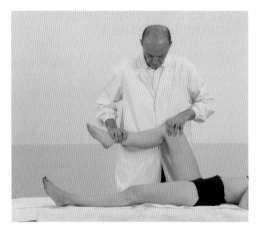 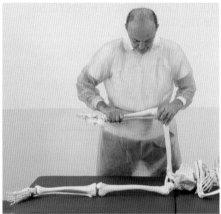

Fig. 6.59 External rotation of the tibia treatment_starting position.

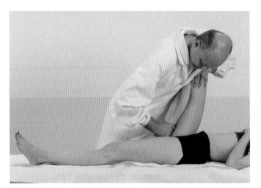 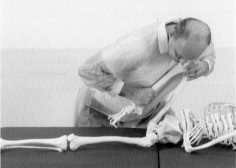

Fig. 6.60 External rotation of the tibia treatment_final position.

Clinical Notes

- Improvement following treatment may turn intense pain to dull pain and then to a feeling of weakness. Should this be the case, the principle of treatment has to be changed as follows. It is no longer necessary to remove Qì stagnation and Blood stasis and expel EPFs, if any; instead, Qì and Blood should be tonified to strengthen tissues and avoid pain exacerbation from physical activities or invasion of EPFs.
- Treatment of the ITBS can ensure excellent results in terms of disappearance of pain and return to daily activities, even sports. Sometimes, temporary worsening of symptoms is observed, especially when cupping is used.
- As far as the ITBS is concerned, pain disappearance or reduction does not necessarily mean that snapping is resolved.

Second Technique

A muscle energy technique (MET) is used. The patient is supine close to the bed edge with the right knee and hip flexed at 90 degrees. The practitioner stands on the patient's right side and holds the patient's ankle with the right hand, while the left hand stabilizes the knee against the chest:

- The practitioner's right hand moves the leg into internal rotation until the restrictive barrier is engaged.
- Then, the patient is asked to dorsiflex the foot and perform an isometric contraction in external rotation against the practitioner's own resistance.
- The position is held for 3 seconds followed by a 3-second postisometric relaxation.
- Afterwards, the practitioner increases internal rotation to engage a new restrictive barrier and again asks the patient to dorsiflex and extrarotate against resistance.

This process needs to be repeated three times (Fig. 6.61; Video 6.21).

Internal Rotation of the Tibia: Treatment

Internal rotation dysfunction: knee internal rotation is better than external rotation.

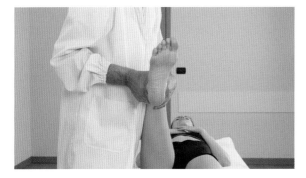

Fig. 6.61 External rotation of the tibia MET treatment_starting position.

We can choose between two techniques.

First Technique

The patient is supine close to the bed edge with the right knee and hip flexed at 90 degrees. The practitioner stands on the patient's right side, holds the patient's ankle with the right hand, and places the web space of the left thumb on the medial femoral condyle.

The patient's knee lies against the practitioner's chest:

- The practitioner moves the tibia into internal rotation and applies a compression force on the tibia with the chest, while extending and externally rotating the knee with the right hand.
- Manipulative treatment (osteopathic manipulative treatment) is performed by extending and forcing the leg into external rotation with the right hand (Figs. 6.62 and 6.63; Video 6.22.

Second Technique

An MET is used. The patient is supine close to the bed edge with the knee and hip flexed at 90 degrees.

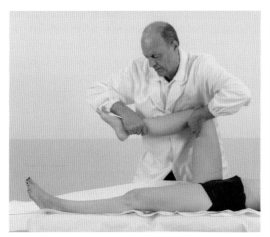

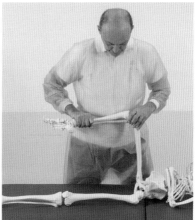

Fig. 6.62 Internal rotation of the tibia treatment_starting position.

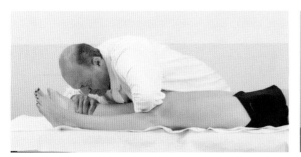

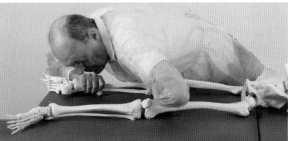

Fig. 6.63 Internal rotation of the tibia treatment_final position.

The practitioner stands on the patient's right side and holds the patient's ankle with the right hand, while the left hand stabilizes the knee against the chest:

- The practitioner's right hand moves the leg into external rotation until the restrictive barrier is engaged.
- Then, the patient is asked to dorsiflex the foot and perform an isometric contraction in internal rotation against the practitioner's own resistance.
- The position is held for 3 seconds followed by a 3-second postisometric relaxation.
- Afterwards, the practitioner increases external rotation to engage a new restrictive barrier and again asks the patient to dorsiflex and intrarotate against resistance.

This process needs to be repeated three times (Fig. 6.64; Video 6.23).

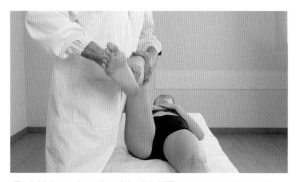

Fig. 6.64 Internal rotation of the tibia MET treatment_starting position.

Adduction of the Tibia: Treatment

Adduction dysfunction: tibial adduction is better than tibial abduction.

The patient is supine close to the bed edge with the right hip and knee slightly flexed and abducted off the bed.

The practitioner stands on the patient's right side and holds the patient's ankle between his thighs to apply distal traction. The thenar eminences and fingers are on the lateral and medial joint spaces and on the popliteal fossa, respectively.

After joint decoaptation and rebalancing, the thrust is performed with the left hand by pushing horizontally and medially (Fig. 6.65; Video 6.24).

Abduction of the Tibia: Treatment

Abduction dysfunction: tibial abduction is better than tibial adduction.

The patient is supine close to the bed edge with the right hip and knee slightly flexed and abducted off the bed.

The practitioner stands on the patient's right side and holds the patient's ankle between his thighs to apply distal traction. The thenar eminences and fingers are on the lateral and medial joint spaces and on the popliteal fossa, respectively.

After joint decoaptation and rebalancing, the thrust is performed with the right hand by pushing horizontally and laterally (Fig. 6.66; Video 6.25).

Anterior Tibia: Treatment

Anterior dysfunction: anterior sliding of the tibia is better than posterior sliding.

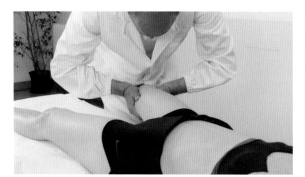

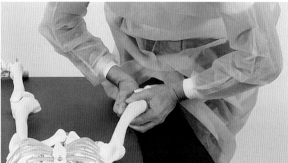

Fig. 6.65 Tibial adduction treatment.

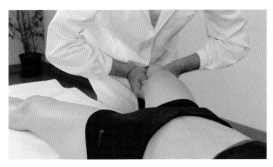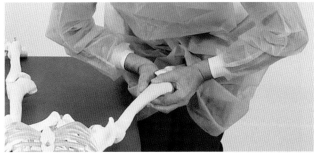

Fig. 6.66 Tibial abduction treatment.

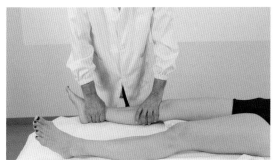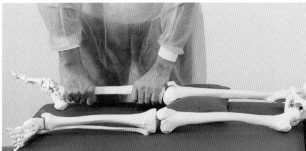

Fig. 6.67 Anterior tibia treatment_starting position.

The patient is supine close to the bed edge with the right knee extended and a pillow under the femur, close to the popliteal fossa.

The practitioner stands on the patient's right side and holds the patient's ankle with the right hand. The left hand is on the anterior tibial tuberosity and the forearm in vertical position with the elbow extended.

While holding the knee in position with the left hand, the right hand slightly extends the knee.

After joint decoaptation and rebalancing, the thrust is performed with the left hand by pushing the anterior tibial tuberosity downward (Figs. 6.67 and 6.68; Video 6.26).

If placing the joint under tension before the thrust is painful, we recommend reevaluation for meniscus tear or ligament sprain before performing the thrust.

Posterior Tibia: Treatment

Posterior dysfunction: posterior sliding of the tibia is better than anterior sliding.

We can choose between two techniques depending on full hip and knee flexion, that is, if it can or cannot be achieved.

First Technique

The patient is supine close to the bed edge with the right knee and hip flexed. The practitioner stands on the patient's right side and holds the patient's ankle with the right hand, while the left hand is placed on the popliteal fossa:

• The practitioner applies a compression force on the tibia with the chest, while flexing the knee with the right hand and creating a wedge with the dorsal surface of the left hand against the femur.

After joint decoaptation and rebalancing, the thrust is performed by forcing the knee and hip into flexion with the right hand, which pushes the tibia toward the gluteal muscles from above downward (Figs. 6.69 and 6.70; Video 6.27).

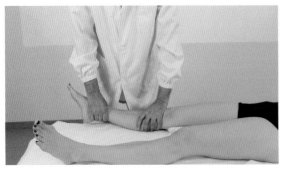
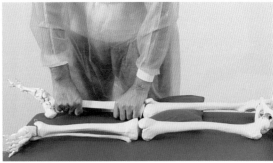

Fig. 6.68 Anterior tibia treatment_final position.

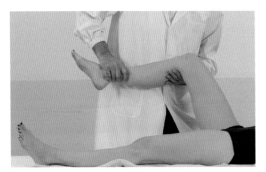
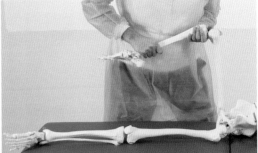

Fig. 6.69 Posterior tibia treatment_starting position.

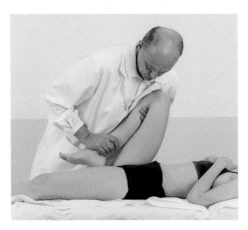
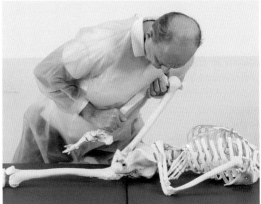

Fig. 6.70 Posterior tibia treatment_final position.

Second Technique

The patient is supine close to the bed edge with knees flexed at 90 degrees and feet flat on the bed.

The practitioner stands on the patient's right side and holds the patient's ankle with the right hand. The left forearm is under the right knee, while the left hand is on the left knee:

- While the right hand pushes the ankle toward the gluteal muscles, the left forearm pulls the proximal tibia backwards a little farther away from the gluteal muscles.

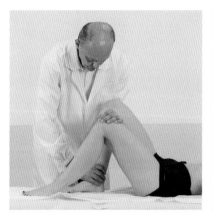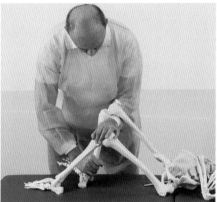

Fig. 6.71 Posterior tibia 2nd technique treatment.

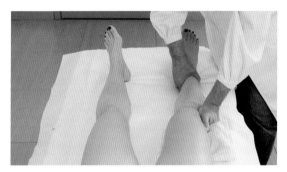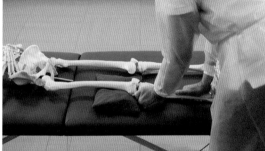

Fig. 6.72 Anterior fibula treatment.

This process needs to be repeated three times without any thrust (Fig. 6.71; Video 6.28).

Somatic Dysfunctions of the Proximal Tibiofibular Joint

Anterior Fibula: Treatment
Anterior dysfunction: anterior sliding of the tibia is better than posterior sliding.

The patient is supine close to the bed edge, the right knee is extended with a pillow under the femur and close to the popliteal fossa.

The practitioner stands on the patient's right side and holds the patient's ankle in internal rotation with the right hand. The thenar eminence of the left hand is on the anterior fibular head and the forearm in vertical position with the elbow extended.

After joint decoaptation and rebalancing, the thrust is performed by vertically pushing the fibular head downward with the left hand (Fig. 6.72; Video 6.29).

Posterior Fibula: Treatment
Posterior dysfunction: posterior sliding of the tibia is better than anterior sliding.

We can choose between two techniques depending on hip and knee flexion, that is, if it can or cannot be achieved.

First Technique

The patient is supine close to the bed edge with the right knee and hip flexed at 90 degrees. The practitioner stands on the patient's right side and holds the patient's ankle with the right hand, while the left hand is on the popliteal fossa with the metacarpophalangeal joint of the index finger placed behind the fibular head:

- The practitioner moves the tibia into internal rotation and then applies a compression force with the chest.
- The knee is then flexed and externally rotated, until a wedge is created with the metacarpophalangeal joint of the left index finger.

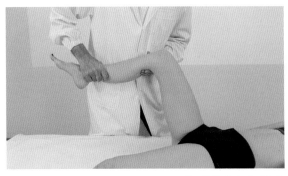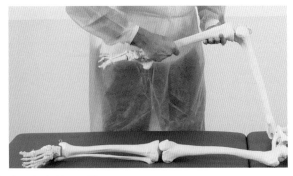

Fig. 6.73 Posterior fibula treatment_starting position.

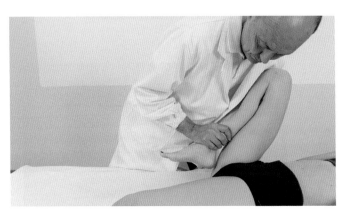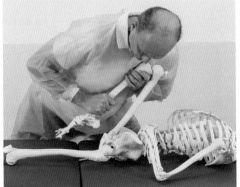

Fig. 6.74 Posterior fibula treatment_final position.

After joint decoaptation and rebalancing, the thrust is performed by flexing the knee and hip and forcing the knee into external rotation with the right hand, which pushes the tibia toward the gluteal muscles from above downward (Figs. 6.73 and 6.74; Video 6.30).

Second Technique

A MET is used. The patient is supine close to the bed edge with the right knee flexed at 90 degrees and foot flat on the bed.

The practitioner sits on the foot to stabilize the leg, holds the tibia with the right hand, while the left thumb, index finger, and middle finger hold the fibular head. The patient is asked to flex the knee against the practitioner's fingers, while the practitioner applies a counterforce. The position is held for 3 seconds and followed by a 3-second period of postisometric relaxation. Afterwards, the practitioner pulls the head of the fibula forward to engage a new restrictive barrier. Then, the patient is asked again to flex the knee against the practitioner's fingers.

This process needs to be repeated three times (Figs. 6.75 and 6.76; Video 6.31).

Somatic Dysfunctions of the Medial Meniscus

Anterior Medial Meniscus: Treatment

Anterior dysfunction: the medial meniscus is not free to move backward and stays fixed in the anterior position.

We can choose between two techniques.

First Technique

The patient is supine close to the bed edge with the right knee flexed at 90 degrees. The practitioner stands on the patient's right side, places the left thumb on the anterior horn of the medial meniscus, and holds the patient's ankle with the right hand:

- The patient's knee lies against the practitioner's chest: pressure applied slightly adducts the hip and abducts the knee.
- The practitioner moves the tibia into internal rotation.

Treatment is performed by abducting, extending, and externally rotating the leg with the right hand,

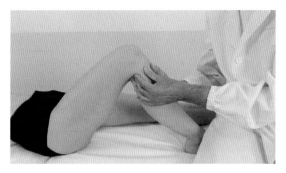 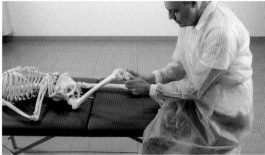

Fig. 6.75 Posterior fibula MET_starting position.

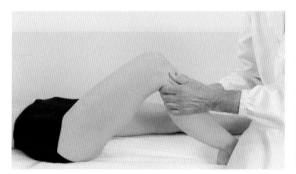 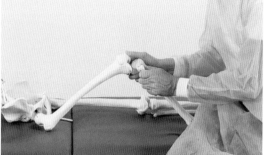

Fig. 6.76 Posterior fibula MET_final position.

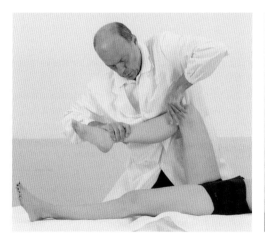 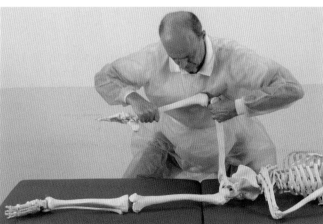

Fig. 6.77 Anterior medial meniscus treatment_starting position.

while the left thumb prevents the meniscus from moving forward and, consequently, forces it to move backward (Figs. 6.77 and 6.78; Video 6.32).

Second Technique
The patient sits on the bed, legs off the edge. The practitioner sits on the right foot and holds the leg in internal rotation and abduction.

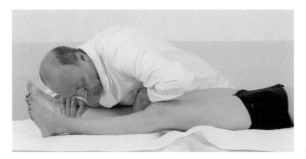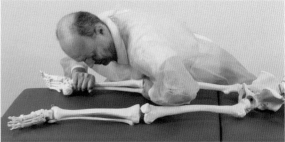

Fig. 6.78 Anterior medial meniscus treatment_final position.

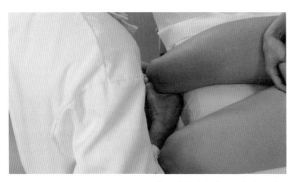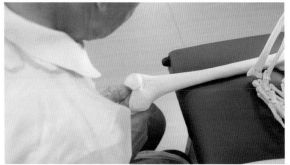

Fig. 6.79 Anterior medial meniscus treatment_2nd_starting position.

Then, the practitioner grasps the knee with both hands and places the thumbs on the anterior horn of the medial meniscus:

- While standing up, the practitioner extends and extrarotates the leg, always keeping the thumbs still on the anterior horn. The aim is to prevent the meniscus from moving forward and, consequently, force it to move backward (Figs. 6.79 and 6.80; Video 6.33).

Somatic Dysfunctions of the Patella

Superolateral Patella: Treatment

Superolateral patellar sliding is better than inferomedial sliding. The patient sits on the bed, legs off the edge. The practitioner sits on the right foot and holds the leg in neutral position.

Then, the practitioner grasps the knee with both hands and places the index fingers on the superior

board of the patella and the thumbs under the inferior board.

While standing up, the practitioner extends the leg and with the index fingers slightly pulls the patella inferiorly and medially (Figs. 6.81 and 6.82; Video 6.34).

Therapeutic Program, Frequency of Sessions

The AcuOsteo method of treatment combines acupuncture and osteopathic manipulations, and, in principle, both therapeutic techniques are used during each session and at the same time.

If the condition is acute or chronic with intense pain, we recommend sessions twice a week for 2 weeks and then once a week for another 2 weeks. If improvement is observed, sessions are then scheduled once a week until complete pain relief or at least reduction by 80% to 90%.

In practice, however, since the osteopathic approach differs from acupuncture in that it follows a

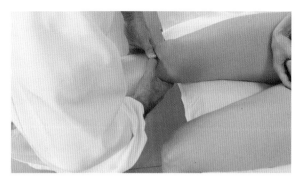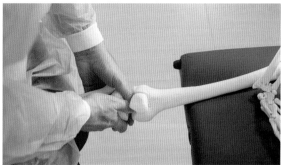

Fig. 6.80 Anterior medial meniscus treatment_2_final position.

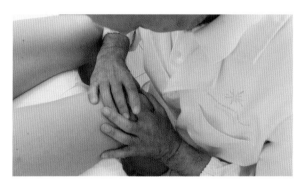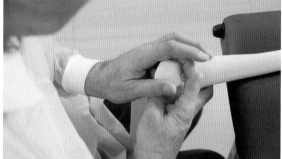

Fig. 6.81 Superolateral patella treatment_starting position.

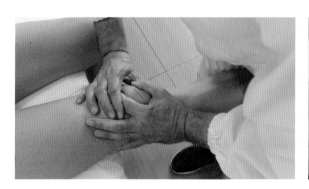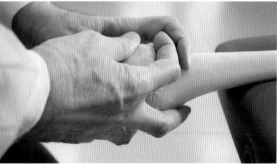

Fig. 6.82 Superolateral patella treatment_final position.

mechanical principle and aims to restore proper joint mobility, we opt for a parsimonious use of osteopathic manipulations over acupuncture; there may be no need to repeat them in every session.

Osteopathic maneuvers are therefore performed in case of persistent somatic dysfunction. That is why the patient should always be reevaluated at the beginning of each session to assess joint conditions and compare them with preexisting dysfunction.

REFERENCE

1. Reaves W, Bong C. *The Acupuncture Handbook of Sports Injuries & Pain*. 3rd ed. Hidden Needle Press; 2013.

BIBLIOGRAPHY

Baldry PE. *Acupuncture, Trigger Points and Musculoskeletal Pain*. 3rd ed. Elsevier; 2005.

Buckup K. *Test Ortopedici*. Verduci Editore; 1997.

Cipriano JJ. *Test Ortopedici e Neurologici*. Verduci Editore; 1998.

Deadman P, Al-Khafaji M, Baker K, Manuale di Agopuntura, Ed. *italiana a cura di Grazia Rotolo e Giulio Picozzi*. CEA (Casa Editrice Ambrosiana); 2000.

De Seze S, Ryckewaert A. *Malattie dell'osso e delle articolazioni*. Aulo Gaggi Editore; 1979.

Audouard M. *Osteopatia, l'Arto Inferiore*. Editore Marrapese; 1989.

Giusti R. *Glossary of Osteophatic Terminology*. 3rd ed. American Association of Colleges of Osteophatic Medicine; 2017.

Greenman PE. *Principles of Manual Medicine*. 2nd ed. Williams & Wilkins; 1996.

Guolo F. *Atlante di Tecniche di Energia Muscolare*. Piccin; 2014.

Hoppenfeld S. *L'Esame Obiettivo dell'Apparato Locomotore*. Aulo Gaggi Editore; 1985.

Legge D. *Close to the Bone*. Sydney College Press; 2010.

Maciocia G. *The Practice of Chinese Medicine*. 3rd ed. Elsevier; 2022.

Misulis KE, Head TC. *Neurologia di Netter*. Elsevier, Masson; 2008.

Nicholas AS, Nicholas EA. *Atlas of Osteophatic Thechniques*. Lippincott Williams & Wilkins; 2012.

Qiao W. Wrist and Ankle and Balance Acupuncture, Italian Chine School of Acupuncture-A.M.A.B. (Association of Medical Acupuncturist of Bologna) Seminar 2007.

Romoli M. *Auricular Acupuncture Diagnosis*. Churchill Livingstone Elsevier; 2009.

Tan RT. Dr. In: Besinger JW ed. *Tan's Strategy of Twelve Magical Points*; 2003.

Tixa S. *Atlas d'Anatomie Palpatoire, tome 2, Membre Inferior*. 3e éd. Elsevier Masson; 2005.

Tixa S, Ebenegger B. *Atlas de Techniques articulaires ostéopathiques, tome 3, Les Membres*. 2e éd. Elsevier Masson; 2016.

Chapter 7

Ankle Pain

Lateral Ankle Sprain and Achilles Tendonitis

Lateral ankle sprain and Achilles tendonitis are the most common ankle musculoskeletal injuries.

Lateral ankle sprain is a sports injury with sudden onset of pain and swelling.

Achilles tendonitis is a multifactorial, inflammatory process, not necessarily caused by a trauma. It presents with pain and peritendinous swelling.

Anatomy and Biomechanics According to Western Medicine

JOINTS AND MUSCLES

The ankle joint, also referred to as the tibiotalar joint, connects the foot to the leg. It is a joint, which mainly allows for dorsiflexion and plantarflexion. Eversion and inversion are mainly produced by other joints of the foot, such as the talocalcaneal joint.

Ankle

The ankle is formed by three bones: the tibia and fibula of the leg and the talus of the foot.

1. The articular medial facet of the lateral malleolus forms the lateral border of the ankle joint.
2. The articular lateral facet of the medial malleolus forms the medial border of the joint.
3. The superior portion of the ankle joint is formed by the inferior articular surface of the tibia and the superior articular surface of the talus.

These surfaces and borders form a bracket-shaped socket, covered in hyaline cartilage known as the mortise.

The body of the talus fits into the mortise. The talus articulates inferiorly with the calcaneus and anteriorly with the navicular bone.

- The upper surface, called the trochlear surface, is somewhat cylindrical and allows for dorsiflexion and plantarflexion of the ankle.
- The talus is broad anteriorly and narrow posteriorly.
- The articulating portion is wedge-shaped and fits between the medial and lateral malleoli.

In dorsiflexion, the anterior part of the talus is held in the mortise, whereas in plantarflexion it is the posterior part. There are two main sets of ligaments in the ankle.

Medial Ligament

Also known as the deltoid ligament, it originates from the medial malleolus. It is made up of four ligaments, which form a triangle and connect the tibia to the talus, calcaneus, and navicular bone. The medial ligament resists overeversion of the foot and prevents subluxation of the ankle joint.

Lateral Ligament

It originates from the lateral malleolus and is formed by the following three separate ligaments, which attach the lateral malleolus to the bones below the ankle joint.

- Anterior talofibular ligament (ATFL): It extends anteromedially, attaches proximally to the anterior border of the lateral malleolus and distally to the lateral surface of the talus. It resists inversion in plantarflexion.
- Posterior talofibular ligament (PTFL): It runs horizontally and medially attaches proximally to the posterior border of the lateral malleolus and distally to the posterior surface of the talus. It resists posterior displacement of the talus.

- Calcaneofibular Ligament (CFL): It runs postero-inferiorly and attaches proximally to the tip of lateral malleolus and distally to lateral surface of calcaneus. It resists inversion.

The lateral ligament resists overinversion of the foot, which is the most common sprain, because the lateral malleolus is longer than the medial malleolus, allowing the talus to invert more than it can revert (Figs. 7.1 and 7.2).

The Muscles

Plantarflexion is produced by the muscles in the posterior compartment of the leg; the two muscles which are primarily responsible for this movement are the triceps surae and posterior tibialis.

The triceps surae is formed by two muscles and three heads: the gastrocnemius, more important and more superficial, and the soleus, situated deep to the gastrocnemius muscle.

The gastrocnemius has a lateral and a medial head, which originate from the lateral and medial femoral condyles, respectively. They fuse to insert onto the posterior surface of the calcaneus through the Achilles tendon.

The soleus originates from the posterior surface of the fibular head and the proximal posterior surface of the tibia. It ends deep in the Achilles tendon.

The tibialis posterior originates from the posterior surface of the inferior tibia, interosseous membrane, and medial surface of the fibula. Then, its tendon runs behind the medial malleolus and attaches distally to the navicular and first cuneiform bones. This muscle allows for plantarflexion and inversion of the ankle.

Dorsiflexion is produced by the muscles in the anterior compartment of the leg; the three muscles which are primarily responsible for this movement are the tibialis anterior, extensor hallucis longus, and extensor digitorum longus.

The tibialis anterior originates from the lateral condyle and proximal third of the tibia, and the interosseous membrane. Then, its tendon attaches distally to the first cuneiform bone and the metatarsus. This muscle allows for dorsiflexion and inversion of the ankle.

The extensor hallucis longus originates from the middle third of the anteromedial surface of the fibula, and the interosseous membrane. Then, its tendon

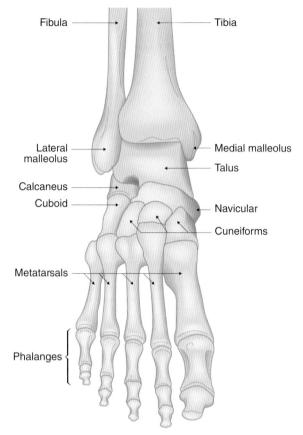

Fig. 7.1 Ankle anatomy: anterior view.

attaches distally to the first toe. This muscle allows for dorsiflexion and inversion of the ankle.

The extensor digitorum longus originates from the lateral condyle of the tibia, interosseous membrane, head and proximal third of the fibula. When its tendon reaches the dorsum of the foot, it divides into four slips that attach distally to the toes 2 to 5. This muscle allows for dorsiflexion and eversion of the ankle.

Eversion is produced by three muscles, the peroneus longus and peroneus brevis, which are found in the lateral compartment of the leg, and the extensor digitorum longus, found in the anterior compartment and already mentioned above.

The peroneus longus originates from the lateral condyle of the tibia, interosseous membrane, and head and proximal two-thirds of the lateral fibula. Then, its tendon runs behind the lateral malleolus, travels

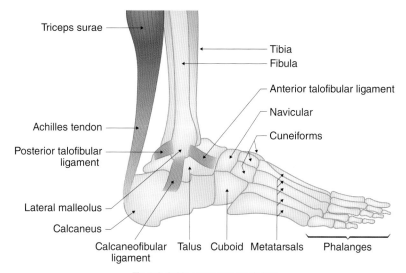

Fig. 7.2 Ankle anatomy: lateral view.

laterally to the sole of the foot, and attaches distally to the first and second metatarsal bones and the first cuneiform bone. This muscle allows for eversion of the ankle.

The peroneus brevis originates from the lateral middle third of the fibula. Then, its tendon runs behind the lateral malleolus, travels anteriorly, and attaches distally to the fifth metatarsal bone. This muscle allows for eversion of the ankle.

ANATOMICAL LANDMARKS

Ankle

The most useful anatomical landmarks are listed below.

- Lateral malleolus: it is the bony prominence projecting from the lateral aspect of the distal fibula.
- Medial malleolus: it is the bony prominence projecting from the medial aspect of the distal tibia.
- Talus: it is located where the tibia and fibula meet, and articulates directly with the medial and lateral malleoli (Figs. 7.3 and 7.4).

JOINT MOVEMENTS

The Physiological Movements of the Ankle

Biomechanics of the ankle is quite complex due to the multiple joints involved in the movements the ankle and foot perform also to walk on uneven terrain.

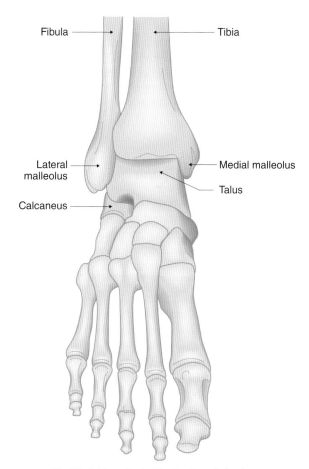

Fig. 7.3 Ankle anatomical landmarks: anterior view.

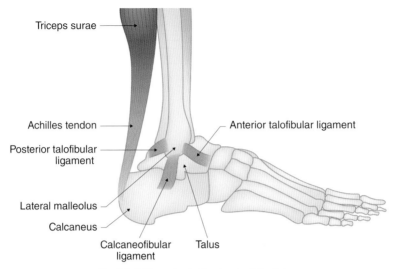

Triceps surae

Achilles tendon

Posterior talofibular
ligament

Anterior talofibular ligament

Lateral malleolus

Calcaneus

Calcaneofibular
ligament

Talus

Fig. 7.4 Ankle anatomical landmarks: lateral view.

This handbook will only focus on the movements more often associated with ankle injuries. As already said, dorsiflexion and plantarflexion are mainly produced by the tibiotalar joint, while inversion and eversion by the talocalcaneal joint.

With the terms inversion and eversion, we refer to the combination of two movements:

- Inversion: supination (internal rotation) and varus (adduction)
- Eversion: pronation (external rotation) and valgus (abduction)

Dorsiflexion and plantarflexion achieve the greatest range of motion. The neutral position of the ankle is with the patient supine, lower limb extended, foot in slightly external rotation (physiological position); this is the starting position to assess.

- Dorsiflexion: the dorsum of the foot moves toward the anterior part of the leg.
- Plantarflexion: the dorsum of the foot moves away from the anterior part of the leg.
- Valgus: the foot moves outward.
- Varus: the foot moves inward.
- Pronation: the foot rotates externally.
- Supination: the foot rotates internally.

The normal range of motion of the ankle from neutral position:

- To dorsiflexion is about 20 to 30 degrees
- To plantarflexion about 30 to 50 degrees
- To valgus 0 to about 20 degrees
- To varus 0 to about 25 degrees
- To pronation 0 to about 20 degrees
- To supination 0 to about 5 degrees

Diagnosis in Western Medicine

LATERAL ANKLE SPRAIN

Lateral ankle sprains are extremely common and damage the ligaments. They occur when the ankle is subjected to traumas. This handbook will only deal with the lateral ligament injuries, which are the most common type of ankle sprains.

The ligaments involved in lateral ankle sprain are mainly the anterior talofibular (ATFL) and the CFL, and they tend to be injured in this order with the ATFL being injured more often.

The most common symptoms are:

- Severe pain under load
- Joint instability
- Swelling
- Range of motion restricted by pain
- Positive inversion stress test

Inversion Stress Test

It is used to assess lateral ankle sprain and stresses the anterior talofibular (ATFL) and/or CFLs.

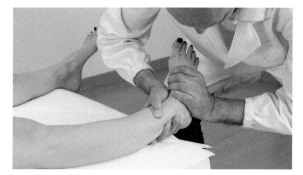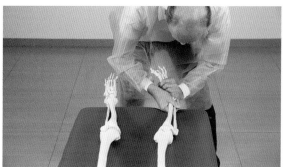

Fig. 7.5 Inversion stress test.

The patient is supine with the right knee extended and foot off the bed edge (Fig. 7.5; Video 7.1).

The practitioner stands close to the bed edge, next to the right foot. The practitioner holds the dorsum of the foot at the level of the neck of the talus with the left hand, while the right hand holds the talus and calcaneus as one unit with the ankle in neutral position. The heel is placed in an inverted position with respect to the tibia. The test is considered positive if the patient reports pain on the lateral ankle ligaments.

ACHILLES TENDONITIS

Achilles tendonitis is inflammation of the Achilles tendon. It can be caused by prolonged mechanical stress upon the tendon, which may or may not be sports-related. This term is used to refer to the more commonly reported midportion tendinopathy and also to the rare insertional tendinopathy.

Tendinopathy occurs in the following three separate stages:
- Reactive tendinopathy
- Tendon disrepair
- Degenerative tendinopathy

The most common symptoms are as follows:
- Morning pain in the tendon and adjacent area
- Swelling
- Thickening of the affected tendon margins
- Stiffer tendon
- Positive test for Achilles tendonitis

Test for Achilles Tendonitis

There is no specific test and consequently the Achilles tendon is examined by palpation. The patient is prone,

feet off the bed edge with dorsiflexion of about 90 degrees. The practitioner stands close to the patient's feet to check if the affected tendon is thicker and more irregular than the other; the more inflamed it is, the more severe and chronic the condition is.

The tendon is then palpated by "pinching" with the thumb and index finger from the lateral and medial sides, starting from the portion proximal to the calf and moving distally to the calcaneal insertion.

The test is considered positive if the patient reports pain over the tendon or calcaneal insertion; the painful area may be 2 to 6 cm wide and located on one or either side.

JOINT PAIN, ARTHRITIS, AND STIFFNESS

Patients with ankle arthritis and postsurgical outcomes usually complain of pain, weakness, and restricted range of motion. Among the most common causes of ankle arthritis are fracture or rheumatoid arthritis; primary osteoarthritis, septic arthritis, and crystal arthropathy are also to be mentioned. Diagnosis is based on the patient's medical history, along with clinical and radiographic examinations.

The most common complications that may occur after surgery or as a result of fracture include:
- Ankle stiffness with possible loss of motion
- Late-onset osteoarthritis
- Failed fusion
- Persistent pain

RED FLAGS IN WESTERN MEDICINE

The presence of heat (calor), redness (rubor), swelling (tumor), pain (dolor) and loss of function

(function laesa) determines the need for diagnostic investigations.

Special attention should be paid if concomitant symptoms are observed, such as numbness, tingling, paresthesia (abnormal sensation), muscle weakness with consequent loss of strength, decreased tendon reflexes and pain, mainly at night.

Patients with rheumatoid arthritis of the ankle usually complain of pain throughout the range of motion, but usually the ankle is not affected. Both fatigue and general discomfort can also be observed.

The use of imaging techniques is mandatory in case of a grade 3 lateral ligaments sprain. Special attention should be paid if concomitant symptoms are observed, such as numbness, tingling, paraesthesia (abnormal sensation), muscle weakness, decreased tendon reflexes and pain, mainly at night.

Abnormalities uncovered on history taking or physical examination may require medical evaluation, laboratory tests, and imaging investigations, such as x-rays, US, CT, and MRI.

Diagnosis in Chinese Medicine

In Chinese Medicine, musculoskeletal pain results from the obstruction of Qì and Blood circulation or inadequate Qì and Blood for the nourishment of the secondary channels, especially the Muscle and Connecting channels.

The Muscle and Connecting channels more often involved in ankle disorders are listed in the following:
- Gall Bladder
- Bladder
- Stomach
- Kidney

The channels affected vary according to pain location:
- Gall Bladder: pain is on the lateral side, the pathology is lateral ankle sprain.
- Bladder: pain is on the lateral and posterior side, with pathologies being lateral ankle sprain and Achilles tendonitis.
- Stomach: pain is on the anterior side, the pathology is ankle pain.
- Kidney: pain is on the medial and posterior side, with pathologies being medial ankle sprain and Achilles tendonitis.

What matters most is to identify the affected channel where pain is located.

Sometimes, it is not so easy to determine it and consequently, the following data concerning the Muscle channels involved in ankle movements should be acquired for a better identification.
- Flexion (dorsiflexion): ST and SP
- Extension (plantarflexion): BL, GB, and KI
- Adduction: KI, LR, and SP
- Abduction: GB and BL
- Internal Rotation: KI, LR, and SP
- External Rotation: GB and BL

Red Flags	Pain	Inspection	Other Signs	Neurological Signs	Recommendations
Inflammation	Pain	Redness, swelling, and heat	–	Functional deficit	Physician evaluation Imaging investigations
Fracture	Spontaneous pain	Deformity and swelling	Movement beyond normal range of motion	Functional deficit	Physician evaluation Imaging investigations
Rheumatoid arthritis	Pain with or without movement	Redness and swelling	Fatigue and general discomfort	Functional deficit	Physician evaluation Imaging investigations Laboratory tests

The information so acquired on the channel, which is likely to be involved, that is, pain location and related movement restriction, can also be integrated with the results from Western Medicine orthopedic tests to identify which muscle, tendon, and joint is affected in the case of:

- Lateral ankle sprain
- Achilles tendonitis

ETIOLOGY

Ankle pain is usually caused by:

- *Overuse, repetitive strain injury*. Through sports (running, tennis or basketball); performing the same movement over and over again causes local Qì stagnation or Qì and Blood deficiency.
- *Trauma, sports injuries*. If mild, they cause local Qì stagnation. If severe, they cause local Blood stasis.
- *Cold and Dampness*. Local invasion causes Qì stagnation or Blood stasis. Previous accidents often predispose the ankle to more frequent invasions of external pathogenic factors (EPFs), especially Cold.

PATHOLOGY

The Muscle and Connecting channels are often affected by Qì stagnation and Blood stasis:

- Qì stagnation manifests itself with widespread pain radiating proximally or distally along the pathway of the Muscle channels and could be associated with muscle contracture and stiffness of the lateral and posterior side of the leg, also perceived upon palpation.
- Blood stasis, usually occurring in the Connecting channels, manifests itself with more intense pain localized in the joint, or more frequently, in the lateral or posterior side of the ankle. It is also perceived upon palpation.

As already mentioned in the Fundamentals of acupuncture for MSK pain in the limbs (see Chapter 1), the term *Connecting channels* includes not only the Connecting channel "proper" but also the Connecting channel "area" that covers the whole pathway of the Main channel.

LATERAL ANKLE SPRAIN

To identify the Muscle and Connecting channels affected, we check location and characteristics of

musculoskeletal pain, palpate the affected area, test the range of motion for each ankle movement and perform orthopaedic tests to elicit pain.

The Pathways of the Gall Bladder Secondary Channels

In case of lateral ankle sprain, the Gall Bladder Muscle and Connecting channels may be involved. The pathways of the Gall Bladder Muscle and Connecting channels explain pain on the lateral aspect of the ankle and distal leg (Fig. 7.6).

The Pathways of the Bladder Secondary Channels

In case of lateral ankle sprain, the Bladder Muscle and Connecting channels may be involved. The pathway of the Bladder Muscle channel explains pain on the lateral and posterior aspect of the ankle, whereas the pathway of the Bladder Connecting channel "proper" doesn't as it doesn't descend to the ankle (Fig. 7.7).

Since we are now referring to the Bladder Connecting channel "area," we regard the Bladder Connecting channels as channels involved.

ACHILLES TENDONITIS

To identify the Muscle and Connecting channels affected, we check location and characteristics of musculoskeletal pain, palpate the affected area, test the range of motion for each ankle movement and perform orthopaedic tests to elicit pain.

The Pathways of the Bladder Secondary Channels

In case of Achilles tendonitis, the Bladder Muscle and Connecting channels are involved. The pathway of the Bladder Muscle channel explains pain on the posterior and lateral aspect of the Achilles tendon, whereas the pathway of the Bladder Connecting channel "proper" does not as it does not descend to the heel (Fig. 7.8).

Since we are now referring to the Bladder Connecting channel "area," we regard the Bladder Connecting channels as channels involved.

The Pathways of the Kidney Secondary Channels

In case of Achilles tendonitis, the Kidney Muscle and Connecting channels may be involved. The pathways of the Kidney Muscle and Connecting channels explain pain on the medial aspect of the Achilles tendon (Fig. 7.9).

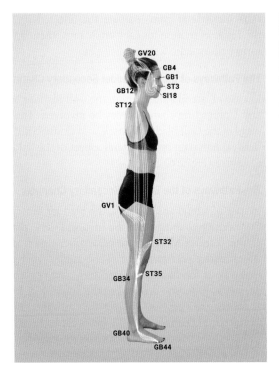

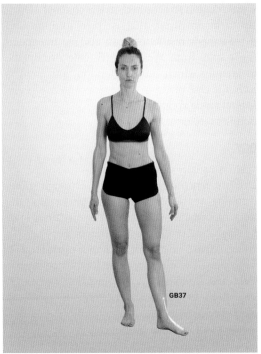

Fig. 7.6 The pathways of the Gall Bladder Muscle and Connecting "proper" channels.

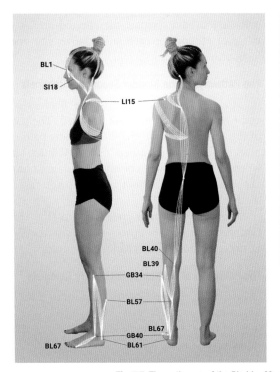

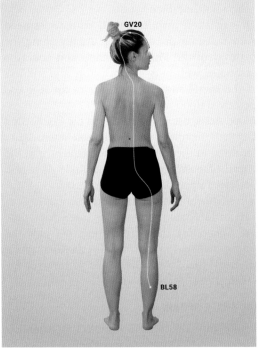

Fig. 7.7 The pathways of the Bladder Muscle and Connecting "proper" channels.

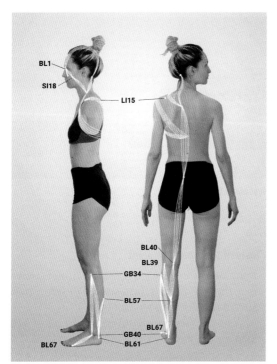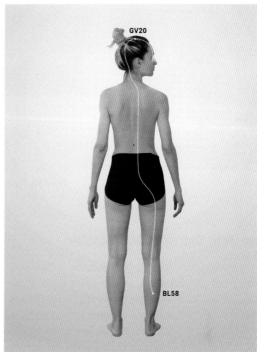

Fig. 7.8 The pathways of the Bladder Muscle and Connecting "proper" channels.

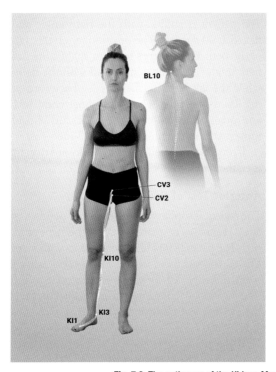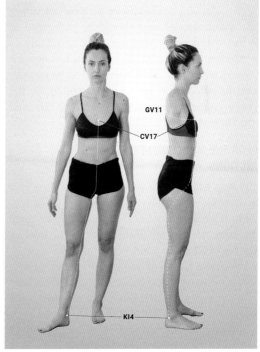

Fig. 7.9 The pathways of the Kidney Muscle and Connecting "proper" channels.

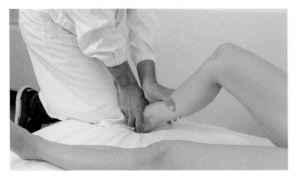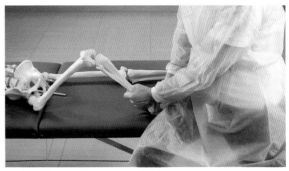

Fig. 7.10 Posterior test of the tibia.

Diagnosis in Osteopathic Medicine

The examination for "somatic dysfunction" is the central concept of the diagnostic process; palpation of the affected area and functionally/anatomically related components of the somatic system is the only way to assess it.

Consequently, the osteopathic diagnostic approach to musculoskeletal ankle pain is based on the identification of joint somatic dysfunctions not only of the ankle but also of the knee and hip.

Regardless of the condition to be treated, be it lateral ankle sprain, Achilles tendonitis, or surgical outcomes, all of the recommended tests should be performed to identify the dysfunctions that occur more frequently.

It is therefore evident that the osteopathic diagnosis is developed regardless of the condition to be treated, therefore the osteopathic tests recommended for the ankle, knee, hip and pelvic girdle will not be repeated when the "injuries" are treated.

TESTS FOR THE MAIN SOMATIC DYSFUNCTIONS

The only way to diagnose somatic dysfunctions of a joint is to assess the passive movements of its articular ends in relation to one another and compare them with the same movements of the joint on the healthy side. Testing of all ankle joints is required.

On the same plane of motion, there is passive mobility quantitatively and qualitatively equal on both sides of a theoretical neutral point that represents the reference point.

When the balance is lost and range and quality of motion are not the same in both directions, then there is somatic dysfunction.

Tests of the Tibiotalar Joint

Commonly known as the tests and dysfunctions of the tibia, they are instead the tests and dysfunctions of the talus in respect to the tibia.

Tests are performed to assess the most common tibial dysfunctions:
- Posterior tibia
- Anterior tibia

Posterior Test of the Tibia

The patient is supine with the right ankle and knee flexed at 90 degrees. The practitioner on the right edge of the bed. The patient's foot lies against the practitioner's thigh. The talus is stabilized with the right hand, while the left hand pushes the leg backward perpendicular to the talus. The practitioner compares range and quality of motion of the backward and forward movements of the tibia (Fig. 7.10; Video 7.2).

If the tibia moves more easily backward than forward, then there is posterior tibial dysfunction, and vice versa.

Anterior Test of the Tibia

The patient is supine with the right ankle and knee flexed at 90 degrees. The practitioner on the right edge of the bed. The patient's foot lies against the practitioner's thigh. The talus is stabilized with the right hand, while the left hand pulls the leg forward perpendicular to the talus. The practitioner compares range and quality of motion of the forward and backward movements of the tibia (Fig. 7.11; Video 7.3).

If the tibia moves more easily forward than backward, then there is anterior tibial dysfunction, and vice versa.

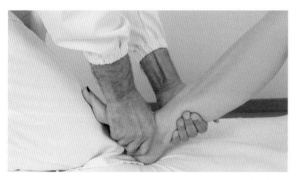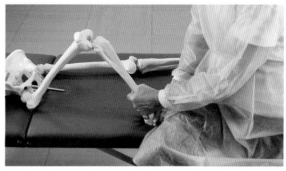

Fig. 7.11 Anterior test of the tibia.

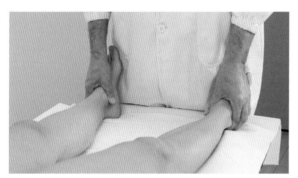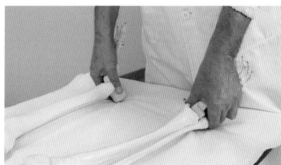

Fig. 7.12 Inferior-superior test of the fibula.

Tests of the Tibiofibular Joint

Tests are performed to assess the most common fibular dysfunctions:

1. Inferior fibula
2. Superior fibula
3. Anterior fibula
4. Posterior fibula

Inferior-Superior Test of the Fibula

The patient is supine with the knees extended and feet close to the bed edge. The practitioner stands close to the bed edge and holds the feet with the hands, positioning the index fingers under the lateral malleolus (Fig. 7.12; Video 7.4).

With the index fingers, the practitioner pushes the lateral malleolus upward along the leg axis and then compares range and quality of motion of the two movements. If the affected fibula does not move easily upward, then there is inferior fibular dysfunction, and vice versa.

Anteroposterior Test of the Fibula

The patient is supine, feet off the bed. The practitioner stands close to the right foot and immobilizes the tibia and talus with the right hand. The practitioner holds the lateral malleolus with the left thumb and index finger, and moves it upward and downward (see Fig. 7.13; Video 7.5).

The practitioner then compares range and quality of motion of the two movements. If the fibula moves more easily upward, then there is anterior fibular dysfunction, and vice versa.

Tests of the Talocalcaneal Joint

A test is performed to assess the most common calcaneal dysfunctions:

- Inversion of the calcaneus
- Eversion of the calcaneus

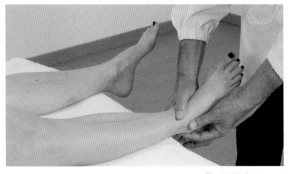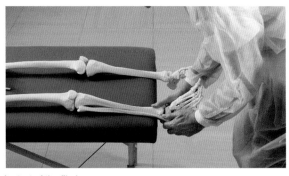

Fig. 7.13 Anteroposterior test of the fibula.

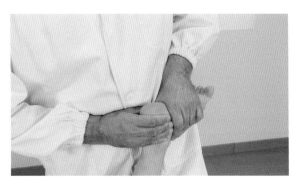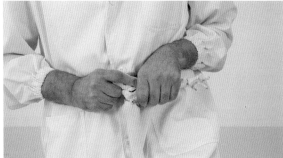

Fig. 7.14 Inversion test of the calcaneus.

Inversion–Eversion Test of the Calcaneus

The patient is prone with the right knee flexed at 90 degrees. The practitioner stands close to the right foot. The practitioner stabilizes the foot in dorsiflexion with the left hand, while the right hand holds the calcaneus, placing the thumb on one side and the index finger on the other side. After applying moderate traction along the axis of the tibia, the practitioner rolls the calcaneus first into eversion and then into inversion, to compare range and quality of motion of the two movements (Figs. 7.14 and 7.15; Video 7.6).

If the calcaneus rolls better into inversion than eversion, then there is calcaneal inversion dysfunction, and vice versa.

Treatment With the AcuOsteo Method: The Choice of an Integrated Approach

The therapeutic approach of the AcuOsteo Method aims to treat those musculoskeletal injuries which do not require consultation with a surgeon or a physician.

Once this fundamental aspect has been defined, treatment envisages the use of acupuncture and osteopathy according to their diagnostic and therapeutic approaches.

We would like to stress that at this point in diagnostic assessment, we do not have to follow the rules of Western Medicine, except for some specific cases, such as arthritis of the ankle, posttraumatic and postsurgical pain, and stiffness, which will be covered later.

In addition, we should not be misled by diagnostic imaging investigations and should rely only on the rules of Chinese and Osteopathic Medicine, which means selecting points according to symptoms and channel pathways and treating all of the somatic dysfunctions encountered.

For didactic purposes, treatment with acupuncture will precede osteopathic treatment, whereas in clinical practice the order is reversed since it may be difficult to perform osteopathic manipulations once the needles have been inserted.

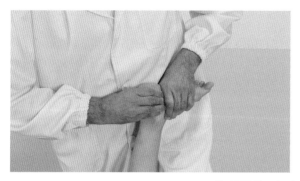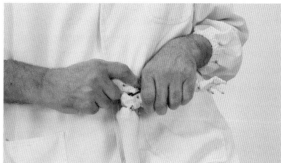

Fig. 7.15 Eversion test of the calcaneus.

An exception to this methodology is represented by those morbidities where marked stiffness prevents joint mobilization as required by osteopathic manipulations. Specifically, we are referring to the outcomes after immobilization following surgery and fractures.

In these cases, we suggest first using acupuncture, especially the bleeding techniques, and then, at the end of the session and after removing the needles, osteopathy.

In any case, it is always the practitioner's clinical experience that will guide them along the most appropriate pathway to treat each patient's condition.

Osteopathic Manipulation in the treatment of "somatic dysfunction" is the central concept of the therapeutic process to treat the affected joints and functionally/anatomically related components of the somatic system.

Consequently, the osteopathic manipulative approach to MSK ankle pain focuses on the treatment of joint somatic dysfunctions not only of the ankle, but also of the pelvic girdle, hip, and knee.

Regardless of the condition to be treated, be it lateral ankle sprain or Achilles tendonitis, all of the dysfunctions diagnosed should be treated.

It is therefore evident that the osteopathic therapeutic approach does not vary with the condition to be treated and thus the osteopathic manipulations described for the ankle, as well as those for the knee, pelvic girdle and hip, will not be repeated under the paragraphs dedicated to the "injuries."

ACUPUNCTURE TREATMENT

Lateral Ankle Sprain

The Five Options and Selection of Acupoints

The approach we suggest is widely described in the section dedicated to the Fundamentals of acupuncture for MSK pain in the limbs (see Chapter 1).

The most important aspect is the identification of the Ah Shi point(s) to determine which channels are affected. In this specific case, the Gall Bladder and Bladder Muscle and Connecting channels are involved and, according to our experience, the Yang Qiao Mai Extraordinary channel may also be involved.

Therefore, when a combination of two points (GB and BL) is presented, the first point to be needled or bled is the GB point, which treats lateral pain, whereas the BL point is the second option to be used in the treatment of lateral and posterior pain. Once the most effective channel is identified, selection of distal points continues along it.

Pricking pain localized on the anterior or inferior side of the lateral malleolus is a sign of Blood stasis to be treated with the bleeding technique, whereas widespread pain radiating proximally to the leg or distally to the foot is a sign of Qì stagnation to be treated with the needling technique. Swelling of the ankle joint is a sign of Dampness to be treated with the bleeding or needling technique.

It is worth reminding that the distal points should be needled one at a time and their effectiveness in terms of pain and range of motion tested after each insertion. The same applies to the local points.

Finally, since both options 1 and 2 consist of several steps, it is important to highlight how selection should be made. Specifically, the practitioner might wonder if all or some of the steps should be followed. The rule we follow is simple; when the result achieved is satisfactory, the remaining steps should be skipped, and the practitioner should move to the following option. Similarly, the use of the points recommended under options 3, 4, and 5 should be carefully evaluated according to the case being treated.

The points and accessory techniques we recommend using are listed below.

The Order of Needling

Option One: Distal Points

First Step: Gall Bladder and Bladder Muscle Channels

GB44 and BL67. These Jing-Well points activate the Gall Bladder and Bladder Muscle channels, and they remove Qì stagnation and Blood stasis with needling and bleeding techniques, respectively.

Second Step: Gall Bladder and Bladder Connecting Channels

GB37 and BL58 (Opposite Side). These Luo points activate the Gall Bladder and Bladder Connecting channels, and they remove Qì stagnation and Blood stasis in acute and chronic conditions from Excess.

LR5 and KI4 (Opposite Side). These Luo points activate the Liver and Kidney Connecting channels. They are also used in chronic Deficiency conditions with dull pain to tonify Qì and Blood in their respective Internally-Externally related channels. In this case, we associate the Yuan point GB40 with the Luo point LR5 and the Yuan point BL64 with the Luo point KI4, that is to say the well-known Luo-Yuan point combination. First, as main point, we needle the Yuan point on the affected side and then, as secondary point, the Luo point on the internally-externally related channel on the opposite side.

Third Step: Empirical Points

There is no point which is classically recommended.

Fourth Step: Opposite Extremity (Upper/ Lower)

TE4 and SI5 (Opposite Side). They are located in the wrist joint that corresponds to the ankle joint on the paired channel according to the Six Stages. Our technique consists of needling the opposite extremity (lower/upper) on the opposite side in acute and chronic conditions. Alternatively, the most tender point on palpation is selected on the same or opposite side.

Fifth Step: Categories of Traditional Points

GB41 (Affected Side) and TE3 (Opposite Side); BL65 (Affected Side) and SI3 (Opposite Side). A good combination includes the Shu-Stream points on the paired channel according to the Six Stages.

First, we needle the Shu-Stream point on the channel involved on the affected side and then the Shu-Stream point on the coupled channel on the opposite side and opposite extremity (upper/lower).

We use this technique in acute and chronic Excess conditions to treat pain and expel or prevent invasion of EPFs.

GB38 and BL60. The Jing-River points are used in acute or chronic Excess conditions due to the invasion of an EPF and they are needled to promote its expulsion from their respective channels. They are also useful to prevent pain exacerbation from seasonal changes or invasion of EPFs.

GB36 and BL63. The Xi-Cleft points are specifically used in acute conditions to treat Blood stasis in their respective channels. However, they are more effective in the Yin rather than in the Yang channels; that is why we would rather avoid using them to treat this condition.

GB40 and BL64. We recommend using these Yuan-Source points in chronic Deficiency conditions with dull pain, in case of weakness, or in the resolution phases of lateral ankle sprain, to tonify Qì and Blood in their respective channels.

In this situation, we can also associate the Yuan point GB40 with the Luo point LR5 and the Yuan point BL64 with the Luo point KI4, that is to say the well-known Luo-Yuan point combination. First, as main point, we needle the Yuan point on the affected side and then, as secondary point, the Luo point on the internally-externally related channel on the opposite side.

Sixth Step: Extraordinary Vessels

In our opinion, no Extraordinary Vessel is effective to treat this disorder.

Option Two: Local Points

First Step: Painful Point(s) (Ah Shi)

Ah Shi Point(s). We identify the most painful point(s) (Ah Shi), usually located anterior to the lateral malleolus on the ATFL or inferiorly on the CFL.

Palpation reveals either the Ah Shi point(s) corresponding to Blood stasis and therefore to be bled or an area of widespread pain corresponding to Qì stagnation and requiring needling. In this area, pain radiates proximally to the lateral or posterior side of the leg, or distally to the lateral side of the foot.

When the bleeding technique is chosen and if the anatomical structure of the ankle allows us to, the cupping therapy should be used to bleed the most painful point(s) (Ah Shi), paying attention not to damage the soft tissues with a too strong cupping.

In the posttraumatic inflammatory phase characterized by intense pain, swelling, and bruises, the use of needles could make pain worse. Therefore their use should be carefully evaluated and the anatomically mirrored points considered as an alternative option, as we will see in Section 1.

In any case, when the Ah Shi point(s) are needled, electroacupuncture stimulation can be taken into consideration and used between two points.

GB40. This is the most important local point in case of lateral ankle sprain, in anatomical terms it corresponds to the tarsal sinus. Deep needling of this point can reach the ankle joint. To make access easier, the ankle can be passively rolled into inversion to select the area with marked depression. Again, this technique should be avoided in the immediately posttraumatic phase.

We also use it because it is an insertion point both of the Gall Bladder and the Bladder Muscle channels in the ankle.

Electroacupuncture stimulation can be taken into consideration and used between this point and one of following two points.

BL62. It can be considered the local point in case of lateral ankle sprain, when pain is located below the lateral malleolus on the Bladder channels.

BL60. It can be considered the local point in case of lateral ankle sprain, when pain is located posterior to the lateral malleolus on the Bladder channels. This point can be considered an adjacent point, if pain is below or in front of the lateral malleolus, as we will see later.

To ensure accuracy and precision of local needle placement and manipulation, we prefer the supine position.

Second Step: Anatomically Mirrored Point(s) (Opposite Side)

The points to be needled are located on the opposite side and should correspond as precisely as possible to the anatomical mirror of the Ah Shi point(s) to be treated. The point(s) may or may not be tender on palpation.

To ensure accuracy and precision of local needle placement and manipulation, we prefer the supine position.

Option Three: Adjacent Points

First Step: Adjacent Points

ST41. This point is located on the anterior side of the ankle and promotes the horizontal flow of local Qì.

BL60. This point is located on the posterior side of the ankle and promotes the horizontal flow of local Qì.

GB34. It is a very important point since it is the insertion point both of the Gall Bladder and of the Bladder Muscle channels in the knee. As such, it promotes the longitudinal flow of Qì in their respective channels, if pain radiates proximally to the leg.

BL61. It is an important point since it is the insertion point of the Bladder Muscle channel in the ankle and as such it promotes the longitudinal flow of local Qì.

Option Four: Etiological Points

First Step: According to Patterns

LI4 and LR3 (Bilaterally). They promote the flow of Qì and help remove Blood stasis. Since LR3 is the Shu/Yuan point of the Liver, it also helps nourish muscles and tendons.

ST36 (Bilaterally). It is used to tonify Qì and Blood in chronic Deficiency conditions or the phases of pain resolution that can turn into muscle weakness.

SP5 and SP9. They are very important points in case of swollen ankle since they resolve Dampness.

Second Step: General Points

GB34 (Bilaterally). It is the Hui-Gathering point of Sinews and is specifically used for ligament sprain. In addition, it promotes the flow of Qì thus contributing to remove Blood stasis.

BL18 (Bilaterally). It treats all Excess and Deficiency conditions of the Liver that may favor the onset or duration of musculotendinous symptoms. It harmonizes the flow of Qì and Blood and enhances treatment of tendons and muscle.

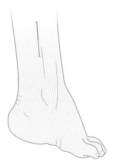

Fig. 7.16 Lower 5.

BL20 (Bilaterally). It transforms "impure" fluids thus contributing to resolve Dampness in case of joint swelling.

Option Five: Microsystems

First Step: Wrist and Ankle Acupuncture
Lower 5. It roughly corresponds to the pathway of the Gall Bladder channels, direction toward the foot (Fig. 7.16).

Lower 6. It roughly corresponds to the pathway of the Bladder channels, direction towards the foot (Fig. 7.17).

Lower 4. It controls lower limb mobility (Fig. 7.18).

Second Step: Ear Acupuncture (Fig. 7.19)
Local point: Ankle
Zang Fu point: Liver
General points: Subcortex and Shenmen

Acute or Chronic Pain From Excess
Intense Pain or Range of Motion Reduced by Pain. Principle of treatment: to remove Qì stagnation and Blood stasis and expel EPFs or IPFs, if any (Box 7.1).

Chronic Pain from Deficiency
Dull Pain or Muscle Weakness. Principle of treatment: to tonify Qì and Blood, strengthen tissues and avoid pain exacerbation from physical activities or invasion of EPFs (Box 7.2).

Therapeutic Program, Frequency of Sessions

The frequency of sessions depends on the clinical condition of the patient. If the condition is acute or chronic with intense pain, we recommend sessions twice a week for 2 weeks and then once a week for another 2 weeks. If improvement is observed, sessions are then scheduled once a week until complete pain relief or at least reduction by 80% to 90%.

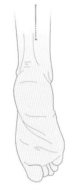

Fig. 7.17 Lower 6.

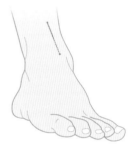

Fig. 7.18 Lower 4.

Response to treatment of lateral ankle sprain may take longer than expected; should this be the case, treatment is to be continued for another week and two more sessions scheduled.

Finally, if the expected outcomes are not achieved, the whole clinical picture should be reconsidered and the patient referred to another specialist.

If the condition is chronic with dull pain, we recommend sessions once a week for four weeks. Afterwards, and if the patient continues to improve, sessions are then scheduled once a week until complete pain relief or at least reduction by 80% to 90%.

Achilles Tendonitis

As indicated in the section dedicated to Western Medicine, we use this term to refer both to midportion tendinopathy and insertional tendinopathy, the only difference between the two of them being pain location. They will be covered together in this chapter, as

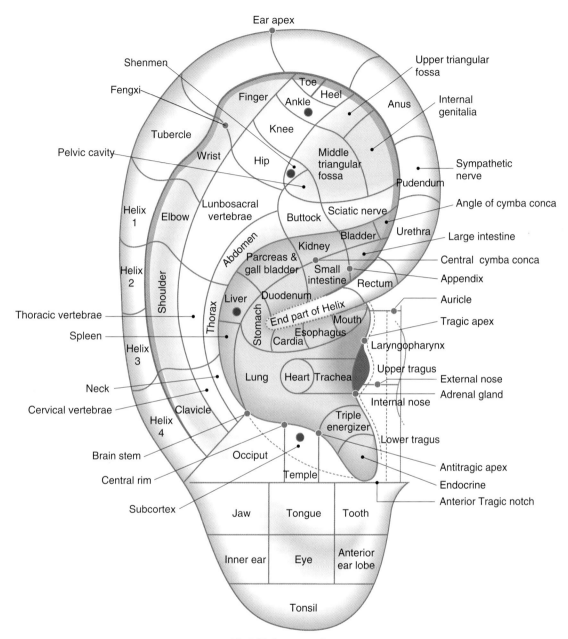

Fig. 7.19 Ear acupuncture.

the therapeutic protocol is always the same as far as distal, adjacent, and etiological points are concerned. Needless to say, the local points and techniques to be used vary according to the different disorders to treat.

The Five Options and Selection of Acupoints

The approach we suggest is widely described in the section dedicated to the Fundamentals of acupuncture for MSK pain in the limbs (see Chapter 1).

BOX. 7.1 ACUTE OR CHRONIC PAIN FROM EXCESS ACUPUNCTURE TREATMENT

Option 1 Distal points	• Jing-Well point GB44 and BL67 • Luo point GB37 and BL58 (opposite side) • Point according to the Six Stages TE4 and SI5 (opposite side) • Jing-River point GB38 and BL60
Option 2 Local points	• Ah Shi • GB40 • BL62 • Anatomically mirrored point(s) (opposite side)
Option 3 Adjacent points	• ST41 • BL60 • Insertion points GB34 and BL61
Option 4 Etiological and general points	• LI4 and LR3 (bilaterally) • SP5 • SP9 • GB34 (bilaterally) • BL18 (bilaterally) • BL20 (bilaterally)

Option 5 Microsystems	• W-A acupuncture
	  • Lower 5
	  • Lower 6
	  • Lower 4
	• Ear acupuncture
	  • Ankle
	  • Liver
	  • Subcortex and Shenmen

BOX. 7.2 CHRONIC PAIN FROM DEFICIENCY ACUPUNCTURE TREATMENT

Option 1 Distal points	• Yuan points GB40 and BL64 • Luo point LR5 and KI4 (opposite side) • Point according to the Six Stages TE4 and SI5 (opposite side) • Jing-River point GB38 and BL60
Option 2 Local points	• Ah Shi • GB40 • BL62
Option 3 Adjacent points	• ST41 • BL60 • Insertion points GB34 and BL61
Option 4 Etiological and general points	• ST36 (bilaterally) • GB34 (bilaterally) • LR3 (bilaterally) • BL18 (bilaterally)

Option 5 Microsystems	• W-A acupuncture
	  • Lower 5
	  • Lower 6
	  • Lower 4
	• Ear acupuncture
	  • Ankle
	  • Liver
	  • Subcortex and Shenmen

The most important aspect is the identification of the Ah Shi point(s) to determine which channels are affected. In this specific case, the Bladder Muscle and Connecting channels are involved, especially when pain is reported in the posterior and lateral tendon or in its calcaneal junction.

According to our experience, the Kidney Muscle and Connecting channels may also be involved when pain is reported in the medial tendon.

Therefore, when a combination of two points (BL and KI) is presented, the first point to be needled or bled is the BL point, which treats posterior and lateral pain, whereas the KI point is the second option, to be used in the treatment of medial pain. Once the most effective channel is identified, selection of distal points continues along it.

Pricking pain on tendon palpation or localized to the Achilles tendinous junction on the posterior calcaneus is a sign of Blood Stasis to be treated with the bleeding technique, whereas any posterior pain radiating along the tendon and calf is a sign of Qì stagnation and therefore needling is the most appropriate technique.

Swelling of the tendon sheath and tissue around the tendon is a sign of Dampness to be treated with a mild bleeding or needling technique.

It is worth reminding that the distal points should be needled one at a time and their effectiveness in terms of pain and range of motion tested after each insertion. The same applies to the local points.

Finally, since both options 1 and 2 consist of several steps, it is important to highlight how selection should be made. Specifically, the practitioner might wonder if all or some of the steps should be followed. The rule we follow is simple; when the result achieved is satisfactory, the remaining steps should be skipped, and the practitioner should move to the following option. Similarly, the use of the points recommended under options 3, 4, and 5 should be carefully evaluated according to the case being treated.

The points and accessory techniques we recommend using are listed below.

The Order of Needling

Option One: Distal Points

First Step: Bladder and Kidney Muscle Channels

BL67 and KI1. These Jing-Well points activate the Bladder and Kidney Muscle channels, and they remove Qì stagnation and Blood stasis with needling and bleeding techniques, respectively (Fig. 7.20; Video 7.7).

BL58 and KI4 (Opposite Side). These Luo points activate the Bladder and Kidney Connecting channels, and they remove Qì stagnation and Blood stasis in acute or chronic conditions from Excess.

The same Luo points are also used in chronic Deficiency conditions with dull pain to tonify Qì and Blood in their respective Internally-externally related channels. In this case, we associate the Yuan point KI3 with the Luo point BL58, and the Yuan point BL64 with the Luo point KI4, that is to say the well-known Luo-Yuan point combination. First, as main point, we needle the Yuan point on the affected side and then, as secondary point, the Luo point on the internally-externally related channel on the opposite side.

Third Step: Empirical Points

There is no point which is classically recommended.

Fourth Step: Opposite Extremity (Upper/Lower)

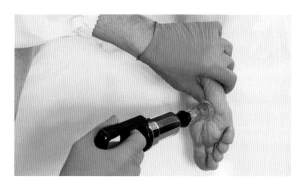

Fig. 7.20 Bleeding of the KI1.

Clinical Notes

....

- Treatment of lateral ankle sprain often ensures excellent outcomes, even when imaging techniques show anatomical changes in joint structures, such as ligament strain or tear.
- Sometimes, temporary worsening of symptoms is observed, especially when cupping or needling are used.

SI5 and HE7 (Opposite Side). They are located in the wrist joint which corresponds to the ankle joint on the paired channel according to the Six Stages.

It is worth remembering that the painful point on the Achilles tendon is not exactly in the ankle joint; it is in fact slightly proximally located and this means we could palpate the forearm in an upward direction along the Small Intestine and Heart Main channels to find another or more tender point(s).

In clinical practice, when treating Achilles tendonitis, the anatomical mirror concept can lead us to select a point, which may be tender or not, on the area corresponding to the distal forearm, along its medial aspect. This area may correspond to the Achilles tendon, although it is not located on the Small Intestine and Heart Main channels, but approximately on the Pericardium Main channel.

In line with our principle of treatment, we first needle SI5 and HE7, or some other more proximal point(s), and then test their effectiveness soon after insertion; if the result is not satisfactory, we remove the needles and move to second option.

Our technique consists of needling the opposite extremity (lower/upper) on the opposite side in acute and chronic conditions.

Alternatively, the most tender point on palpation is selected on the same or opposite side.

Fifth Step: Categories of Traditional Points

BL65 (Affected Side) and SI3 (Opposite Side); KI3 (Affected Side) and HE7 (Opposite Side). A good combination includes the Shu-Stream points on the paired channel according to the Six Stages. First, we needle the Shu-Stream point on the channel involved on the affected side and then, the Shu-Stream point on the coupled channel on the opposite side and opposite extremity (upper/lower). We use this technique in acute and chronic Excess conditions to treat pain and expel or prevent the invasion of EPFs. It is worth reminding that in the Yin channels the Shu-Stream point corresponds to the Yuan-Source point. That is why KI3 could also be used in chronic Deficiency conditions, as we will see later.

BL60 and KI7. The Jing-River points are used in acute or chronic Excess conditions due to the invasion of an EPF and they are needled to promote its expulsion from their respective channels. They are also useful to prevent pain exacerbation from seasonal changes or invasion of EPFs. However, they are more effective in the Yang rather than in the Yin channels; that is why we use BL60 and would rather avoid using KI7 to treat this condition.

BL63 and KI5. The Xi-Cleft points are specifically used in acute conditions to treat Blood stasis in their respective channels. However, they are more effective in the Yin rather than in the Yang channels; that is why we use KI5 and would rather avoid using BL63 to treat this condition.

BL64 and KI3. We recommend using these Yuan-Source points in chronic Deficiency conditions with dull pain, in case of weakness, or in the resolution phases of Achilles tendonitis, to tonify Qì and Blood in their respective channels.

In this situation, we can also associate the Yuan point BL64 with the Luo point KI4, and the Yuan point KI3 with the Luo point BL58, that is to say the well-known Luo-Yuan point combination. First, as main point, we needle the Yuan point on the affected side and then, as secondary point, the Luo point on the Internally-Externally related channel on the opposite side.

Sixth Step: Extraordinary Vessels

In our opinion, no Extraordinary Vessel is effective to treat this disorder.

Option Two: Local Points

First Step: Painful Point(s) (Ah Shi)

Ah Shi Point(s). With the pinching palpation technique, we identify the most painful point(s) (Ah Shi), which is usually located at the level of the midportion of the tendon or on the tendon calcaneal junction (Fig. 7.21; Video 7.8).

Palpation reveals the Ah Shi point(s) corresponding either to Blood stasis or to an area of widespread pain radiating proximally to the calf or distally to the heel, that is to say the point(s) to be bled or needled, respectively.

When the bleeding technique is chosen and if the anatomical structure of the ankle allows us to, the cupping therapy should be used to bleed the most painful point(s) (Ah Shi), paying attention not to damage the soft tissues with a too strong cupping.

Alternatively, a choice can be made between two needling techniques, according to the location of pain:

- Pain on the midportion of the tendon: one to three pairs of lateral and medial needles are inserted obliquely and inferiorly at an angle of about 45 degrees. The needles are inserted anteriorly and close to the tendon and its sheath. Attention should be paid to avoid the risk of needling the tendon.

   Electroacupuncture stimulation can be taken into consideration and used between the pairs of needles.
- Pain on the tendon calcaneal junction: needles are inserted perpendicularly to the required depth to reach the periosteum.

We use 0.25 × 25 mm or 0.30 × 40 mm needles; the diameter and length of the needle to be used depend on the patient physique.

In acute or exacerbation of chronic conditions, a moxa stick or moxa on the needle can be added to move local Qì and Blood and help reduce swelling. Attention should be paid since too much heat can increase the ongoing inflammatory process.

BL60. It can be considered the local point to treat midportion Achilles tendonitis on the lateral side.

This point promotes the longitudinal flow of local Qì in the Bladder channels. As described in the fifth step, being a Jing-River point, it is also useful to expel EPFs and prevent pain exacerbation from their invasion.

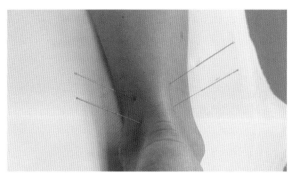

Fig. 7.21 Needling of the Ah Shi point(s).

BL59. It can be considered a local point to treat midportion Achilles tendonitis on the lateral side. This point promotes the longitudinal flow of local Qì in the Bladder channels.

BL61. It can be considered a local point to treat Achilles insertional tendonitis on the lateral aspect of the bone-tendon junction. It is the insertion point of the Bladder Muscle channel in the ankle and as such it promotes the longitudinal flow of local Qì in the Bladder channels.

KI3. It can be considered the local point to treat midportion Achilles tendonitis on the medial side.

This point promotes the longitudinal flow of local Qì in the Kidney channels. As described in the fifth step, being a Yuan-Source point, it is also useful to tonify local Qì and Blood in chronic Deficiency conditions.

We also use it because it is an insertion point of the Kidney Muscle channel in the ankle, as we will see later.

KI7. It can be considered a local point to treat midportion Achilles tendonitis on the medial side.

KI5. It can be considered a local point to treat Achilles insertional tendonitis on the medial aspect of the bone-tendon junction. This point promotes the longitudinal flow of local Qì in the Kidney channels. As described in the fifth step, being a Xi-Cleft point, it is also specifically used in acute conditions to treat Blood stasis.

To ensure accuracy and precision of needle placement and manipulation, we prefer the prone position, feet off the bed edge.

Second Step: Anatomically Mirrored Points (Opposite Side)

The points to be needled are located on the opposite side and should correspond as precisely as possible to the anatomical mirror of the Ah Shi point(s) to be treated. The point(s) may or may not be tender on palpation.

To ensure accuracy and precision of needle placement and manipulation, we prefer the prone position, feet off the bed edge.

Option Three: Adjacent Points

First Step: Adjacent Points

BL57. It is an important point since it corresponds to the musculotendinous junction of the calf muscles.

In addition, it is an insertion point of the Bladder Muscle channel in the calf. Since it promotes the longitudinal flow of local Qì in the Bladder channels, it can also release tension of the calf, which in turn improves postural balance of the ankle and reduces tendon inflammation and pain.

BL40. It is the insertion point of the Bladder Muscle channel in the knee and as such it promotes the longitudinal flow of local Qì. In addition, it removes Blood stasis from the posterior leg.

KI3. It is the insertion point of the Kidney Muscle channel in the ankle and as such it promotes the longitudinal flow of local Qì.

Option Four: Etiological Points

First Step: According to Patterns

LI4 and LR3 (Bilaterally). They promote the free flow of Qì and help remove Blood stasis. Since LR3 is the Shu/Yuan point of the Liver, it also helps nourish muscles and tendons.

ST36 (Bilaterally). It is used to tonify Qì and Blood in chronic Deficiency conditions or the phases of pain resolution that can turn into muscle weakness.

SP5 and SP9. They are very important points to treat peritendinous swelling, since they resolve Dampness.

Second Step: General Points

GB34 (Bilaterally). It is the Hui-Gathering point of Sinews and is specifically used for tendon disorders. In addition, it promotes the flow of Qì, thus contributing to remove Blood stasis.

BL18. It treats all Excess and Deficiency conditions of the Liver that may favor the onset or duration of musculotendinous symptoms. It harmonizes the free flow of Qì and Blood and enhances treatment of tendons and muscle.

Option Five: Microsystems

First Step: Wrist and Ankle Acupuncture

Lower 6. It roughly corresponds to the pathway of the Bladder channels, direction toward the foot (Fig. 7.22).

Lower 1. It roughly corresponds to the pathway of the Kidney channels, direction toward the foot (Fig. 7.23).

Second Step: Ear Acupuncture (Fig. 7.24)

Local point: Ankle
Zang Fu point: Liver
General points: Subcortex and Shenmen

Acute or Chronic Pain From Excess.

Intense Pain or Range of Motion Reduced by Pain. Principle of treatment: to remove Qì stagnation and Blood stasis and expel External or Internal Pathogenic Factors, if any (Box 7.3).

Chronic Pain From Deficiency.

Dull Pain or Muscle Weakness. Principle of treatment: to tonify Qì and Blood, strengthen tissues and avoid pain exacerbation from physical activities or invasion of EPFs (Box 7.4).

Therapeutic Program, Frequency of Sessions

The frequency of sessions depends on the clinical condition of the patient. If the condition is acute or chronic with intense pain, we recommend sessions twice a week for two weeks and then once a week for another two weeks. If improvement is observed, sessions are then scheduled once a week until complete pain relief or at least reduction by 80% to 90%. Treatment of Achilles tendonitis may not achieve the expected results within the expected timeframe. Should this be the case, then sessions should be scheduled twice a week for one more week.

If the expected improvement is not observed, then the whole clinical picture should be reconsidered and the patient referred to another specialist.

If the condition is chronic with dull pain, we recommend sessions once a week for four weeks. Afterwards, and if the patient continues to improve, sessions are then scheduled once a week until complete pain relief or at least reduction by 80% to 90%.

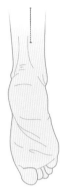

Fig. 7.22 Lower 6.

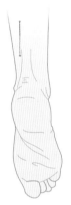

Fig. 7.23 Lower 1.

CLinical Notes

- Improvement following treatment may turn intense pain to dull pain and then to a feeling of weakness. Should this be the case, the principle of treatment has to be changed as follows; it is no longer necessary to remove Qì stagnation and Blood stasis and expel EPFs, if any; instead, Qì and Blood should be tonified to strengthen tissues and avoid pain exacerbation from physical activities or invasion of EPFs.
- Sometimes, temporary worsening of symptoms is observed, especially when cupping is used.
- Finally, results may not meet our expectations. An explanation for the poorer outcome could be the fact that Achilles tendonitis may be caused not only by ankle dysfunctions, but also dysfunctions of the knee, hip, and pelvic girdle. Further investigations are therefore mandatory.

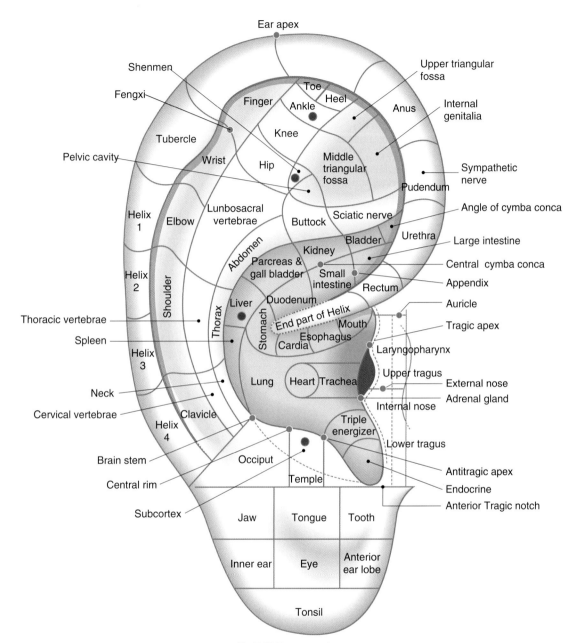

Fig. 7.24 Ear acupuncture.

OSTEOPATHIC MANIPULATIVE TREATMENT

This section will deal with osteopathic manipulations to treat ankle joint dysfunctions.

As already mentioned in the section dedicated to the Fundamentals of osteopathy for MSK pain in the limbs (see Chapter 1), the key point of the osteopathic therapeutic process is the treatment not only of the

BOX. 7.3 ACUTE OR CHRONIC PAIN FROM EXCESS
ACUPUNCTURE TREATMENT

Option 1 Distal points	• Jing-Well points BL67 and KI1 • Luo points BL58 and KI4 (opposite side) • Point according to the Six Stages SI5 and HE7 (opposite side) • Shu-Stream points BL65 and KI3 (affected side) and SI3 and HE7 (opposite side) • Jing-River points BL60 • Xi- Point KI5
Option 2 Local points	• Ah Shi • BL60 • BL59 • BL61 • KI3 • KI7 • KI5 • Anatomically mirrored point(s) (opposite side)
Option 3 Adjacent points	• Insertion points BL57, BL40, and KI3
Option 4 Etiological and general points	• LI4 and LR3 (bilaterally) • GB34 (bilaterally) • BL18 (bilaterally) • SP5 • SP9

Option 5 Microsystems	• W-A acupuncture
	  • Lower 6
	  • Lower 1
	• Ear acupuncture
	  • Ankle
	  • Liver
	  • Subcortex and Shenmen

BOX 7.4 CHRONIC PAIN FROM DEFICIENCY
ACUPUNCTURE TREATMENT

Option 1 Distal points	• Yuan points BL64 and KI3 • Luo points KI4 and BL58 (opposite side) • Point according to the Six Stages SI5 and HE7 (opposite side) • Jing-River point BL60
Option 2 Local points	• Ah Shi • BL60 • BL59 • BL61 • KI3 • KI7 • KI5
Option 3 Adjacent points	• Insertion points BL57, BL40, and KI3
Option 4 Etiological and general points	• LI4 and LR3 (bilaterally) • GB34 (bilaterally) • BL18 (bilaterally)

Option 5 Microsystems	• W-A acupuncture
	  • Lower 6
	  • Lower 1
	• Ear acupuncture
	  • Ankle
	  • Liver
	  • Subcortex and Shenmen

somatic dysfunctions of the ankle but also of those which are functionally and anatomically related.

Consequently, the osteopathic manipulative approach to musculoskeletal ankle pain is based on the identification of joint somatic dysfunctions not only of the ankle, but also of the knee, hip, and pelvic girdle.

Regardless of the condition to be treated, be it lateral ankle sprain, Achilles tendonitis, arthritis of the ankle or surgical outcomes, all of the dysfunctions identified should be treated.

Somatic Dysfunctions of the Tibiotalar Joint

Anterior Tibia: Treatment
Anterior dysfunction: anterior sliding is better than posterior sliding.

First technique

The patient is supine with the right knee extended (Fig. 7.25; Video 7.9).

The practitioner stands close to the right ankle. The practitioner holds the calcaneus with the right hand, while the plantar aspect of the foot lies against

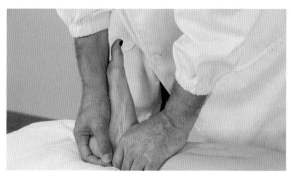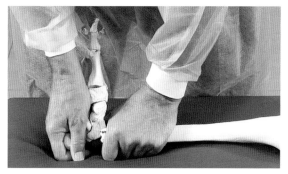

Fig. 7.25 Anterior tibia treatment.

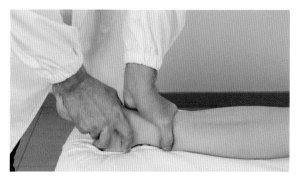

Fig. 7.26 Anterior tibia MET treatment.

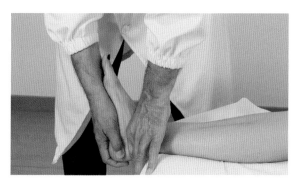

Fig. 7.27 Posterior tibia MET treatment.

the forearm and the left hand is positioned on the tibia next to the tibiotalar joint. With the foot in dorsiflexion, a progressive downward force is applied on the tibia and the restrictive barrier engaged. After joint decoaptation and rebalancing, a vertical thrust is performed by pushing the tibia downward.

Second technique

A muscle energy technique (MET) is used (Fig. 7.26; Video 7.10).

The patient is supine with the right knee extended. The practitioner stands close to the right ankle. The practitioner holds the dorsum of the foot at the level of the talar neck with the right hand, while the left hand holds the tibia next to the tibiotalar joint. The practitioner engages the restrictive barrier bringing the foot into plantarflexion.

The patient is asked to bring the foot into dorsiflexion and perform an isometric contraction against the practitioner's own resistance (the force exerted by the patient should not overcome the practitioner's resistance).

The position is held for 3 seconds followed by a 3-second postisometric relaxation before a new restrictive barrier is engaged. This process needs to be repeated three times.

Posterior Tibia: Treatment

Posterior dysfunction: posterior sliding is better than anterior sliding.

A muscle energy technique (MET) is used. The patient is supine with the right knee extended (Fig. 7.27; Video 7.11).

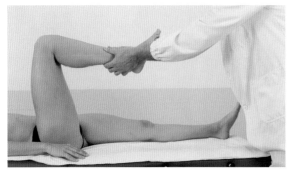

Fig. 7.28 Inferior fibula treatment: starting position.

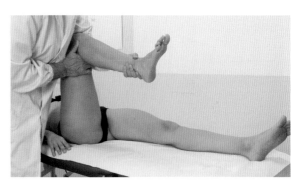

Fig. 7.30 Superior fibula treatment: starting position.

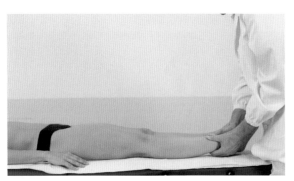

Fig. 7.29 Inferior fibula treatment: final position.

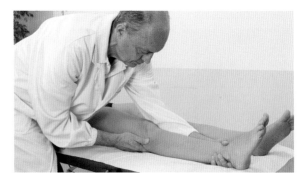

Fig. 7.31 Superior fibula treatment: final position.

The practitioner stands close to the right ankle.

The practitioner holds the calcaneus with the right hand, while the plantar aspect of the foot lies against the forearm; the left hand holds the ankle with the web of the thumb and index finger on the talar neck.

The practitioner engages the restrictive barrier bringing the foot into dorsiflexion.

The patient is asked to bring the foot into plantarflexion and perform an isometric contraction against the practitioner's own resistance (the force exerted by the patient should not overcome the practitioner's resistance).

The position is held for 3 seconds followed by a 3-second postisometric relaxation before a new restrictive barrier is engaged. This process needs to be repeated three times.

Somatic Dysfunctions of the Tibiofibular Joint

Inferior Fibula: Treatment
Inferior dysfunction: superior sliding on the affected side is worse than on the unaffected side.

The patient is supine with the right knee and hip flexed at 90 degrees.

The practitioner stands close to the edge of the bed and holds the ankle, placing the thenar eminences under both malleoli (Figs. 7.28 and 7.29; Video 7.12).

The patient is asked to push against the practitioner's hands to extend the knee, while the practitioner applies a counterforce which slowly allows for progressive extension of the knee. The patient is then returned to the starting position. This process needs to be repeated three times.

Superior Fibula: Treatment
Superior dysfunction: superior sliding on the affected side is better than on the unaffected side.

The patient is supine with the right knee and hip flexed at 90 degrees.

The practitioner stands close to the right edge of the bed and holds the ankle with the left hand, placing the right thumb proximal to the fibular head (Figs. 7.30 and 7.31; Video 7.13).

The patient is then asked to extend the hip and knee on the bed, while the practitioner pushes distally on the fibular head.

Afterwards, the patient is asked to flex the hip and knee, while the practitioner applies a counterforce that slowly allows for progressive flexion of the knee. This process needs to be repeated three times.

Anterior Fibula: Treatment

Anterior dysfunction: anterior sliding is better than posterior sliding.

The patient is supine, feet off the bed, a foam roller under the right ankle (Fig. 7.32; Video 7.14).

The practitioner stands close to the right foot and immobilizes the tibia and talus with the right hand, while the left thenar eminence is placed on the anterior side of the lateral malleolus.

After joint decoaptation, rebalancing, and reaching a point of tension, a vertical thrust is performed by pushing the malleolus downward.

Posterior Fibula: Treatment

Posterior dysfunction: posterior sliding is better than anterior sliding.

The patient is prone, feet off the bed, a foam roller under the right ankle (Fig. 7.33; Video 7.15).

The practitioner stands close to the right foot and immobilizes the tibia anteriorly with the left hand, while the right thenar eminence is placed on the posterior side of the lateral malleolus.

After joint decoaptation, rebalancing, and reaching a point of tension, a vertical thrust is performed by pushing the malleolus downward.

Somatic Dysfunctions of the Talocalcaneal Joint

Inversion of the Calcaneus: Treatment

Calcaneal inversion dysfunction: the calcaneus rolls better into inversion than eversion.

The patient is prone with the right knee flexed at 90 degrees.

The practitioner stands close to the right foot (Fig. 7.34; Video 7.16).

The practitioner stabilizes the foot in dorsiflexion with the left hand, while the right hand holds the calcaneus, placing the thumb on one side and the index finger on the other side.

After applying moderate traction along the axis of the tibia, the practitioner progressively moves the calcaneus into eversion, meaning that the calcaneus rolls outward (pronation) and turns into valgus. This process needs to be repeated three times.

Eversion of the Calcaneus: Treatment

Calcaneal eversion dysfunction: the calcaneus rolls better into eversion than inversion.

The patient is prone with the right knee flexed at 90 degrees (Fig. 7.35; Video 7.17).

The practitioner stands close to the right foot.

The practitioner stabilizes the foot in dorsiflexion with the left hand, while the right hand holds the calcaneus, placing the thumb on one side and the index finger on the other side.

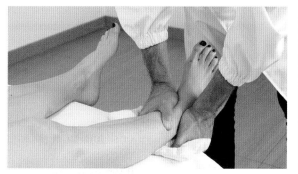
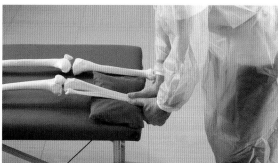

Fig. 7.32 Anterior fibula treatment.

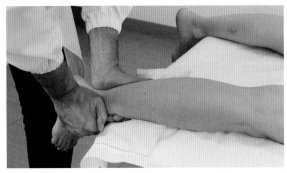
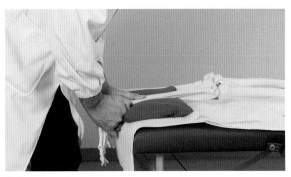

Fig. 7.33 Posterior fibula treatment.

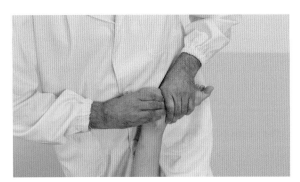
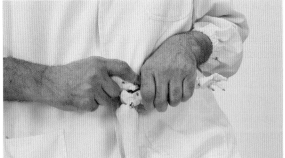

Fig. 7.34 Inversion of the calcaneus treatment.

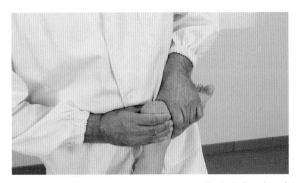
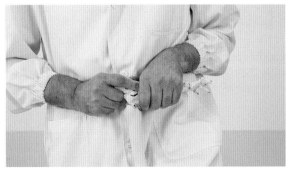

Fig. 7.35 Eversion of the calcaneus treatment.

After applying moderate traction along the axis of the tibia, the practitioner progressively moves the calcaneus into inversion, meaning that the calcaneus rolls inward (supination) and turns into varus. This process needs to be repeated three times.

Therapeutic Program, Frequency of Sessions

The AcuOsteo Method of treatment combines acupuncture and osteopathic manipulations and, in principle, both therapeutic techniques are used during each session and at the same time.

If the condition is acute or chronic with intense pain, we recommend sessions twice a week for two weeks and then once a week for another two weeks. If improvement is observed, sessions are then scheduled once a week until complete pain relief or at least reduction by 80% to 90%.

In practice, however, as the osteopathic approach differs from acupuncture in that it follows a mechanical principle and aims to restore proper joint mobility, we opt for a *parsimonious* use of osteopathic manipulations over acupuncture; there may be no need to repeat them in every session.

Osteopathic manoeuvres are therefore performed in case of persistent somatic dysfunction. That is why the patient should always be reevaluated at the beginning of each session to assess joint conditions and compare them with preexisting dysfunction.

BIBLIOGRAPHY

Baldry PE. *Acupuncture, Trigger Points and Musculoskeletal Pain*. 3rd ed. Elsevier; 2005.
Buckup K. *Test Ortopedici*. Verduci Editore; 1997.
Cipriano JJ. *Test Ortopedici e Neurologici*. Verduci Editore; 1998.
Deadman P, Al-Khafaji M, Baker K, Manuale di Agopuntura Ed. *italiana a cura di Grazia Rotolo e Giulio Picozzi*. CEA (Casa Editrice Ambrosiana); 2000.
De Seze S, Ryckewaert A. *Malattie dell'osso e delle articolazioni*. Aulo Gaggi Editore; 1979.
Audouard M. Osteopatia, l'Arto Inferiore. Editore Marrapese, Roma 1989.
Giusti R. *Glossary of osteophatic terminology*. 3rd ed. American Association of Colleges of Osteophatic Medicine; 2017.
Greenman PE. *Principles of manual medicine*. 2nd ed. Williams & Wilkins; 1996.
Guolo F. *Atlante di Tecniche di Energia Muscolare*. Piccin; 2014.
Hoppenfeld S. L'Esame Obiettivo dell'Apparato Locomotore. Aulo Gaggi Editore, 1985
Legge D. *Close to the bone*. Sydney College Press; 2010.
Maciocia G. *The practice of chinese medicine*. 3rd ed. Elsevier; 2022.
Misulis KE, Head TC. *Neurologia di Netter*. Elsevier, Masson; 2008.
Nicholas AS, Nicholas EA. *Atlas of osteophatic thechniques*. Lippincott Williams & Wilkins; 2012.
Qiao W. *Wrist and ankle and balance acupuncture, Italian Chine School of Acupuncture-A.M.A.B. (Association of Medical Acupuncturist of Bologna)*. Seminar; 2007.
Reaves W, Bong C. *The acupuncture handbook of sports injuries & pain*. 3rd ed. Hidden Needle Press; 2013.
Romoli M. *Auricular acupuncture diagnosis*. Churchill Livingstone Elsevier; 2009.
Tan RT. In: Besinger JW, ed. *Dr. Tan's strategy of twelve magical points*. 2003.
Tixa S. *Atlas d'Anatomie Palpatoire, tome 2, Membre Inferior*. 3e éd. Elsevier Masson; 2005.
Tixa S, Ebenegger B. *Atlas de Techniques articulaires ostéopathiques, tome 3, Les Membres*. 2e éd. Elsevier Masson; 2016.

Wrist-Ankle Acupuncture

Wrist-ankle acupuncture (WAA) was developed in China between 1966 and 1977 by Professor Zhang Xinshu, a physician who graduated in Western medicine and specialized in neurology and psychology.

This relatively new technique is indicated for pain management, specifically musculoskeletal (MSK) pain. That is why we associate it with somatic acupuncture. However, it can also be successfully used in the treatment of internal medicine diseases and psychological disorders, both of which will not be covered by this book.

It is based on the selection of six points in the wrist and another six in the ankle. These points are used to treat conditions localized in six different regions of the body. The six regions, which are bilateral and develop longitudinally, are numbered one to six: three are found in the "yin" (medial or anterior) zone, and the remaining three in the "yang" (lateral or posterior) zone.

These six regions are divided horizontally into two halves by the diaphragm: the upper half above the diaphragm and the lower half below.

In the sagittal plane, the midline running from front to back divides the body into right and left sides, and thus separating the six symmetrical zones.

Selection of the point(s) to needle is very easy and made according to the longitudinal zones where the symptom manifests itself. The division of the body into two halves, upper and lower, is particularly significant, since the points located around the wrist will be mostly used to treat disorders in the upper zone, whereas those around the ankle are to treat disorders in the lower zone (Figs. A1.1–A1.3).

The Benefits of Wrist-Ankle Acupuncture

- It is a particularly safe technique, since the needle is inserted tangential to the skin into the subcutaneous tissue.

- No manipulation of the needle is required and, consequently, it is a painless technique, which explains why it is easily accepted by patients.
- Only 12 points are used and therefore it is easy to memorize them.
- Treatment consists of just three steps:
  - Localization of the affected area or Ah Shi point(s)
  - Localization of the related WAA point(s)
  - Insertion of the needle to be directed towards the region to treat.
- More combinations of points can be used to treat diseases of the upper or lower zone, but also to treat different conditions located in both zones.
- In addition to being extremely effective in pain management, it is useful for a better identification of the painful region or Ah Shi point(s), when pain is widespread, and identification of the channel involved is difficult.

Side Effects

- Subcutaneous hematoma
- Fainting due to vasovagal syndrome

Point Localization

Anatomical landmarks in the wrist (upper) and ankle (lower).

Upper 1–6

The wrist points (upper) are located two fingers proximal to the wrist crease.

UPPER 1–3 are on the palmar aspect of the forearm; upper 4 is located along the radial border of the forearm: upper 5 and 6 are on the dorsal aspect of the forearm.

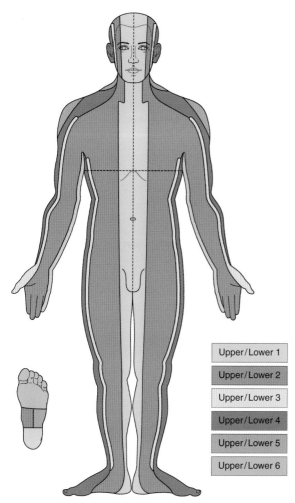

Fig. A1.1 The six regions: anterior view.

| Upper/Lower 1 |
| Upper/Lower 2 |
| Upper/Lower 3 |
| Upper/Lower 4 |
| Upper/Lower 5 |
| Upper/Lower 6 |

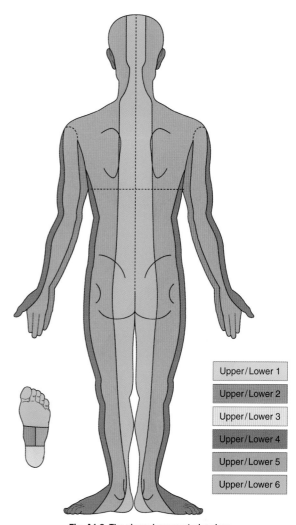

Fig. A1.2 The six regions: posterior view.

| Upper/Lower 1 |
| Upper/Lower 2 |
| Upper/Lower 3 |
| Upper/Lower 4 |
| Upper/Lower 5 |
| Upper/Lower 6 |

Lower 1–6

The ankle points (Lower) are located 3 fingers proximal to the apex of the lateral or medial malleolus.

Lower 1–3 are on the medial aspect of the leg; lower 4 is on the front aspect; lower 5 and 6 are on the lateral aspect.

Main Indications

Below is a description of the points and indications for the treatment of MSK pain with specific reference to some of the diseases which will be covered in this manual.

Upper 1

It is located between the ulna and the tendon of the flexor carpi ulnaris (Fig. A1.4).

Indications

INDICATIONS   Medial   elbow   pain   (medial epicondylitis).

Upper 2

It is located in the center of the volar surface of the forearm, between the tendons of the palmaris longus

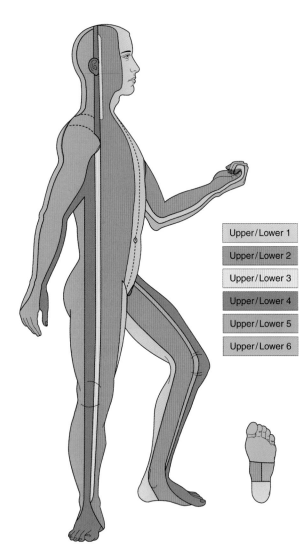

Fig. A1.3 The six regions: lateral view.

Upper/Lower 1
Upper/Lower 2
Upper/Lower 3
Upper/Lower 4
Upper/Lower 5
Upper/Lower 6

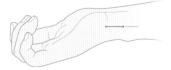

Fig. A1.4 Upper 1.

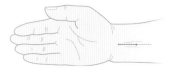

Fig. A1.5 Upper 2.

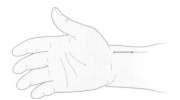

Fig. A1.6 Upper 3.

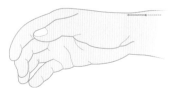

Fig. A1.7 Upper 4.

and the flexor carpi radialis. It is very similar to but not quite the same as PC6 (Fig. A1.5).

INDICATIONS There are no specific diseases that will be covered in this book.

Upper 3

It is located between the internal border of the radius and the radial artery (Fig. A1.6).

INDICATIONS Anterior shoulder pain (LHB).

Upper 4

It is located on the radial border. To locate it, place the index fingers on the sides of the radius: the point lies in between the two sides (Fig. A1.7).

INDICATIONS Anterior shoulder pain (LHB), lateral elbow pain (lateral epicondylitis), and lateral wrist pain (radial styloiditis).

Upper 5

It is located in the center of the dorsal surface of the forearm, between the radius and the ulna. To locate it, place the index fingers on the sides of the radius and the ulna. It is very similar to, but not quite the same as, TE5 (Fig. A1.8).

INDICATIONS Lateral shoulder pain (infraspinatus and supraspinatus tendonitis), dorsal wrist pain (extensor tenosynovitis), and motor impairment and sensory deficits of the upper limbs.

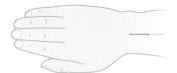

Fig. A1.8 Upper 5.

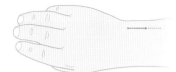

Fig. A1.9 Upper 6.

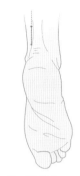

Fig. A1.10 Lower 1.

Upper 6

It is located on the dorsal surface of the forearm, between the ulna and the extensor carpi ulnaris tendon (Fig. A1.9).

INDICATIONS Posterior shoulder pain (infraspinatus tendonitis), medial elbow pain (medial epicondylitis), and medial wrist pain (ulnar styloiditis).

Lower 1

It is located near the inner border of the Achilles tendon (Fig. A1.10).

INDICATIONS Medial calf muscle pain (Achilles tendonitis).

Lower 2

It is located in the center of the medial surface of the leg, near the inner border of the tibia. It is very similar to, but not quite the same as, SP6 (Fig. A1.11).

INDICATIONS Hip pain on the medial side and knee pain (meniscus tear and medial collateral ligament sprain).

Lower 3

It is located about 1 cm medial to the anterior crest of the tibia (Fig. A1.12).

INDICATIONS Knee pain (patellar pain on the medial side).

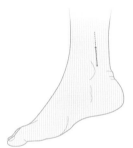

Fig. A1.11 Lower 2.

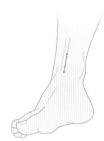

Fig. A1.12 Lower 3.

Lower 4

It is located midway between the anterior crest of the tibia and the anterior border of the fibula (Fig. A1.13).

INDICATIONS Hip pain on the anterior side, knee pain (patellofemoral pain syndrome and joint pain), anterior ankle pain, and motor impairment and sensory deficits of the lower limbs.

Lower 5

It is located in the center of the lateral surface of the leg, in a groove between the posterior border of the fibula and the peroneus longus tendon (Fig. A1.14).

INDICATIONS Hip and thigh pain on the lateral side (trochanteric bursitis, iliotibial band syndrome), and knee and ankle pain on the lateral side (insertional tendonitis of biceps femoris, lateral ankle sprain).

Lower 6

It is located near the lateral border of the Achilles tendon (Fig. A1.15).

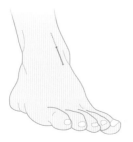

Fig. A1.13 Lower 4.

INDICATIONS Tendon pain (insertional tendonitis of biceps femoris, Achilles tendonitis on the posterior and lateral side).

Needle Insertion Technique

After shaving and cleaning the skin, the needle is inserted at an angle of 15 to 30 degrees, directed towards the target region. Then the needle is slid slowly and tangentially to the skin into the subcutaneous tissue until its whole length is inserted.

We recommend using 0.25–25-mm needles, or 0.20 × 15 mm, to be secured in place by an adhesive plaster.

Needles should be removed after one or two days, even though leaving them in place just for a couple of hours ensures their lasting effectiveness (Fig. A1.16).

If performed correctly, the practitioner feels the needle sliding smoothly and the patient reports neither pain nor discomfort. No needle manipulation is required. The practitioner should not elicit De Qì. The patient should not feel the needle inserted at all. Blood vessels, scars, skin lesions, and bony prominences should be avoided. If pain is reported, the needle should be removed.

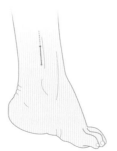

Fig. A1.14 Lower 5.

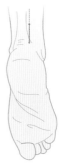

Fig. A1.15 Lower 6.

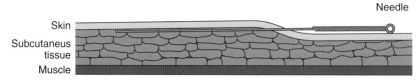

Fig. A1.16 Needling technique.

Red Flag

Upper 1 should not be used during periods of the first trimester of pregnancy.

CLINICAL NOTES

- Both patient and practitioner should be in a comfortable position throughout needle insertion.
- It is worth reminding that the given dimensions refer to the patient's fingers, either two or three.
- When the condition to treat is distal to the upper or lower points, the needle is inserted targeting the region to be treated. Therefore, once the upper or lower point has been located, needle insertion will be more proximal, so that the tip reaches exactly the upper or lower point selected.
- After inserting the needle, the wrist or ankle should be moved in all directions to be sure that the patient feels no pain at all.

BIBLIOGRAPHY

CEA (Casa Editrice Ambrosiana). *Trattato di Agopuntura e Medicina Cinese, a cura di Lucio Sotte, Agopuntura Cinese, AA vari.* 2007.

Qiao W. *Wrist and Ankle and Balance Acupuncture, Italian Chine School of Acupuncture-A.M.A.B. (Association of Medical Acupuncturist of Bologna).* Seminar; 2007.

Yajuan Wang. *Micro-Acupuncture in Practice.* Churchill Livingstone Elsevier; 2009.

Ear Acupuncture

Ear acupuncture is a technique that involves the stimulation of specific points on the auricle.

Although the Huang Di Nei Jing describes a system of channels converging in the ear ("the ear is the place where all the channels meet"), it was not until 1950 when a group of scholars from different nations focused on this subject, and a technique integrating Chinese and Western medicine was developed.

In particular, Paul Nogier, a French MD, further investigated the relationship between the ear and internal organs. After conducting a thorough study, he described the ear as being similar to an inverted fetus; the acupuncture points on the ear corresponded to the body parts of the fetus, organized into tissues, organs, and systems, including those that modulate pain perception.

In 1987 the nomenclature and localization of auricular points were standardized according to the scheme suggested by the China Association of Acupuncture and Moxibustion.

Characteristics

Ear acupuncture can be a stand-alone technique, but this handbook will illustrate its application on musculoskeletal (MSK) pain when associated with somatic acupuncture. It has proved to be effective in the treatment of excess-related and deficit-related painful conditions. The ear is divided into two surfaces: anterior and posterior.

The Anterior Surface Presents Four Ridges

The helix is the prominent rim of the auricle with a helicoid shape contouring three-quarters of the ear. It includes the root of helix, the apex, the auricular tubercle, and the lobe (Fig. A2.1).

Antihelix, the curved ridge, which is bigger than the helix. It arises from the helix and runs concentrically.

It is separated from the helix by the scaphoid fossa. It is a Y-shaped ridge consisting of two branches (upper and lower, or short branches of the "Y") and a body (the long branch of the "Y").

Tragus, a small, curved flap located latero-anterior to the external auditory meatus. It presents two palpable protrusions: the superior apex, also known as the supratragic tubercle, and the inferior apex.

Antitragus, a small tubercle, located opposite to the tragus and above the earlobe.

4 fossae: Scaphoid fossa, the groove between the helix and the antihelix

Triangular fossa, the triangular groove between the upper and lower branches of the antihelix

Concha (upper and lower), a fossa bounded by the antitragus, the body and the inferior branch of the antihelix. The root of the helix divides it into two parts: an upper part, called the superior concha, and a lower part, called the inferior concha.

The lobe is the soft, fleshy, lower part of the auricle. The earlobe is variable in size and shape.

The Posterior Surface Presents Less Evident Ridges And Grooves

Ridges and grooves correspond to those located on the anterior surface. The regions of the posterior surface will not be further investigated as we only use the posterior points to "reinforce" the action of the corresponding ear point located on the anterior surface and identified to treat the painful area.

Below is the location of those points relevant to this handbook, according to the standardization by the China Association of Acupuncture and Moxibustion.

Specifically,
- The areas located in the scaphoid fossa, which correspond to the upper limbs
- The areas located in the upper and lower branches of the antihelix, which correspond to the lower limbs, glutes, and sciatic nerve

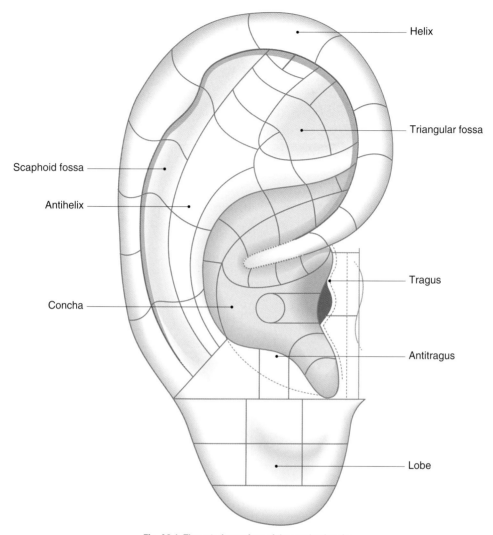

Fig. A2.1 The anterior surface of the ear: landmarks.

Our approach to the treatment of musculoskeletal disorders with ear acupuncture includes:
1. Locating the anatomical area affected
2. Identifying the organ involved from the perspectives of both Chinese and Western medicine
3. Using points modulating pain perception

The Upper and Lower Limb

The upper limb is located in the scaphoid fossa, which is divided into five areas, listed below from top to bottom (Fig. A2.2).

Fingers: in the first area
Wrist: in the second area
Elbow: in the third area
Shoulder: in the fourth area
Clavicle: in the fifth area

The lower limb is located in the upper branch of the antihelix, which is divided into four areas, listed below from top to bottom (Fig. A2.3).

Toes and heel: both in the first area, which is divided into the posterior and anterior region
Ankle: in the second area
Knee: in the third area
Hip: in the fourth area

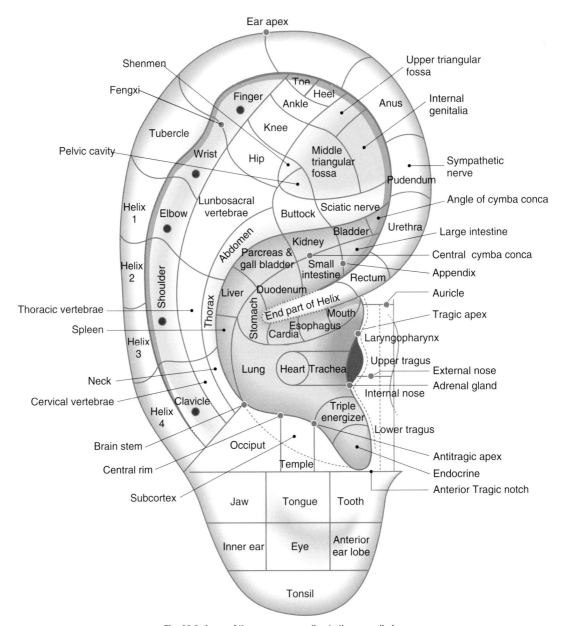

Fig. A2.2 Areas of the ear corresponding to the upper limbs.

Liver

The Liver is the only organ we use to treat osteoarticular diseases, on account of its physiological relation with muscles and tendons. The Liver is found at the level of the upper concha, in the posteroinferior area (Fig. A2.4).

Shenmen and Subcortex

The Shenmen is located in the triangular fossa, above the bifurcation between the upper and lower branches of the antihelix. It calms the Shen and relaxes the muscles.

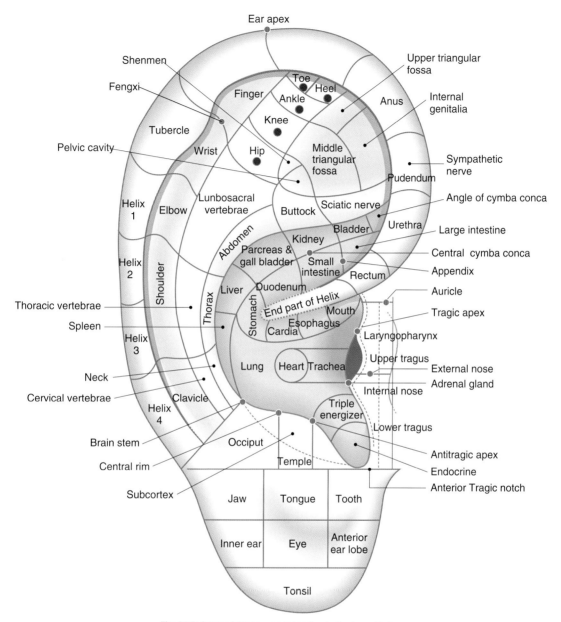

Fig. A2.3 Areas of the ear corresponding to the lower limbs.

Stimulation of Auricular Areas

The Subcortex is located in the middle of the lower third of the inner side of the antitragus. It calms the Shen, promotes the flow of Qì and Blood, and regulates the excitatory-inhibitory function of the cerebral cortex (Fig. A2.5).

Auricular areas may be stimulated with needles, either left in situ or not, or seeds from the Vaccaria plants, or magnets, which are secured on the selected areas with an adhesive plaster.

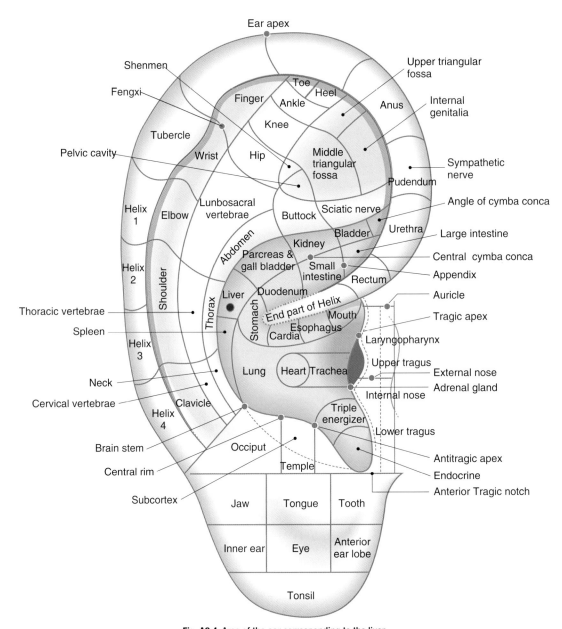

Fig. A2.4 Area of the ear corresponding to the liver.

We recommend choosing the most sensitive point in the selected area: the point can be located using a palpatory, a device specifically designed for this purpose.

Our preferred technique is the application of magnetic beads. They are applied after disinfecting the skin and then are left in place, secured with an adhesive plaster for 4 to 5 days.

Side Effects and Contraindications

In rare cases, ear acupuncture can cause palpitations, dizziness, nausea, fatigue, sleepiness, or local

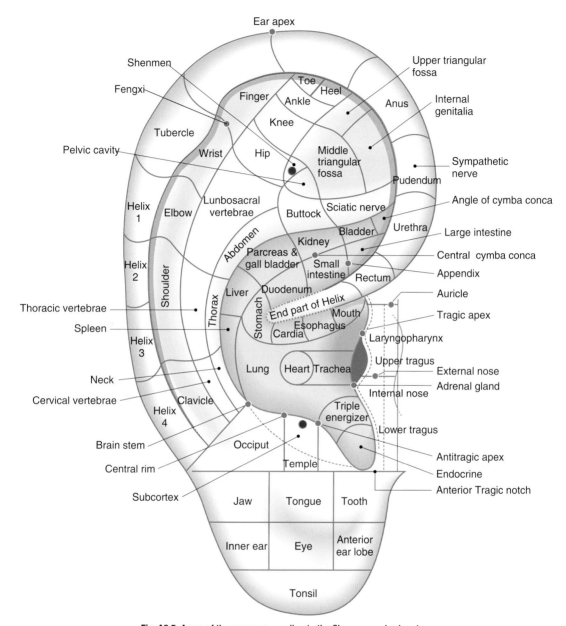

Fig. A2.5 Areas of the ear corresponding to the Shenmen and subcortex.

symptoms, such as heat, excessive pain, itching, small blisters, ecchymoses, and sometimes local infections.

Low-grade side effects disappear in a few hours or the day after. Severe side effects require suspension of treatment. No specific contraindications to the stimulation of auricular points with magnets have been reported. However, it is worth a reminder that patients with diabetes or psoriasis or elderly patients might have thinner, and therefore more sensitive, skin. Special attention should be given to these cases. This technique should not be performed when the skin is damaged.

BIBLIOGRAPHY

CEA (Casa Editrice Ambrosiana). *Trattato di Agopuntura e Medicina Cinese, a cura di Lucio Sotte, Agopuntura Cinese, AA vari*. 2007.

Romoli M. *Auricular Acupuncture Diagnosis*. Churchill Livingstone Elsevier; 2009.

Yajuan Wang. *Micro-Acupuncture in Practice*. Churchill Livingstone Elsevier; 2009.

Bleeding

Bloodletting consists of making capillaries under the skin slightly bleed, thus causing soft bleeding in various parts of the body.

Bleeding techniques were first described in the *Lingshu* and *Suwen*.

Major Therapeutic Aims of Bloodletting in Musculoskeletal Disorders

- It can drain excess from the channels, for example, the external pathogenic factors, such as Heat.
- It can remove obstacles to the flow, as happens with Blood stasis.
- It can invigorate the flow of Blood. In the case of paresthesia/numbness, it activates/improves microcirculation, and also nourishes Blood in deficiency conditions.
- It can reduce swelling by improving microcirculation.

Suitable Areas to Bleed Described in This Handbook

- Specific acupoints: distal Jing points: the fingertip or toe tip is to be gently
- Other regions of the body: Ah Shi points, with or without cupping, if the area to treat is suited for cupping

With regards to the number of drops to elicit, we prefer to follow the classical rule, for example we make it bleed until blood turns from dark red, a sign of Blood stasis, to bright red, a sign of definite removal of Blood stasis.

The bleeding technique can also be used in the case of bilateral pain since it neither prevents patient's movements nor causes pain.

However, this technique may prevent us from immediately testing the effectiveness of our treatment, since the type of tissue area involved may cause the needle insertion to be painful. This could be the case when treating a joint to move for assessment of the range of motion.

Bleeding Technique

JING-WELL POINTS

- Wear medical latex gloves
- Gently pinch the fingertip or toe tip between the thumb and index finger to promote venous pooling
- Keep the distal phalanx of the finger firm
- Use a sterile lancet to quickly prick to the shallow depth of 0.1 cun proximal to the corner of the hand or nail bed of the foot
- Pinch the distal phalanx to elicit drops of blood
- Alternatively, in our opinion, the number of drops can be intuitively calculated according to the proximal distance between the pain site and the Jing-Well point; for example, if pain is located in the foot or ankle, we elicit 10 drops; in the knee 20; in the hip 30.
- If it is difficult to achieve adequate blood loss and the same point can be pricked to a deeper depth; alternatively, if the patient is lying supine, place their hand or foot lower than the bed to use gravitational force (Fig. A3.1).

AH SHI(S) POINTS

The bleeding technique is easy to apply: the Ah Shi point(s) is pricked quickly and superficially with a sterile lancet (Fig. A3.2).

- Wear medical latex gloves.
- A lancet is used if the pain is pricking or localized in a small area.
- We use a plum blossom needle if the painful area is wider.

If the body area to treat is suited for cupping, this therapy should be associated to further promote blood flow; otherwise, tissues should be gently pinched with the thumb and index finger to elicit blood drops.

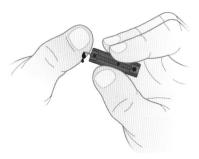

Fig. A3.1 Jing-Well point: bleeding technique.

BIBLIOGRAPHY

CEA (Casa Editrice Ambrosiana). *Trattato di Agopuntura e Medicina Cinese, a cura di Lucio Sotte, Agopuntura Cinese, AA vari*. 2007.
Qiao W. *Blood-Letting Therapy*. Italian Chine School of Acupuncture-A.M.A.B. (Association of Medical Acupuncturist of Bologna) Seminar; 2014.

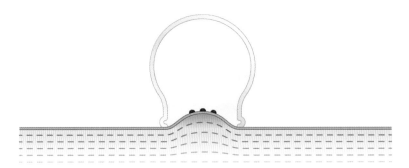

Fig. A3.2 Ah Shi point: bleeding cupping technique.

Cupping

Cupping therapy is a form of traditional medicine that belongs to different cultures, including Traditional Chinese Medicine, and is used by practitioners from different medical specialties.

This chapter will only cover those aspects related to musculoskeletal (MSK) pain and, in general, its use on the Ah Shi point(s).

Materials of Cups

Cups may be made of different materials. Classically, bamboo or glass cups are used. The air inside is vacuumed out by means of a flame. We prefer using plastic cups with an outlet valve and pistol grip, where suction is created by engaging a hand pump directly on the cup. They are the safest since there is no risk of burning.

Cleaning

After every use, cups are washed and soaked in a disinfectant solution for surgical instruments for the time required by the product.

Mechanisms of action

The main actions are the following:
- Promoting Qì and Blood flow in the channels.

Cupping therapy, especially when associated with bleeding, allows the removal of Qì stagnation and Blood stasis, thus eliminating pain.
- Expels external and internal pathogenic factors such as Wind, Cold, Dampness, and Heat.

Cupping therapy helps expel the Cold and resolves Dampness, which leads to Qì stagnation and Blood stasis. However, we prefer using moxibustion to expel the Cold, whereas to resolve Dampness we would rather associate cupping with bleeding, which better promotes the circulation of fluids. Cupping with bleeding is also our preferred technique to clear the Heat.

Methods of Cupping

Cupping therapy varieties (Fig. A4.1) can be classified as follows:
- Light cupping
- Mild cupping: it is the method we use. It removes Qì stagnation and Blood stasis and eliminates both external and internal pathogenic factors.
- Strong cupping

Cupping Techniques

BLEEDING CUPPING

When treating MSK pain, and if the anatomical structure of the area to treat allows us to, we prefer associating cupping with bleeding (Fig. A4.2) to remove Qì stagnation and Blood stasis, to resolve Dampness, and clear Heat in the case of inflammation.

Procedure
- Use gloves and disinfect the skin before and after cupping.
- After making the selected point bleed, the cup is placed on the skin.
- To remove blood stasis, blood is drawn into the cup until its color turns from dark to light red. To resolve Dampness and clear Heat, suction draws out a smaller quantity of blood and the volume depends on the patient's general conditions.

Red Flags

- During cupping therapy, the patient should never be left alone to avoid damage to the skin or underlying structures.
- Contraindications: infections, wounds, cracked skin, and extremely thin skin, patients on long-term corticosteroid treatment, geriatric patients, and debilitated patients.

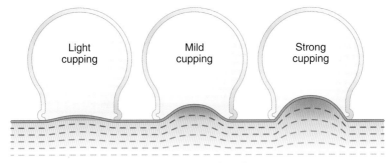

Fig. A4.1 Methods of cupping.

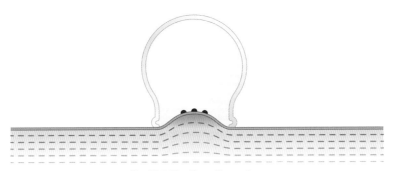

Fig. A4.2 Bleeding with cupping.

Clinical Notes

- Cupping creates a mild suction, and the skin rises just a little inside the cup.
- Duration of cupping depends on the patient's tolerability and underlying skin conditions.
- During the procedure, the skin may appear red and ecchymosis may occur. Blisters should never be observed. Counseling should be done with the patient about posttreatment marks that can last for several weeks.
- Utmost attention should always be paid to avoid damaging the tendinous or soft tissues with cupping that is too strong.
- The anatomical structure of the affected region or the patient's weak body structure may not allow the use of cupping for bleeding; for example, in the wrist in the case of radial styloiditis. Should this be the case, gently pinch the tissue between the thumb and index finger to promote venous pooling.

- Contraindications to local cupping: fracture, grade III muscle tear, or complete tendon tear.
- Preinvestigations before bleeding and cupping: check the medical history to see if the patient takes drugs that affect bleeding time, such as new oral anticoagulants, oral anticoagulant therapy, or medications with similar effects.

BIBLIOGRAPHY

Chirali IZ. Terapia di coppettazione in Medicina Tradizionale Cinese, traduzione dalla 3rd edition a cura di Roberto Palasciano, Shiatsu Milano Editore. 2021.

Marmori F. *Tecniche associate all'agopuntura*. Italian Chinese School of Acupuncture-A.M.A.B. (Association of Medical Acupuncturists of Bologna) Seminar; 2017.

Qiao W. *Acupuncture Treatment for Pain-Relieving*. Italian Chine School of Acupuncture-A.M.A.B. (Association of Medical Acupuncturist of Bologna) Seminar; 2014.

CEA (Casa Editrice Ambrosiana). *Trattato di Agopuntura e Medicina Cinese, a cura di Lucio Sotte, Agopuntura Cinese, AA vari*. 2007.

Moxibustion

The word 灸, translated into English is moxibustion, and means "to burn."

It is a form of therapy that aims at relieving a variety of conditions using heat and entails burning various types of leaves, including mugwort (*Artemisia vulgaris*) leaves. Heat penetrates through the skin into the deep tissues and warms the Main and Secondary channels.

Basically, it includes direct and indirect moxibustion:

- Direct moxibustion: moxa cones are placed directly on the skin.
- Indirect moxibustion: the burning moxa does not touch the skin.

We only use indirect moxibustion on the acupoints or Ah Shi points.

Main Functions of Moxibustion Therapy in the Management of Musculoskeletal Pain

- Warming channels and expelling Cold

External Cold can cause Qì and Blood flow to slow down, thus leading to Qì stagnation and Blood stasis. Heat applied to acupoint(s) or Ah Shi point(s) expels the external pathogenic factor (Cold) and eliminates pain. Moxibustion is also indicated in the case of external or internal Dampness because it can remove it.

- Warming Spleen and Kidney Yang

Some types of Bi syndromes, such as some forms of arthritis, are often associated with Spleen and Kidney Yang deficiency. In this case, a moxa box is used to treat BL20, BL23, and GV4.

- Tonifying Qì and Blood

In chronic Deficiency conditions and resolution phases of musculoskeletal (MSK) pain, mild moxibustion can also be useful to promote Qì and Blood flow in the affected area.

Moxibustion Techniques

INDIRECT MOXIBUSTION

The burning moxa does not actually touch the skin.

Moxa Stick
Dried mugwort leaves are rolled into a cigar-shaped stick (Fig. A5.1) that can be used to treat the following:
Excess conditions:

- Sparrow pecking: the moxa stick is held close to the skin and then moved up and down quickly, like a sparrow pecking, for a couple of minutes. The aim of this treatment is to expel the internal or external pathogenic factor.

Deficiency conditions:

- Circular moxa: the moxa stick is held close enough to the skin to generate heat. It hovers over the point(s) with slow circular movements until the area to treat is warmed up. The aim of this stimulation is to tonify Qì and Blood in the affected tissues.

Moxa Box
It is usually made of wood and contains an inner grid for a variable number of moxa cigars (Fig. A5.2), depending on the intensity of the heat to be generated. We use it on the Back-Shu points of the spleen and kidney to tonify Yang deficiency in the case of arthritis with Cold and Dampness.

Moxa on the Needle
After inserting the needle into an acupoint, the handle of the needle is wrapped in a moxa cylinder and ignited (Fig. A5.3). We use it to promote the flow of local Qì and Blood. We also use it on major joints, such as the shoulder, hip, and knee, to make the heat penetrate deep into the joint and have the Cold or Dampness expelled.

Fig. A5.1 Moxa stick.

Fig. A5.2 Moxa box.

Fig. A5.3 Moxa on the needle.

Red Flags

- During moxibustion, the patient should never be left alone, and the practitioner should oversee the whole procedure to avoid any burns or injuries to the skin.
- Special attention should be paid if the patient's medical history mentions diabetes or any condition that might reduce sensitivity to heat or pain. Should this be the case, moxibustion should be reconsidered.
- An allergy to mugwort or plants belonging to the Asteraceae or Compositae family is a contraindication to moxibustion.

Clinical Notes

- When using moxa on the needle, the handle should not touch the skin to avoid burns. A thin piece of cardboard should be placed around the needle to cover the surrounding area for protection against falling of moxa ashes.
- In the management of MSK pain, moxibustion generally aims at removing Qì stagnation and Blood stasis and expels external and internal pathogenic factors, which are mainly Cold or Dampness. However, attention should be paid because too much heat can increase the ongoing inflammatory process.
- Moxibustion is usually well accepted by patients.

- Special attention should be paid to geriatric and pediatric patients, whose skin is definitively more sensitive and delicate.
- Skin lesions and infections are contraindications to moxibustion.

BIBLIOGRAPHY

Marmori F. *Tecniche associate all'agopuntura*. Italian Chinese School of Acupuncture-A.M.A.B. (Association of Medical Acupuncturists of Bologna) Seminar; 2017.

Qiao W. *Acupuncture Treatment for Pain-Relieving*. Italian Chine School of Acupuncture-A.M.A.B. (Association of Medical Acupuncturist of Bologna) Seminar; 2014.

CEA (Casa Editrice Ambrosiana). *Trattato di Agopuntura e Medicina Cinese, a cura di Lucio Sotte, Agopuntura Cinese, AA vari*. 2007.

Arthritis

Arthritis in Western medicine is an umbrella term often used to describe conditions characterized by progressive damage to joints (bone, cartilage, synovial layer, and joint capsule). Common symptoms include inflammation, swelling, redness, stiffness, and restricted range of motion in joints.

There is no corresponding term in TCM. The condition described above is referred to as the Bì syndrome or painful obstruction syndrome, meaning the obstruction of the channels due to the invasion of external pathogenic factors (EPFs), mainly Wind, Cold, and Dampness. The term *Bì* is very old and was first used in Chapter 43 of the Su Wen.

This disease typically affects the channels and only reaches the Zang Fu after some time. The invasion of EPFs results from a preexisting and temporary deficiency of Qì and Blood that allows the Wind, Cold, and Dampness to invade the body.

It should be stressed that such a deficiency is relative and depends on the strength of the EPFs and the body's Qì. When the EPFs are temporarily stronger than the Qì, then they can penetrate the body and result in painful obstruction syndrome. Therefore this deficiency is not absolute. If that was the case, it would mean that anyone who suffers from Qì or Blood deficiency would develop painful obstruction syndrome, and vice versa, which doesn't happen.

The main channels to be invaded by the EPFs are the Muscle and Connecting channels. If the condition is not treated in the correct way, the EPFs penetrate deeper and can reach the Main channels and the inner layers, thus affecting the Zang Fu.

The main cause of Bì syndrome is the invasion of the EPFs, such as Wind, Cold, and Dampness, which are briefly described below.

Wind

Wind is regarded as the most dangerous of the EPFs and usually combines with other factors. It is commonly considered an etiological factor, that is, a rapid and sudden shift in weather, rather than standard weather conditions, outpacing the body's ability to adapt to the attack.

Cold

Cold is a very common cause of Bì syndrome. It mainly contracts and congeals; consequently, it is a cause of Qì stagnation and Blood stasis, resulting in intense pain that is usually located in one single joint.

Dampness

Dampness is another very common cause of painful obstruction syndrome. It can result from the exposure to damp outdoor or indoor environments.

Consequently, each factor corresponds to a painful syndrome, notably:

- Wind painful obstruction syndrome: it is characterized by soreness and pain of muscles and joints, limitation of movement, and pain wandering from muscle to muscle and joint to joint.
- Cold painful obstruction syndrome: it is characterized by severe pain with limitation of movement, and it usually affects one single joint.
- Damp painful obstruction syndrome: it is characterized by pain, soreness, and swelling of muscles and joints, associated with a feeling of heaviness and numbness of the limbs. Pain is fixed in one place and aggravated by damp weather.
- Heat painful obstruction syndrome: it originates from any of the previous clinical pictures when the EPF turns into heat in the interior. There is usually an underlying Yin deficiency. It is characterized by heat, redness, and swelling in the joints, with a limitation of movement and severe pain.
- Bony painful obstruction syndrome: it only develops in chronic conditions and originates from any

of the types mentioned above. It is typical of the elderly with painful joints with swelling and bone deformities.

Chronic Bì syndrome: it is characterized by:

General Qì and Blood deficiency: muscle weakness

Phlegm in the joints: swelling and deformity of joints and bones, muscle atrophy

Blood stasis: often resulting from a persistent Qì stagnation, it manifests with more intense pain, mainly at night, and marked stiffness

Liver and Kidney deficiency: pain and stiffness (tendons and cartilages are not adequately nourished) and bone degeneration (bones are not adequately nourished) resulting in phlegm accumulation in the joints.

Treatment

Before describing treatment of arthritis, a short introduction should be made.

As widely described in this handbook, MSK pain is mainly a sign of Qì stagnation and Blood stasis. Therefore arthritis should always be treated following the five options thoroughly described in the previous chapters, whether its onset or acute relapse depends or not on a shift in weather.

Below, instead, we describe the basic etiologic treatment of the patient with arthritis. When pain is acute or chronic from Excess, the therapy we suggest is a treatment option to further support our five options protocol. Treatment is tailored to the patient and specifically targets the joint or MSK structure affected to help relieve pain.

Treatment of Bì syndromes in acute, exacerbated, and chronic Excess conditions aims to expel the predominant pathogenic factor and promote the circulation of local Qì and Blood: it mainly acts on the channel(s) involved. This approach has already been described in the chapter dedicated to acupuncture treatment (see Chapter 1).

However, when Bì syndrome becomes chronic, the internal organs should also be treated.

- Wind Bì syndrome: expels Wind and tonifies Blood, in particular Liver Blood. Uses BL12, BL17, BL18, SP10, TE6, GB31, GB39, and GV14.
- Cold Bì syndrome: expels Cold and tonifies Yang, in particular Kidney Yang. Uses BL23, ST36, KI3, CV4, CV6, GV4, GV14, and moxa.
- Dampness Bì syndrome: resolves Dampness and tonifies the Spleen, in particular spleen Qì. Uses SP9 SP6, ST36, GB34, and BL20.
- Heat Bì syndrome: clears Heat. Uses GV14 with bleeding, ST43, LI4, and LI1.
- Bony Bì syndrome: uses the points related to the bones. Uses BL11 and GB39.

Chronic Bì syndrome: uses points related to:

Blood and Qì deficiency: BL20, BL23, ST36, SP6, LR8, and CV4.

Phlegm (in the joints): BL20, CV12, CV9, ST40, SP9, and SP6.

Blood stasis: BL17, SP10, SP6, and LI11.

Liver and Kidney deficiency: BL11, BL18, BL23, LR8, KI3, ST36, SP6, GB34, and GB39.

Clinical Notes

- In Bì syndrome, pain varies with weather conditions. In particular, it gets worse with the pathogenic factor underlying the syndrome (Wind, Cold, and Dampness).
- Bì syndromes can be differentiated according to the pathogenic predominant factor over the others, but all the factors (Wind, Cold, and Dampness), if present, should be treated.

BIBLIOGRAPHY

Maciocia G. *The Practise of Chinese Medicine*. 3rd ed. Elsevier; 2022.

Qiao W. *Acupuncture Treatment for Pain-Relieving*. Italian Chine School of Acupuncture-A.M.A.B. (Association of Medical Acupuncturist of Bologna) Seminar; 2014.

Postsurgical Musculoskeletal Pain

In this context, we should also mention limb surgery. Though well performed, they can result in pain, restriction of joint movements, and stiffness. They cause Qì stagnation and Blood stasis, possible damage to the channels, and scar formation, all factors that could lead to obstruction of Qì and Blood flow in the channels.

In addition, if the fracture is intraarticular or in the case of malunion, secondary arthritis is likely to occur. Postsurgical arthritis or following fracture also leads to cartilage damage and bone erosion, which may be associated with swelling and osteophytes.

According to TCM, these conditions can be attributed to

- Blood and Yin deficiency (cartilage damage and bone erosion)
- Dampness and Phlegm (swelling and osteophytes)

Therefore the principle of treatment will be the mobilization of Qì and Blood to remove stagnation and stasis, as recommended by the five options described in this handbook, along with the specific treatment of the pattern or pathogenic factor involved.

- Blood and Yin deficiency: BL11, BL18, BL23, KI3, ST36, SP6, GB39, and LR8
- Dampness and Phlegm: BL20, CV12, CV9, ST36, ST40, SP9, and SP5.

It is worth a reminder that Cold is an EPF that can easily penetrate the body in the case of arthritis. Should this be the case, moxibustion is recommended (see Appendix 5).

Clinical Notes

- Local bleeding is very important because it promotes Qì and Blood flow, and it improves range of motion. This technique is to be used when signs of stasis are observed in the Secondary channels, specifically:
  Ah Shi point(s)
  Spider veins
  Redness or painful scars.
- To promote the flow of Qì and Blood, sometimes it can be useful to "direct the flow" by inserting needles under the scar. Insertion starts from an area where the skin is intact, with the needle being inserted either longitudinally and tangentially, or transversely from oblique to transverse, depending on the area to be treated.

BIBLIOGRAPHY

Maciocia G. *The Practise of Chinese Medicine*. 3rd ed. Elsevier; 2022.

Qiao W. *Acupuncture Treatment for Pain-Relieving*. Italian Chine School of Acupuncture-A.M.A.B. (Association of Medical Acupuncturist of Bologna) Seminar; 2014.

Index

Note: Page numbers followed by *f* indicate figures and *b* indicate boxes.

Radial styloiditis (*Continued*)
    Ah Shi point(s), 119, 119*f*, 120*f*
    LI5, 119–120
   microsystems, acupuncture, 120–122
    dull pain/muscle weakness, 121
    intense pain/range of motion, 121
    Upper 4, 120, 120*f*
    Upper 5, 120–121, 120*f*
Radial styloid process, 106, 108
Radial tuberosity, 75
Radiocarpal joint, 106–108, 114–116, 131–135
   anterior carpus, 114–115, 115*f*, 131–133, 133*f*, 134*f*
   carpus compression, 133–134, 134*f*
   posterior carpus, 115–116, 116*f*, 131, 133*f*
Radioulnar joint, 104
   anterior radial head, 103*f*, 104
   posterior radial head, 104, 104*f*
Range of motion (ROM), 26, 142
Range of passive motion, 27–28, 28*f*
Resisted knee flexion test, 187, 187*f*
Restrictive barrier, 25
Reverse Cozen test, 80, 80*f*
Rheumatoid arthritis, 188–189, 236
Rolling test, 150, 150*f*

S

Sacroiliac joint, 150–152, 170–172
   anterior rotation of the ilium, 170–171, 170*f*, 171*f*
   iliac torsion, 171–172
   posterior rotation of the ilium, 171, 171*f*, 172*f*
   upslip treatment, 172, 172*f*
Sacrum, 136
Sartorius, 139
Scaphoid fossa, 266
Scapula, 33
Scapulothoracic (ST) joint, 33
Semimembranosus, 181
Semitendinosus, 181
Shoulder arthritis, 39
Shoulder joints, 33–74
   anatomical landmarks, 34, 36*f*
   joints and muscles, 33–34
   pain, 39
   physiological movements, 34–36
   planes of motion, 37*f*
Shoulder pain
   acromioclavicular joint, 45–46

Shoulder pain (*Continued*)
   AcuOsteo method, 49–74
   anatomy and biomechanics, Western medicine, 33–36, 35*f*
   diagnosis
    in Chinese medicine, 41–44
    in osteopathic medicine, 44–49
    in Western medicine, 36–41
   etiology, 41
   first rib, 48–49
   glenohumeral joint, 46–48
   long head of biceps, 48
   pathology, 41
   sternoclavicular joint, 44–45
Shoulder stiffness, 39
Shu-Stream points, 15, 16*b*
Shu transporting points, 15
Small intestine, 41–43, 43*f*, 50, 82–83, 83*f*, 110, 112, 113*f*
Snapping hip syndrome (SHS), 143
Soft tissue techniques, 26, 31
Soleus muscle, 232
Somatic dysfunctions, 28, 29*f*
   ankle pain
    osteopathic diagnostic approach, 240
    osteopathic manipulation, 243
    talocalcaneal joint, 241–242, 257–258
    testing for, 240–242
    tibiofibular joint, 241, 256–257
    tibiotalar joint, 240–241, 254–256
   elbow pain
    humeroulnar joint, 100–104
    radioulnar joint, 104
   hip pain
    hip joint, 173–175
    pubic symphysis, 172–173
    sacroiliac joint, 170–172
   humeroulnar joint, 84–86
   knee pain
    medial meniscus, 198–199, 226–228
    patella, 199, 228
    proximal tibiofibular joint, 196–198, 225–226
    testing, 194–199
    tibiofemoral joint, 194–196, 218–225
   osteoarticular disorder, 25–26
   proximal radioulnar joint, 86–87
   sacroiliac joint, 150–152
   shoulder pain